CONTROL OF GENE EXPRESSION

ADVANCES IN EXPERIMENTAL MEDICINE AND BIOLOGY

m.e'. "Oholo" Biological Conference on Strategies for the Control of Gene Expression, 18th, Zikhron Ya'aqov, Israel, 1973.

CONTROL OF GENE EXPRESSION

Edited by

Alexander Kohn

Director
Israel Institute for Biological Research
Ness Ziona, Israel
and
Tel Aviv University Medical School
Tel Aviv, Israel

and

Adam Shatkay

Deputy Scientific Director
Israel Institute for Biological Research
Ness Ziona, Israel

PLENUM PRESS • NEW YORK AND LONDON

Library of Congress Cataloging in Publication Data

"Oholo" Biological Conference on Strategies for the Control of Gene Expression,
   18th, Zikhron Ya'aqov, Israel, 1973.
   Control of gene expression; [proceedings]

   (Advance in experimental medicine and biology, v. 44)
   Includes bibliographical references.
   1. Genetic regulation—Congresses. 2. Gene expression—Congresses. I. Kohn,
Alexander, ed. II. Shatkai, Adam, ed. III. Title. IV. Series. [DNLM: 1. Genetics,
Biochemical—Congresses. 2. Genetics, Microbial—Congresses. W1AD559 v. 44
1974 / QH431 039 1973c]
QH450.047   1973   575.1'2   74-3157
ISBN 0-306-39044-2

Proceedings of the Eighteenth Annual "OHOLO" Biological Conference
on Strategies for the Control of Gene Expression held March 27-30,
1973, at Zichron Yaakov, Israel

© 1974 Plenum Press, New York
A Division of Plenum Publishing Corporation
227 West 17th Street, New York, N.Y. 10011

United Kingdom edition published by Plenum Press, London
A Division of Plenum Publishing Company, Ltd.
4a Lower John Street, London W1R 3PD, England

Printed in the United States of America

ORGANIZING COMMITTEE

PROF. N. GROSSOWICZ, Hebrew University, Jerusalem

PROF. A. KEYNAN, Hebrew University, Jerusalem

PROF. M. A. KLINGBERG, Israel Institute for
Biological Research, Ness Ziona

PROF. A. KOHN, Israel Institute for Biological
Research, Ness Ziona

PROF. M. REVEL, Weizmann Institute of Science,
Rehovoth

PROF. M. SELA, Weizmann Institute of Science,
Rehovoth

DR. A. SHATKAY, Israel Institute for Biological
Research, Ness Ziona

PREFACE

The OHOLO Conferences have been convened annually from the
Spring of 1956; the wide areas they have covered, from different
and overlapping disciplines, can be seen from the following list:

1956 Bacterial Genetics (not published)
1957 Tissue Cultures in Virological Research (not published)
1958 Inborn and Acquired Resistance to Infection in Animals
      (not published)
1959 Experimental Approach to Mental Diseases (not published)
1960 Cryptobiotic Stages in Biological Systems*
1961 Virus-Cell Relationships**
1962 Biological Synthesis and Function of Nucleic Acids**
1963 Cellular Control Mechanism of Macromolecular Synthesis**
1964 Molecular Aspects of Immunology**
1965 Cell Surfaces**
1966 Chemistry and Biology of Psychotropic Agents
      (not published)
1967 Structure and Mode of Action of Enzymes**
1968 Growth and Differentiation of Cells *In Vitro***
1969 Behaviour of Animal Cells in Culture**
1970 Microbial Toxins**
1971 Interaction of Chemical Agents with Cholinergic
      Mechanisms**
1972 Immunity in Viral and Rickettsial Diseases***

The participants who attend these Conferences are drawn from different scientific institutions in Israel and from many foreign
countries; they are engaged in fields of study which represent
widely divergent approaches to biology. Thus a distinguishing
feature of the OHOLO meetings has been their multi-disciplinary
nature.

---

*   Published by Elsevier Publishing Co., Amsterdam (1960).
**   Published by the Israel Institute for Biological
         Research, Ness Ziona.
***   Published by Plenum Press, New York (1972).

These small international conferences are also characterized by their relaxed atmosphere, with ample time for informal as well as formal discussions.

The present volume contains almost all the papers presented at the Eighteenth OHOLO Biological Conference, devoted to Strategies for the Control of Gene Expression, held at Zichron-Yaakov, Israel, on March 27-30, 1973.

In order to obtain an overview of the broad spectrum of knowledge in the field, and to summarize a considerable number of closely related topics, noted investigators were invited to discuss and analyze together the goals already achieved and to speculate on future trends in the study of gene expression.

More than 200 participants (including some twenty from overseas) took part in this meeting, and the twenty-four papers presented summarize much data gathered in extensive studies.

We have pleasure in thanking the Chairman of the Sessions and the Moderator of the Round Table Discussion, the participants who presented papers, and all those who joined in the discussions and so willingly cooperated in contributing to this record of the Conference.

We believe that this meeting provided an opportunity for the cross fertilization and stimulation of ideas between scientists in the various disciplines. The information gathered in this volume shows how much has already been done and what prospects lie ahead.

The Editors gladly take this opportunity of expressing their thanks to the Organizing Committee for their efforts and dedication in preparing the meeting, and to Mrs. Ilana Turner and Mr. Hanoch Yorav for their help. We also gratefully acknowledge the efficient assistance of Mrs. Myra Kaye in editing the papers, of Mrs. LaVerne Binstock in the technical preparation of the manuscript for publication, and the financial assistance of EMBO and the U.S. European Research Office.

Alexander Kohn

Adam Shatkay

CONTENTS

CONTROL OF GENE EXPRESSION

OPENING ADDRESS

        Alexander Kohn

        Israel Institute for Biological Research

        Ness-Ziona, Israel

    I have the honor and the pleasure of welcoming all partici-
pants to this conference on the "Strategies for the Control of
Gene Expression", and I extend our special greetings to our distinguished guests and colleagues from abroad.

    Right at the beginning, I should like to explain why we call
a conference which takes place in Zichron Yaakov, the OHOLO Conference. It is not for the same reason that Humpty-Dumpty gave to
Alice, that he uses a word to mean what he wants it to mean....

    Oholo is an educational institution operated by an autonomous
unit of the General Federation of Labor, situated on the shores of
the Lake of Galilee near Kibbutz Kinereth; we have held our biological conferences there 15 out of 18 times. It is named after Berl
Katzenelson, one of the leaders of the Zionist socialist movement,
and the literal translation of "Oholo" is "his tent". Because the
large number of participants could not have been accomodated at
Oholo, this year again we have the conference in one of the oldest
pioneer settlements of the modern era (it is 90 years old). Zichron
Yaakov means Jacob's Memorial named after the father, James, of
Baron Rothschild who supported the settlers here. Zichron is also
a place suited for this conference because here, at the start of
the century, while still under the Turkish rule, was founded the
first research institute of genetics. I refer to the Agricultural
Research Station established by Aharon Aharonson, who became known
as the discoverer of the wild precursor of wheat in this region.

    The Oholo conferences were originated by the late Professor
Hestrin, and Professors Grossowicz and Keynan, and are organized
by the Israel Institute for Biological Research at Ness-Ziona.

The Institute's scientists are engaged in basic and applied research in various fields of biology and chemistry. The purpose of these conferences is to foster interdisciplinary communication between Israeli scientists and their colleagues abroad. This year's conference is devoted to the problem of Control of Gene Expression.

Just ten years ago we held a conference directly related to the subject of the present meeting. Its topic was Cellular Control Mechanisms in Macromolecular Synthesis. In these ten years, continuing research has led to a wealth of fruitful and challenging information contributing greatly to the solution of the central problem of how DNA controls the sequence of amino acids in proteins. It should be remembered that the "central dogma" was proposed only about 20 years ago, and it was less than 30 years ago that Beadle and Tatum stated that discrete genes were the basic units of all living things. Within a cell, great variation exists in the number of the diverse protein molecules. It is therefore clear that there must exist in cells devices for selective synthesis of these proteins, which are needed in large numbers. The biological assembly line must be extremely flexible and must be able to adjust itself not only to momentary changes and shortages of particular raw materials, but also to a number of environmental signals important for the survival of the organism. Misquoting George Orwell I would say: "All proteins are equal, but some are more equal than others"; the more equal are of course the proteins with catalytic properties, the enzymes, the perfect biological representatives of Maxwellian demons. In a most complicated mixture of molecules in a cell, the enzyme recognizes one particular molecular species to catalyse a specific chemical reaction. The fact that during the complicated and intricate process of protein synthesis, the insertion of amino acids into polypeptide chains occurs with less than one error per 1000 amino acids stresses the sophistication of nature at the molecular level. During the past, the problem of how this fantastic accuracy is achieved was met with ignorance and speculation, but now our attitude to it has become more hopeful and even self assured.

We try hard to follow Jean Perrin's statement that in the world of living "Il s'agit toujours d'expliquer du visible compliqué par de l'invisible simple".

Let us therefore hope that by the end of this conference we shall have clearer concepts of how gene expression is controlled in the steps of transcription from DNA to RNA, translation from RNA to protein, and how viral infection, the action of hormones and aging, affect the regulation of diverse essential processes in the living cell.

I should like to end by giving some advice to our speakers by again quoting from Lewis Carroll: "Begin at the beginning - the King said gravely - and go on till you come to the end. Then stop."

So, I stop and let the conference commence with the opening lecture of Dr. Bautz:

"Initiation of Transcription by RNA Polymerase of E. coli and Phage 3."

INITIATION OF TRANSCRIPTION BY RNA POLYMERASES OF E. COLI AND PHAGE T3.

E.K.F. Bautz, W.T. McAllister, H. Küpper, E. Beck
and F.A. Bautz

Institut für Molekulare Genetik Universität Heidelberg
69 Heidelberg/West Germany

INTRODUCTION

Unlike eukaryotes, bacteria possess only a single species of RNA polymerase which is responsible for the expression of the entire genetic information of the cell. Evidence for a single enzyme comes from the action of the drug rifampicin, which interacts with RNA polymerase and upon addition to a cell culture eliminates the synthesis of ribosomal, transfer and messenger RNA. A single-step mutation of rifampicin resistance restores the ability to synthesize all RNA species in the presence of the drug (1).

The control of gene expression in bacteria appears to occur largely at the level of transcription. Operationally, we can differentiate between three different types of genes:

1) those that are nearly always expressed at optimal rates, e.g. the rRNA genes

2) those that are always expressed at very low levels, e.g. the i-gene coding for the lac repressor

and 3) those genes subject to repression and induction (e.g. catabolite operons).

The difference between genes of type one and two appears exclusively in the structure of their promotors, the RNA polymerase having a very high affinity for the first and a very low affinity for the second class. An example is the i^Q mutation which results

in an increased production of lac repressor. This mutation has
been interpreted as a promotor mutation that results in a DNA
sequence for which the RNA polymerase has an increased affinity.

Repression and induction in the classical sense, via repressor molecules, is now called negative control: the repressor
blocks initiation of transcription by occupying a site near to or
overlapping the promotor; the presence of an inducer removes such
blocks. Some operons, such as the lac operon, can additionally
be regulated through positive control elements, auxiliary factors,
which increase the affinity of RNA polymerase for the promotor.
One example is the cyclic AMP receptor protein (called CRP or CAP
factor) which, together with cAMP, is required for optimal transcription of the lac operon.

Thus most questions concerning the regulation of transcription in bacteria center on 1) the interaction of RNA polymerase
with promotor sites, 2) the interaction of auxiliary factors
with RNA polymerase and/or promotor sites, and 3) the interaction
of repressors with operator sites. Therefore, in order to obtain
more detailed information on gene expression, it is essential that
we know as much as possible about the structure of RNA polymerase
as well as the DNA region it recognizes, and also about the mechanisms of the reactions involved in the initiation of RNA chains.

RNA polymerase isolated from E.coli cells consists of 5 sub-
units $\alpha_2\beta\beta'\sigma$ having a combined molecular weight of approximately
470,000 daltons (2). Except for the two α polypeptides, the subunits are non-identical. This means that nearly 9×10^6 daltons
of DNA is required to code for all the subunits. Thus, elucidating the structure and obtaining detailed information about this
enzyme should prove rather difficult. In order to produce an RNA
chain, the enzyme has to perform a series of different reactions
which can be divided into 3 steps: initiation, chain elongation,
and termination. While the α, β and β' subunits are required for
all   steps, the σ protein was found to be required for initiation only and it was therefore of interest to study the function
of this subunit in initiation (3). The data obtained in this
laboratory, some of which are given below, as well as results
obtained in other laboratories, have led to the conclusion that
the σ protein is an allosteric effector, drastically increasing
the affinity of the enzyme for specific binding sites which we
define here operationally as the equivalents to the genetically
defined promotors.

While the E.coli RNA polymerase appears to work in two different conformational states, determined by the presence or absence

of the σ protein, another RNA polymerase, produced after infection
with phages T3 or T7, does not require a specific protein factor
for initiation of RNA chains (4,5). This enzyme in fact consists
of only one single polypeptide chain (MW ≈ 110,000 daltons) and
yet it appears to perform all functions at least as efficiently as
the far bigger bacterial enzyme. It was therefore of interest to
compare the analogous functional steps of the two structurally
different RNA polymerases. In this paper we summarize our work
on the σ dependent binding of RNA polymerase to promotor sites
and we compare the biochemical properties of the E.coli and T3 RNA
polymerases.

Initiation by E.coli RNA Polymerase

The sequence of events leading to the synthesis of an RNA
chain can be outlined as follows:

1) $Enzyme + DNA \longrightarrow Enzyme \cdot DNA$)
) Association
2) $Enzyme \cdot DNA \underset{15°C}{\overset{20°C}{\rightleftarrows}} Enzyme^+ \cdot DNA$)

3) $Enzyme^+ \cdot DNA + NTP_1 + NTP_2 \longrightarrow Enzyme^+ \cdot DNA \cdot NTP_1 \cdot NTP_2$)
) Initiation
4) $Enzyme^+ \cdot DNA \cdot NTP_1 \cdot NTP_2 \longrightarrow Enzyme^+ \cdot DNA \cdot NTP_1 - NMP_2 + PP_i$)

5) Translocation of enzyme on DNA template   )
)
6) $Enzyme^+ \cdot DNA \cdot NTP_1 - NMP_2 + NTP_3 \longrightarrow Enzyme^+ \cdot DNA \cdot NTP_1 - NMP_2 - NMP_3 + PP_i$)

                                                        Polymerization

The initial association (step 1) with DNA is non-specific; both
holoenzyme $(\alpha_2\beta\beta'\sigma)$ and core enzyme $(\alpha_2\beta\beta')$ can form complexes
and there are only partial limitations as to the number of enzyme
molecules which can associate with DNA. If an enzyme is bound to
a promotor site, there is a transition to a highly stable complex
(step 2) which forms only in the presence of the σ factor. In
addition, formation and maintenance of the tight complex requires
temperatures above 17° (and low ionic strength). These complexes
are specific as they seem to form only at genuine promotor sites.
The promotor-bound holoenzyme is partially resistant to rifampicin
and totally resistant to polyanions like heparin or polyinosinic
acid (poly I) (6,7). The next step requires the addition of the
first and second substrate molecules into the initiation and chain
elongation sites. Binding to the initiation site appears to be

purine-specific, with a K_m several fold higher than that of the
second site (8). From the second nucleoside-triphosphate, PP_i is
then split off to yield the first phosphodiester bond. From here
on the enzyme enters the catalytic cycle, involving a translocation
step (5), with the initiation site becoming the product terminus
site holding the 3' terminal nucleotide of the growing chain and
the chain elongation site becoming free to accept a new substrate
molecule (step 6).

When we realized that polyanions having a higher affinity
for the enzyme than native DNA could remove all nonspecifically
bound enzyme molecules from the DNA, but that they could not remove enzyme already bound to a promotor site, it became obvious
that this resistance should be able to be utilised as a tool to
isolate the tight enzyme binding sites of DNA. The experimental
scheme is analogous to the isolation of ribosome-binding sites as
carried out by Steitz (9), involving digestion of unprotected DNA
with DNase, followed by gel filtration of the enzyme-promotor complex to separate it from the digestion products. Using DNA highly
labelled with ^{32}P from phages T3 or T7 and incubating with 10
enzymes per genome, followed by competition with poly I, about
0.2 percent of the input DNA became resistant against pancreatic
DNase. This amount corresponds to approximately 2 promotors per
genome (assuming one promotor to consist of 35 - 40 base pairs).
If one omits competition by poly I, the amount of DNA protected
is directly proportional to the number of enzyme molecules. Very
little DNase-resistant ^{32}P label was observed to cosediment with
the RNA polymerase when σ was omitted in the initial binding, even
without poly I competition (Fig. 1). Fingerprinting of the
resistant material after conversion to apurinic acid shows that
the sequences obtained are nonrandom, suggesting that specific
DNA sequences had been selected by the enzyme during formation
of the tight DNA-enzyme complexes.

On the basis of these data, and also of data obtained by
others (10,11) it is possible to deduce the following simplified
functional model (Fig. 2). Whereas holoenzyme has a low affinity
for regions of DNA which do not contain initiation signals (promotor sites), the association with a promotor region results in
the formation of a very tight complex. Core enzyme, on the other
hand, appears not to discriminate between the two types of sequences but has an intermediate affinity. It binds to promotor
sites much less strongly than the holoenzyme, but shows a somewhat
higher affinity for non-promotor regions than the holoenzyme.
Thus one can view the function of σ as that of an allosteric
effector causing the core enzyme to undergo a conformational
change which enables it to search out initiation signals very
effectively.

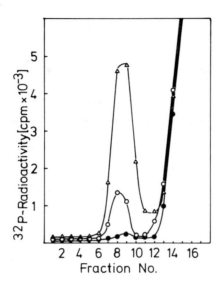

Fig. 1.   Protection of promotor sequences of T7 DNA by E.coli RNA
polymerase.
Eighty μg of ^{32}P-labelled T7 DNA (1 x 10^7 CPM) were incubated at
37° with 16 μg of E.coli RNA polymerase in a 1.0 ml reaction mixture containing 10 mM Tris HCl, pH 8.0, 10 mM 2-mercaptoethanol
and 10 mM MgCl$_2$. After 20 minutes, 80 μg poly-inosinic acid was
added and incubation was continued for another 60 minutes. Unprotected DNA was then digested by adding 100 μg pancreatic DNase and
continuing the incubation for a further 10 minutes. The last step
was repeated, and the reaction mixture was then loaded on to a
Sephadex G x 100 column (40 x 1.6 cm) and eluted with 10 mM Tris
HCl, pH 8.0, 5 mM 2-mercaptoethanol and 1 mM EDTA.

Δ ——— Δ - holoenzyme, no poly I
o ——— o - holoenzyme, with poly I
● ——— ● - core enzyme without poly I

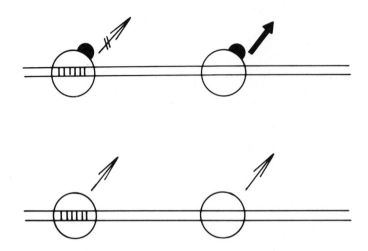

Fig. 2.   Effect of sigma on the binding of E.coli RNA polymerase
to DNA.
Holoenzyme containing the sigma subunit (◗) binds very tightly
to promotor regions (cross-hatched areas) of double stranded DNA,
but has a low affinity for non-promotor regions. Core enzyme, on
the other hand, exhibits an intermediate affinity for both promotor
and non-promotor regions.

Initiation of RNA Chains by T3 RNA Polymerase

      The data above give some information about the binding of RNA
polymerase, but do not indicate much concerning the further steps
in the initiation reaction which involve the addition of the first
and second nucleoside triphosphates. For this purpose, the RNA
polymerase made after bacteriophage T3 infection is a good object
for study as it appears to have a high degree of template specificity. After infection, the early region of the T3 phage genome
is transcribed by the RNA polymerase of the host. This region
comprises about 20 percent of the total genome and is demarcated

by a strong termination signal past which the E. coli polymerase
cannot read. The late region (the other 80 percent of the genome)
is transcribed by the protein product of gene 1. This enzyme is
less complicated in structure than the host enzyme and consists of
only one polypeptide chain having a MW of 110,000 daltons.

To determine the dependence of enzyme activity on the concentration of the nucleoside triphosphates which serve as substrates, one can vary the concentration of one triphosphate and
keep that of the other three at a high level. The results of such
experiments can be graphically displayed in a Lineweaver-Burk plot
in which the inverse of the initial velocity (1/V) of the reaction
is plotted against the inverse concentration (1/S) of the variable
substrate. Varying the concentration of either ATP, CTP, or UTP
resulted in a linear dependence of activity on substrate concentration; changing the concentration of GTP gave a curvilinear plot
which became linear when plotted as $1/V$ vs $1/S^2$ (Fig. 3). This
suggests that the simultaneous addition of two GTP moieties is
required at some stage during the synthetic reaction. Studies on
the exchange of pyrophosphate (PP_i), which measures the reverse
reaction of synthesis, support the contention that this unusual
dependence of enzyme activity on the concentration of GTP reflects
initiation with the sequence pppGpG, i.e. the fact that one ob-
tains high levels of PP_i exchange in the presence of only GTP as
substrate indicates that the sequence of at least the first two
nucleotides is GG (12). In contrast, with T7 DNA as template,
almost no PP_i exchange was observed with GTP alone but only when
GTP and ATP were both present, suggesting that, in this case, an
adenylic acid residue occupies one of the first two positions at
the 5' end of the message (12).

Checking the dependence of enzyme activity on the concentration of each of the substrates with T7 DNA template, variation of
the concentration of only GTP did not give the type of curvilinear
plot observed with T3 DNA; a curvilinear plot was obtained only if
the concentrations of both GTP and ATP were varied simultaneously
(Fig. 4). This finding supports the PP_i exchange data, indicating
that, indeed, the T3 RNA polymerase is forced to start RNA chains
with another sequence on T7 DNA than on the closely related T3 DNA.
The T7 RNA polymerase, however, appears to be able to start with
GG on both T7 and T3 DNA templates (12).

The T3 RNA polymerase is sensitive to either the rifampicin
derivative AFO/13 or to heparin. Binding of enzyme to DNA does
not render it resistant to heparin, and, unlike E.coli RNA polymerase (7), the T3 enzyme remains sensitive to heparin or high
salt concentrations even after the formation of the first dinucleotide, since preincubation with GTP alone does not render

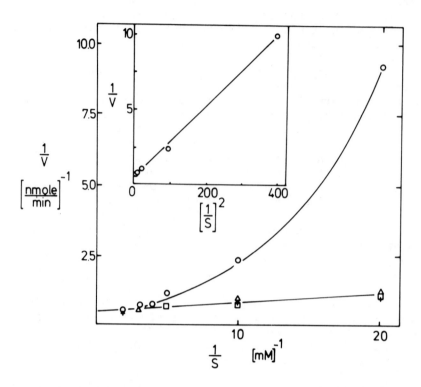

Fig. 3. The effect of varying the concentration of a single
nucleoside triphosphate on the rate of nucleotide incorporation by
the T3 RNA polymerase.

Reaction mixtures contained in 0.25 ml: 0.04 M Tris-HCl, pH 7.9,
0.01 M $MgCl_2$, 0.05 M KCl, 0.01 M 2-mercaptoethanol, 0.1 mM-Na_3-
EDTA, 12 µg T3 DNA, 0.5 mg/ml bovine serum albumin, and three of
the four nucleoside triphosphates at a concentration of 0.4 mM.
The concentration (S) of the fourth nucleoside triphosphate was
varied as indicated. Synthesis was initiated by the addition of
enzyme (to a final concentration of 5 µg/ml) and after 5 min at
37° the reactions were terminated by the addition of 2 ml of 5
percent trichloroacetic acid. Terminated reactions were filtered
through Whatman GF/A filters which were washed with 20 ml of 5
percent TCA, dried, and counted in a toluene-based liquid scintillation system. The initial rate of synthesis (V) has been calculated as nmoles (^{3}H)-UMP incorporated/min. The variable substrates
were: GTP (O), CTP (□), ATP (Δ), and ATP (+).

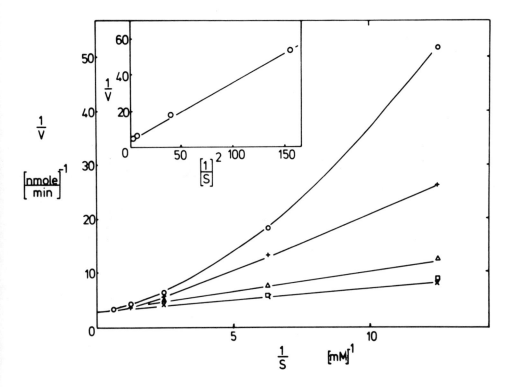

Fig. 4.   Kinetics of RNA synthesis by the T3 RNA polymerase on
a T7 DNA template.
The effect of varying the concentration of either one or two
nucleoside triphosphates on the rate of nucleotide incorporation
was examined as described in Fig. 3.   The concentration of T7
DNA in the reaction mixtures was 50 μg/ml.   The variable substrates were: GTP (+), ATP (□), CTP (X), GTP and ATP (O), ATP
and CTP (Δ).

the enzyme resistant (Table 1).   If preincubated with GTP and
ATP, however, the enzyme becomes almost fully resistant to heparin.
It was therefore of interest to determine the size of the products
that accumulate under the two conditions, i.e., incubation with
GTP alone or with GTP and ATP.   The results were rather clear cut
(12); incubation with GTP alone resulted in the production of
almost exclusively the dinucleotide pppGpG, whereas incubation with
both GTP and ATP yielded a tetranucleotide as the major product,
and tri- and penta-nucleotides as minor components.   These results

TABLE 1

RESISTANCE OF ENZYME-DNA COMPLEX TO HEPARIN AFTER INCUBATION WITH VARIOUS NUCLEOTIDES

Preincubation conditions[+]	Time of addition of heparin (80 μg/ml)	^{3}H-UMP incorporated (nmoles)	
No substrate present	---	1.16	(100 percent)
	- 15 sec	0.03	(3 ")
	0 "	0.02	(2 ")
	+ 15 "	0.82	(71 ")
	+ 30 "	1.22	(105 ")
Enzyme + DNA preincubated with:			
GTP	- 15 "	0.06	(5 ")
GTP + ATP	"	0.85	(73 ")
GTP + UTP	"	0.08	(7 ")
GTP + CTP	"	0.06	(5 ")
GTP + ATP + CTP	"	1.20	(103 ")
GTP + CTP + UTP	"	0.09	(8 ")

+ Standard assay mixtures containing the substrates indicated were preincubated for 5 min at 18°. Synthesis was started at 0 time by the addition of the remaining triphosphates and incubation was continued for 3 min at 18°.

indicate that most RNA chains start with the sequence pppGpGpAp$_G^A$.
Quantitatively, there are many more dinucleotides produced during
incubation with GTP alone than tetranucleotides when ATP is also
present, indicating that the enzyme recycles much more quickly
if it can produce only dinucleotides. Thus, during polymerization
the T3 RNA polymerase is more tightly bound to DNA than during
initiation.

CONCLUSIONS

The sequence of events which are involved in the synthesis of
RNA by the E.coli RNA polymerase have been characterized in some
detail. The investigations described in this report have dealt
with the mechanism whereby this complex enzyme is able to recognize the correct initiation signals on the DNA template. The
sigma factor is required for this step, and acts as an allosteric
effector which increases the affinity of the enzyme for promotor
regions and decreases the affinity of the enzyme for non-promotor
regions. The latter characteristic of the sigma factor offers an
explanation for the "sigma cycle" (13) in that, following initiation, loss of the sigma factor would facilitate binding of the
enzyme to non-promotor regions of the DNA which are subsequently
transcribed.

The bacteriophage T3 RNA polymerase, although considerably
simpler in structure than the host enzyme, does not appear to
require an initiation factor for accurate transcription (4).
Kinetic analyses have shown that on a T3 DNA template, this enzyme initiates all RNA chains with the sequence pppGpG. The
apparent K_m for GTP determined from these experiments is about 5
times that for other nucleotides which are involved only in chain
elongation. On a T7 DNA template, where the starting sequence is
pppGpA, the K_m for ATP was no different than for CTP (which again,
is involved only in polymerization). Since K_m values are an indication of the affinity of an enzyme for its substrate, these
findings suggest that there are only two substrate binding sites
on the T3 enzyme. The first, or initiation site (site I) is
filled by GTP and the K_m for this site is 5 - 7 times that of the
second, or polymerization site (site II). Such a model assumes
that after the formation of a phosphodiester bond, the enzyme
translocates on the DNA template, and that the 3' terminal nucleotide of the growing product then occupies the initiation site.
The polymerization site (site II) thus continues to function in
the same manner during the successive addition of all subsequent
nucleotides. A similar two-site model for the E.coli RNA polymerase has been proposed by Goldthwait et al. (8). It is interesting to note that the first site of the host enzyme also

exhibits a K_m value that is higher than that of the second site, and that the 5' terminal nucleotide is always a purine.

In a reaction mixture containing GTP alone as a substrate, the T3 RNA polymerase continuously catalyzes the formation of dinucleotides without the formation of a stable transcription complex. In contrast, it has been found that the host enzyme becomes resistant to the effects of high salt concentrations after the formation of the first phosphodiester bond (14). The T3 polymerase becomes resistant to high salt concentrations (or the polyanion heparin) only after the formation of an RNA chain 3 - 4 nucleotides long. Whether these differences reflect dissimilarities in the manner in which the enzymes undergo conformational changes that result in a tighter binding to the template, or in the tightness of binding of the enzyme and template itself, is not known. However, in both cases the enzymes are more tightly bound to DNA during polymerization than during initiation.

Unlike the host RNA polymerase (6), incubation of the T3 RNA polymerase and template in the absence of substrates does not lead to a complex which is resistant to heparin (Table 1). This result indicates that the polyanion is able to inactivate free enzyme molecules as well as any DNA-bound enzyme molecules that may be present. While we have not directly measured the binding of enzyme to DNA, indirect evidence suggests that a relatively stable complex is formed. For example, after incubation of the T3 RNA polymerase with T3 DNA, it is possible to isolate fragments of DNA which remain resistant to DNase for over 10 min at 37° (Beck and Bautz, unpublished observations). In addition, although the T3 RNA polymerase is unable to initiate on T4 DNA, it remains tightly bound to this template during a subsequent incubation period in the presence of T3 DNA and substrate (5). Moreover, a DNA-cellulose column containing T4 DNA is routinely used as a purification step in the isolation of the T3 DNA polymerase. The salt-dependent elution of the RNA polymerase from this column indicates that the binding to DNA is reversible at ionic strengths greater than 0.15 M KCl. The binding of the E.coli RNA polymerase to template is also inhibited at higher ionic strengths (11) although in this case the range of salt concentrations at which the effect is observed is somewhat higher.

With the sizable amount of information now available, it is interesting to compare the T3 and E.coli RNA polymerases. To facilitate this, a summary is presented in Table 2 giving the results of these, and other, findings. It is apparent that although the two enzymes differ markedly in their physical structure they have many biochemical features in common. It will be of

TABLE 2

PORPERTIES OF THE T3 AND E. COLI RNA POLYMERASES

	T3	E. coli
Enzyme structure	1) MW = 110,000 daltons	1) MW = 470,000 daltons
	2) only 1 protein species in SDS-gels	2) has 5 subunits ($\beta\beta'\alpha_2\sigma$)
	3) probably active as monomer	3) probably active as monomer
	4) requires no protein factors for accurate transcription	4) requires σ factor for accurate initiation and ρ factor for termination
	5) two substrate binding sites: K_m for initiation site = 5 x K_m for polymerization site	5) two substrate binding sites: K_m for initiation site = 10 x K_m for polymerization site
Binding to DNA	1) complex relatively stable	1) complex highly stable above 20°
	2) complex not resistant to heparin or high salt concentration	2) complex resistant to heparin, but not high salt concentration
	3) enzyme does not bind to heparin or DNA at high salt concentrations	3) enzyme does not bind well to DNA at salt concentrations > 0.2 M

(Table 2 continued)

	T3	E.coli
Initiation	1) starts with: pppGpG on T3 DNA / pppGpA on T7 DNA	1) always starts with a purine, usually has pyrimidine in second position
	2) inhibited at salt concentrations > 0.1 M KCl	2) inhibited at salt concentrations > 0.2 M
	3) formation of dinucleotide (pppGpPu) does not give resistance against heparin or high salt concentration; formation of tetranucleotide is sufficient to give stabilization against high salt concentration	3) formation of first phosphodiester bond gives stable complex resistant to high salt concentration
Polymerization	1) chain elongation rate = 170 nucleotides/sec at 37°	1) chain elongation rate = 20 - 50 nucleotides/sec at 37°
	2) size of products identical at 0.05 M KCl and 0.15 M KCl, or in presence of ρ factor	2) size of products altered above 0.20 M KCl or by presence of ρ factor
	3) E_a = 23 Kcal/mole	3) E_a = 23 Kcal/mole

interest to see if RNA polymerases isolated from other organisms exhibit some of the same characteristics.

REFERENCES

1. YURA, T., IGARASHI, K. & MASUKATA, K. (1970). In Lepetit Colloquium on RNA Polymerase and Transcription (Silvestri, ed.) p.71, North Holland Publ.Co., Amsterdam.
2. BURGESS, R.R. (1969). J.Biol.Chem. 244, 6168.
3. BURGESS, R.R., TRAVERS, A.A., BAUTZ, E.K.F. & DUNN, J.J. (1969). Nature, 221, 43.
4. CHAMBERLIN, M., McGRATH, J. & WASKELL, L. (1970). Nature, 228, 227.
5. DUNN, J.J., BAUTZ, F.A. & BAUTZ, E.K.F. (1971). Nature New Biol. 230, 94.
6. ZILLIG, W., ZECHEL, K., RABUSSAY, D., SCHACHNER, M., SETHI, V.S., PALM, P., HEIL, A., & SEIFERT, W. (1970). Cold Spring Harbor Symp.Quant.Biol. 35, 47.
7. BAUTZ, E.K.F., BAUTZ, F.A. & BECK, E. (1972). Mol.Gen.Genet. 118, 199.
8. GOLDTHWAIT, D.A., ANTHONY, D.D. & WU, C-W (1970). In Lepetit Colloquium on RNA Polymerase and Transcription (Silvestri, ed) p.10, North Holland Publ.Co., Amsterdam.
9. STEITZ, J.A. (1969). Nature, 224, 957.
10. MUELLER, K. (1971). Mol.Gen.Genet. 3, 273.
11. HINKLE, D.C. & CHAMBERLIN, M. (1972). J.Mol.Biol. 70, 157.
12. McALLISTER, W.T., KÜPPER, H. & BAUTZ, E.K.F. (1973). Eur.J. Biochem. 34, 489.
13. TRAVERS, A.A. & BURGESS, R.R. (1969). Nature, 222, 537.
14. SO, A.G. & DOWNEY, K.M. (1970). Biochemistry, 9, 4788.

IN VIVO AND IN VITRO INITIATION OF TRANSCRIPTION

W. Szybalski

McArdle Laboratory for Cancer Research, University of
Wisconsin, Madison, Wisconsin, U. S. A.

We have been trying to identify the sites of initiation of
transcription in bacteriophage λ and to characterize the elements
that control the transcription. The mRNAs were prepared both in
vivo, by pulse labeling the phage-infected or induced lysogenic
cells, and in vitro, by using the λ DNA template and Escherichia
cell RNA polymerase together with ^{32}P-labeled nucleoside triphosphates. The promoter-proximal mRNA sequences were determined. The
following observations were based on refs. 1-5.

1) The promoter and operator regions are not transcribed into
RNA. Promoter p and operator o are defined by mutations that impair
their function.

2) Synthesis of RNA begins at the starting point designated s,
which is located downstream from the promoter and operator. In one
case it was found that the distance between the p, o and s sites was
about 200 nucleotides long.

3) The starting points, as defined by the 5'-terminal deoxynucleoside triphosphate and the initial sequences, up to 200 nucleotides, were determined for four mRNAs. Sequences initiated in vivo
are identical to those synthesized in vitro. The four mRNAs comprise
two major long messages initiated at the p_L and p_R promoters, and
two self-terminating short RNA species.

4) Both self-terminating RNAs contain the UUUUUUA-OH 3'-termi-
nal sequence. One, designated oop, is 80 nucleotides long, transcribed leftward near the ori site (origin of λ DNA replication),
and is probably involved in the priming of the leftward λ DNA

23

replication. The other is almost 200 nucleotides long, and transcribed rightward in the Q-S-R region of λ.

5) In the in vitro experiments, initiation of transcription
in the immunity region was not observed, although such messages
were initiated in vivo.

6) The transcriptional controls that operate during development of phage λ are strongly interlocked and coupled to DNA replication.

REFERENCES

1. BLATTNER, F.R. & DAHLBERG, J.E. (1972). Nature [New Biol.]
    237, 227.

2. BLATTNER, F.R., DAHLBERG, J.E., BOETTIGER, J.K., FIANDT, M. &
    SZYBALSKI, W. (1972). Nature [New Biol.] 237, 232.
3. LOZERON, H.A., FUNDERBURGH, M.L., DAHLBERG, J.E., STARK, B.P.
    & SZYBALSKI, W. (1972). Abst. Ann. Meet. Am. Soc. Microbiol.
    p. 237.
4. DAHLBERG, J.E., LOZERON, H.A. & SZYBALSKI, W. Bacteriophage
    Meeting, Cold Spring Harbor, N.Y., p. 86.
5. SZYBALSKI, W. (1972). In: LEDOUX, L.G.H. (Ed.), "Uptake of
    informative molecules by living cells." Amsterdam, North
    Holland Publishing Co. p. 59.

BACILLUS CEREUS OUTGROWTH "EARLY PROTEINS" AND THEIR POSSIBLE

ROLE IN CONTROL OF TRANSCRIPTION

Z. Mazor, H. Ben-Ze'ev, Z. Silberstein and
Amikam Cohen

Department of Microbiological Chemistry, The Hebrew
University-Hadassah Medical School, Jerusalem, Israel

INTRODUCTION

When dormant spores of Bacillus cereus are heat activated
and then exposed to germination inducers, transcription is initiated and is followed by the synthesis of a small number of
protein species (1). If, in addition to germination inducers,
other necessary nutrients are added to the medium, the rate of
RNA synthesis increases and the sequential appearance of protein
species is observed (2). It has been shown that the sequential
synthesis of these protein species is controlled on the transcription level (3).

The development of bacteriophage following bacterial infection is also controlled by sequential transcription of the phage
genome. "Early" genes are transcribed by the host transcription
system (4); some of the "early" phage gene products may modify
host RNA polymerase (5), interact with host control elements (6),
or may replace host polymerase (7) or some of its subunits (8).
These functions result in a change of the specificity of the
bacterial transcription system and implement the synthesis of
"late" phage RNA species.

If sequential transcription of DNA of outgrowing spores is
controlled by a mechanism similar to that which controls phage
development, one may expect the proteins which are synthesized
immediately following induction of germination to play a decisive
role in the control of sequential transcription observed during
spore outgrowth.

25

THE ROLE OF EARLY PROTEINS IN TRANSCRIPTION

Inhibition of protein synthesis at early stages of B. cereus spores outgrowth of chloramphenicol or puromycine reduces the rate of RNA synthesis by ten to twenty fold (9). When these antibiotics are added to vegetative cells or to spores at a later stage of outgrowth they have little effect on the rate of RNA synthesis. Thus, by adding protein synthesis inhibitors to outgrowing spores at different time intervals following induction of germination, and determining the effect of time of exposure to these antibiotics on the rate of RNA synthesis, the time of synthesis of the protein (or proteins) required for later transcription can be estimated. The data presented in Fig. 1 indicate that this protein is synthesized between 6 and 12 minutes following induction of germination. This synthesis is observed in a medium containing both germination inducers and amino acids, which permit normal outgrowth, as well as in a medium containing only germination inducers, which allow the synthesis of a limited number of protein species (1). The synthesis of this protein coincides immediately with or follows spore germination.

The effect of inhibition of protein synthesis on the population of pulse labeled RNA species was studied by RNA-DNA competitive hybridization experiments. A number of RNA species pulse labeled at a late stage of outgrowth are not present in RNA extracted from outgrowing B. cereus spores at an earlier stage (10). Accordingly, RNA extracted 7 min following induction of germination does not compete against RNA pulse labeled at 30 min for sites on B. cereus DNA as well as does RNA extracted 30 min following induction (Fig. 2b). On the other hand, both 7 min RNA and 30 min RNA compete equally well against RNA pulse labeled 7 min following germination induction (Fig. 2a). When RNA of spores outgrowing in the presence of chloramphenicol was pulse labeled at 30 min following germination induction and assayed, by competitive hybridization experiments, against 7 min and 30 min unlabeled RNA, for sites on B. cereus DNA, both preparations of unlabeled RNA competed equally well (Fig. 2c). These experiments suggest that inhibition of protein synthesis at an early stage of spore outgrowth affects both the rate of RNA synthesis and the sequence of transcription.

In order to determine whether protein synthesis is required for transcription of phage DNA, we have studied the effect of protein synthesis inhibitors on phage CP-51 DNA transcription in outgrowing B. cereus spores. When sporulating B. cereus cells are infected by CP-51 bacteriophage, phage DNA enters the newly formed spore but the lytic cycle does not proceed. Instead,

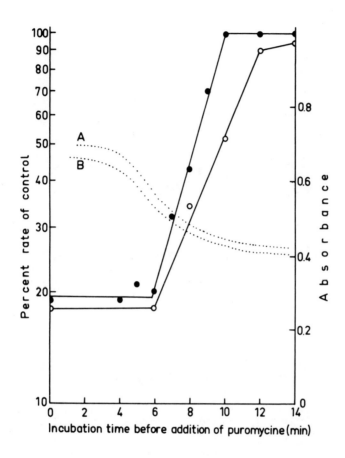

Fig. 1. The effect of time of addition of puromycine on the rate of RNA synthesis.
Puromycine (100 μg/ml) was added to incubation mixtures in germination medium (o), or CDGS-glucose (●) (9), at different times following initiation of germination. ^{3}H-uracil was added 20 min after initiation to each of the mixtures and the rate of incorporation of radioactivity to acid insoluble material was determined. Control-incubation mixture without puromycine. (A) Absorbancy of suspension in medium CDGS-glucose. (B) Absorbancy of suspension in germination medium.

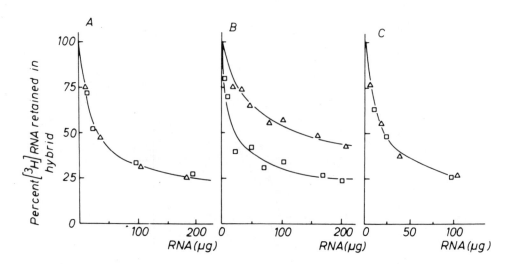

Fig. 2. Competitive hybridization to B. cereus DNA of RNA synthesized in the presence or absence of chloramphenicol.
RNA of outgrowing spores was pulse labeled with ^{3}H-uracil at 7 (A)
or 30 min (B) following induction of germination. RNA of spores
outgrowing in the presence of 200 μg/ml chloramphenicol was pulse
labeled at 30 min after induction of germination (C). All preparations of pulse labeled RNA were hybridized to CP-51 DNA in the
presence of the indicated amounts of unlabeled RNA extracted from
outgrowing spores at 7 (Δ) or 30 (□) min after germination induction.

    Hybridization reaction mixtures (14) contained (A) 3.2 μg,
(B) 1.5 μg or (C) 1.9 μg ^{3}H RNA, 4 μg heat denatured B. cereus
DNA and the indicated amounts of unlabeled RNA, in a total volume
of 100 μl of 0.9 M sodium chloride and 0.09 M sodium citrate.

    Twelve percent of the input ^{3}H RNA pulse labeled at 7 min,
following induction of germination, 14 percent of the input [3]H
RNA pulse labeled at 30 min and 9 percent of the input ^{3}H RNA of
spores outgrowing in the presence of chloramphenicol and pulse
labeled at 30 min after induction of germination, hybridized in
the absence of competitors.

phage DNA is trapped in the spore until outgrowth, when phage development is initiated (11).

Spores harboring phage DNA were heat activated and incubated in medium supplemented with germination inducers. B. cereus RNA labeled at different periods was prepared and assayed for percent of label hybridizable to CP-51 DNA. ·Only 0.2-0.3 percent of total labeled RNA was hybridizable to CP-51 DNA when pulses were given during the first 40 min following induction of germination. (The efficiency of hybridization in this system, as measured by percent of in vitro prepared CP-51 RNA hybridizable to CP-51 DNA, was 70 percent.)   An increase in the percent of pulse labeled RNA hybridizable to CP-51 DNA was observed at 45 min following induction of germination. After this stage, phage development proceeds at a rate similar to that observed in infected vegetative cells (12). The low percent of label hybridizable to CP-51 DNA observed when RNA was pulse labeled at early stages of outgrowth may be due to a low level of phage RNA synthesis or to nonspecific retention of label on the filters. To resolve between these alternatives, RNA labeled at early outgrowth was eluted from the filters and rehybridized to B. cereus or CP-51 phage DNA. While 50 percent of the label rehybridized to CP-51 DNA, only 2 percent hybridized to B. cereus DNA, confirming there is a low rate of phage RNA synthesis before the increase observed at 45 min.

If early outgrowth proteins are required for phage DNA transcription, inhibition of protein synthesis will result in the elimination of the increase in rate of phage RNA synthesis at 45 min. If, on the other hand, early outgrowth proteins are not required for phage RNA synthesis, the decrease in total RNA synthesis in the presence of protein synthesis inhibitors should result in a 10-20 fold increase in the proportion of phage RNA present in total RNA, pulse labeled at early stages of outgrowth. The results presented in Fig. 3, fit the second· alternative. Thus, a protein which is synthesized early during outgrowth is required for B. cereus DNA transcription but not for phage DNA transcription.

CELL AND SPORE RNA POLYMERASE

Speculating on the nature of the early outgrowth protein, it may be RNA polymerase, one of its subunits, a factor required for transcription of B. cereus DNA, or another element of transcription control. If the structure and specificity of B. cereus RNA polymerase change during outgrowth, one may expect differences between spore and vegetative cell enzymes. B. cereus RNA polymerase consists of at least two peptide subunits, one of molecular weight 140,000 daltons which has polymerase activity with

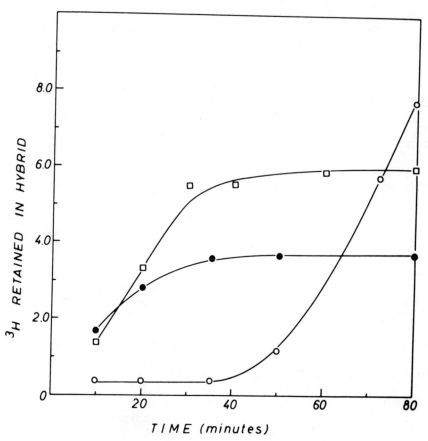

Fig. 3. Effect of chloramphenicol and puromycine on CP-51 RNA
synthesis in outgrowing B. cereus spores harboring CP-51 DNA.
RNA was pulse labeled with ³H-uracil during the outgrowth of
spores harboring CP-51 DNA in the presence of 200 µg/ml chloramphenicol (□) or 200 µg/ml puromycine (●) which were added to
the suspensions of outgrowing spores before induction of germination. Spores outgrowing in the absence of antibiotics (o).
     Hybridization of pulse labeled RNA to membrane bound de-
natured DNA was carried out according to Gillespie and Spiegelman
(15) with 40 µg heat denatured DNA bound to 25 mm 0.45 µ Sartorius
membrane filters. Filters were suspended in Denhardt solution
(16) before hybridization to reduce background. Hybrid retained
on filters is expressed as percent of labeled RNA added to the
hybridization mixture.

poly [d(A-T)] template, and one of 29,000 daltons which is needed for phage DNA transcription. Both peptides are present in both vegetative and spore enzymes and have similar electrophoretic mobilities in sodium dodecyl sulfate polyacrylamide gel electrophoresis. Unlike the vegetative cell enzyme, spore enzyme subunits dissociate from each other upon purification by DEAE cellulose chromatography and glycerol gradient centrifugation (13).

Template specificity of B. cereus vegetative cell and spore RNA polymerase was studied using poly [d(A-T)] and CP-51 phage DNA (Fig. 4). Partially purified enzyme preparations of spores or vegetative cells can transcribe CP-51 DNA or poly [d(A-T)] at low or high (0.15 M KCl) salt concentrations. Purification of the enzymes by DEAE cellulose chromatography reduces the ability of both spore and cell enzymes to transcribe CP-51 DNA at low ionic strength. Activity with phage DNA template is retained if the column is not washed with 0.15 M KCl prior to enzyme elution. Enzyme preparations of spores and vegetative cells have similar ratios of activity with CP-51 DNA to activity with poly [d(A-T)] when the assay is conducted at high ionic strength. High salt concentration does not increase the activity of enzyme purified by phosphocellulose chromatography with CP-51 DNA template (Fig.4).

The fidelity of in vitro transcription of these enzymes was determined by competitive hybridization to CP-51 phage DNA of tritium labeled RNA, synthesized in vitro, against unlabeled RNA purified from vegetative cells after infection by CP-51 phage in the presence of chloramphenicol. The results presented in Fig. 5 indicate that RNA synthesized by either vegetative cell or spore enzymes is homologous to early CP-51 RNA synthesized in vivo by the host transcription system.

The observation that spore RNA polymerase can transcribe phage CP-51 DNA is consistent with the finding that phage DNA transcription is initiated in spores outgrowing in the presence of chloramphenicol or puromycine. These two results suggest that the peptide which is synthesized at early stages of outgrowth and is necessary for transcription of cellular DNA is not one of the known RNA polymerase subunits which are required for CP-51 DNA transcription.

THE MISSING FACTOR

The components of the B. cereus transcription system which are present in the dormant spores must be complemented by a protein factor which is synthesized at early stages of outgrowth in order to support sequential transcription of the bacterial genome

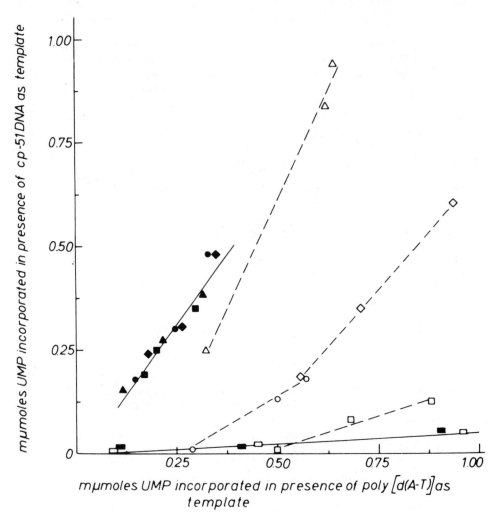

Fig. 4.　Effect of KCl concentration on activity of B. cereus
spore of vegetative cell RNA polymerase with CP-51 phage DNA or
poly [d(A-T)].
Enzyme purification and assay methods are as described elsewhere
(13) except that 0.5 mg/ml bovine serum albumin was present in
the assay mixtures.　Enzyme preparations from spores (□,■ , o,
●) and from vegetative cells (◇, ◆ , △, ▲) were purified by passage through a DEAE cellulose column, with (□,■ , ◇, ◆), or
without (o, ●, △, ▲) a 0.15 M KCl wash before elution of the
enzyme from the column.　Assays were conducted in the absence
(□, o, ◇ , △) or presence (■, ●,◆ , ▲) of 0.15 M KCl.
　　　Activity of enzyme purified by phosphocellulose chromatography (17) in the presence (■) or absence (□) of 0.15 M KCl.

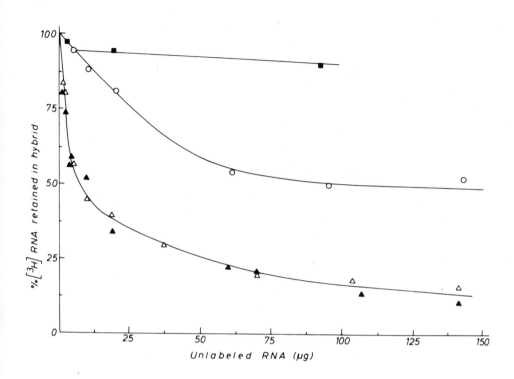

Fig. 5. Competitive hybridization to CP-51 DNA of in vitro synthesized ^{3}H-RNA and RNA of infected cells.
^{3}H-RNA was synthesized by B. cereus spores (▲, ■) or vegetative
cell RNA polymerase (Δ, o) in the presence of 0.15 M KCl (for
assay conditions see Fig. 4, save that the ^{3}H-UTP concentration was
reduced to 0.075 mM and its specific activity increased to
200 Ci/mmole). After synthesis, RNA was purified by phenol extraction, DNase (10 µg/ml) and pronase (25 µg/ml) treatments, additional phenol extraction and dialysis.
    RNA was prepared from cells infected by CP-51 phage in the
presence of chloramphenicol (100 µg/ml) 30 min following infection
(Δ, ▲), from infected cells in the absence of chloramphenicol 45
min after infection (o) and from uninfected cells (■).
    The hybridization reaction mixture (as described in legend to
Fig. 2) contained ^{3}H in vitro synthesized RNA (20,000 cpm), 0.6 µg
heat denatured CP-51 DNA and the indicated amounts of unlabeled RNA
in a total volume of 100 µl of 0.9 M sodium chloride and 0.09 M
sodium citrate.
    RNA retained in hybrid is expressed as percent of labeled re-
tained in the absence of competitor RNA; under these conditions, 8
percent of the input ^{3}H-RNA were hybridized.

during the development of the spore to a vegetative cell. While
this factor has not yet been isolated, and its activity was not
demonstrated in vitro, in vivo studies predict the following biological properties:

1. It should enhance transcription activity of B. cereus DNA,
    but not of phage CP-51 DNA.
2. It should be present in outgrowing spores, but not in spores.
3. It is not one of the known B. cereus RNA polymerase subunits.
4. It is synthesized during the first minutes of germination in
    outgrowth medium and in germination medium.

    Heat activated spores incubated in germination medium synthe-
size a small number (5-6) of protein species (1). Thus, unless
the investigated transcription factor is synthesized at a level
not detectable by autoradiography of the gel electrophoretogram,
it should be one of the 5 protein species synthesized under these
conditions. This possibility is presently under investigation.

REFERENCES

1. A. TORRIANI & C. LEVINTHAL (1967). J.Bacteriol. 94, 176-183.
2. W. STEINBERG & H.O. HALVORSON (1968). J.Bacteriol. 95,
        469-478.
3. Y. KOBAYASHI, W. STEINBERG, A. HIGA, H.O. HALVORSON &
        C. LEVINTHAL (1965). Spore III (Halvorson, H.O.,
        Hanson, R. & Campbell, L.L., eds.). Am.Soc.Microbiol.,
        Washington, pp.200-212.
4. M. CHAMBERLIN (1970). Cold Spring Harbor Symp. Quant.Biol.
        35, 851-873.
5. G. WALTER, W. SEIFERT & W. ZILLIG (1968). Biochem.Biophys.
        Res.Commun. 30, 240-247.
6. Y.W. ROBERTS (1970). Cold Spring Harbor Symp.Quant.Biol.
        35, 121-127.
7. M. CHAMBERLIN, Y. McGRATH & L. WASKELL (1970). Nature, 228,
        227-231.
8. A. STEVENS (1970). Biochem.Biophys.Res.Commun. 41, 367-373.
9. A. COHEN & A. KEYNAN (1970). Biochem.Biophys.Res.Commun. 38,
        744-749.
10. J.N. HANSON, G. SPIEGELMAN & H.O. HALVORSON (1970). Science,
        168, 1291-1298.
11. C.B. THORNE (1968). J.Virol. 2, 657-662.
12. A. COHEN, H. BEN-ZE'EV & J. YASHOUV (1973). J.Virol.
        (in press).

13. A. COHEN, Z. SILBERSTEIN & Z. MAZOR (1973). *Biochim.Biophys. Acta. 294*, 442-449.
14. R. BOLLE, H. EPSTEIN, W. SALSAR & E.P. GEIDUCHEK (1968). *J.Mol.Biol. 31*, 325-348.
15. D. GILLESPIE & S. SPIEGELMAN (1965). *J.Mol.Biol. 12*, 829-842.
16. D.T. DENHARDT (1966). *Biochem.Biophys.Res.Commun. 23*, 641-646.
17. A. COHEN, Z. SILBERSTEIN & Z. MAZOR (1972). Spore V (Halvorson, H.O., Hanson, R. & Campbell, L.L. eds.). *Am.Soc.Microbiol., Washington*, pp. 247-253.

IN VITRO TRANSCRIPTION OF E. COLI tRNA GENES CARRIED BY

TRANSDUCING PHAGES

Violet Daniel, J.S. Beckmann, Sara Sarid, J. Grimberg
and U.Z. Littauer

Biochemistry Department, Weizmann Institute of Science
Rehovot, Israel

Transducing phages have proved very useful in studies involving specific bacterial genes carried by the phage DNA; because of their smaller size, the DNA of these phages is highly enriched in specific bacterial genes as compared with the bacterial chromosome and may be used as template for in vitro RNA transcription. In order to study the transcription of a bacterial tRNA molecule, we have used the transducing phage $\phi 80 psu_3^+$ (1). The su_3^+ gene carried by the $\phi 80$ phage is the structural gene which specifies a tRNA^{Tyr} molecule that enables the amber codon, UAG, to be read as tyrosine (2,3). There are two types of tyrosine tRNA's (I and II) in E.coli, differing by two nucleotides in the variable loop. The main species in E.coli cells is tRNA^{Tyr} II; the minor species tRNA^{Tyr} is specified by two identical genes, one of which can undergo a mutation resulting in a single base change in the anticodon region of the tRNA (su_3^+). The two tRNA^{Tyr} I genes are located near the $\phi 80$ attachment site on the bacterial chromosome and can be transduced by the $\phi 80$ bacteriophage as a single or a tandem double copy.

IN VITRO TRANSCRIPTION OF $\phi 80 psu_3^+$ BY E. COLI RNA POLYMERASE

Transcription of RNA requires that both initiation and termination of the reaction take place at their proper sites. E.coli RNA polymerase is composed of several subunits ($\alpha_2\beta\beta'$ and σ). The subunit σ, which can be separated from the core enzyme ($\alpha_2\beta\beta'$) by chromatography on phosphocellulose, is believed to be required for initiation of RNA synthesis at the correct sites on the DNA template. It was observed that $\phi 80 psu_3^+$ phage DNA was a

37

poor template for core polymerase and that the transcription on this DNA could be increased 10 fold by the addition of σ subunit. The φ80psu$_3^+$ phage DNA was transcribed in vitro by the holoenzyme and the tRNA^{Tyr} sequences in the synthesized-RNA were identified by their ability to compete with E.coli ^{32}P-tRNA for hybridization sites on the φ80psu$_3^+$ DNA (Fig.1) (4). The results clearly show that φ80psu$_3^+$ RNA synthesized in vitro contains polynucleotide chains homologous to those found in the in vivo transfer RNA molecules. The competition is specific since RNA transcribed on φ80 phage DNA (which does not carry the tRNA^{Tyr} gene) does not compete with E.coli ^{32}P-tRNA. From such experiments, and knowing the amount of ^{32}P labeled tRNA^{Tyr} in the hybridization mixture, one can calculate the amounts of tRNA^{Tyr} sequences in the in vitro synthesized RNA. It was found that only small amounts of tRNA^{Tyr}-like polynucleotide chains (∿ 1 percent) are synthesized by core polymerase alone. The relative amounts of tRNA^{Tyr} sequences in the transcribed RNA are increased when synthesis is conducted in the presence of the σ subunit to about 3-10 percent. An additional 2 to 3 fold increase in the amount of tRNA^{Tyr} sequences is obtained when transcription is conducted by holoenzyme in the presence of the termination factor.

The size of the transcribed RNA was analyzed by sedimentation through sucrose density gradients (Fig. 2). Holoenzyme transcribes φ80psu$_3^+$ DNA with the production of large RNA molecules; transcription in the presence of ρ factor results in a reduction of the average size distribution of the total synthesized RNA, particularly with respect to molecules having sedimentation constants of 16S or higher. The effects of σ and ρ factors on the size distribution of tRNA^{Tyr} like chains transcribed on φ80psu$_3^+$ DNA were examined in the in vitro synthesized RNA fractionated by centrifugation through sucrose gradients. Each gradient was divided into four regions containing RNA of different sizes (Roman numbers, Fig. 2), and the location of the tRNA^{Tyr}-sequences was then identified by their ability to compete with E.coli ^{32}P-tRNA for hybridization to φ80psu$_3^+$ DNA. It was observed that tRNA^{Tyr} chains synthesized with core enzyme (lacking σ) have a wide size distribution, since all four fractions show similar competing activity. The size of tRNA^{Tyr}-like chains synthesized in the presence of σ and ρ is reduced and maximal amounts are observed in fraction III which represent molecules of size 5-8S. From these results it can be concluded that the in vitro transcription of tRNA^{Tyr} by purified RNA polymerase requires the presence of σ subunit and ρ factor but does not produce a molecule of the size of tRNA. The transcribed tRNA^{Tyr} was larger than a mature tRNA molecule, and was observed to be cleaved to 4.5-4S molecules by an E.coli ribonuclease P isolated by the procedure of Robertson et al., (5).

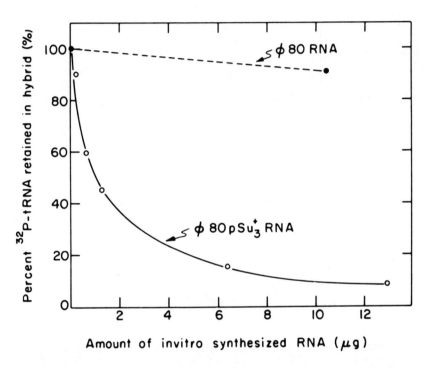

Fig. 1.   Competition of RNA transcribed <u>in vitro</u> on φ80psu$_3^+$ and
          φ80 DNAs with <u>E.coli</u> ^{32}P-tRNA.
The hybridization mixture contained 2 µg of the light strand of
φ80psu$_3^+$ DNA, 0.9 µg of ^{32}P-tRNA (1.6x10^6 cpm/µg), and different
amounts of <u>in vitro</u> synthesized φ80psu$_3^+$ or φ80 RNA in a total
volume of 0.3 ml 2 x SSC. Mixtures were incubated for 2 hr at
68°C, loaded on filters, washed with 50 ml of 2 x SSC on each side,
treated with pancreatic RNase (25 µg/ml in 2 x SSC), washed again
and counted. The radioactivity remaining on the filter was expressed as percentage of control which contained no competing RNA.

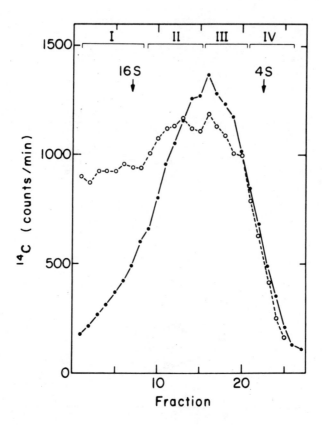

Fig. 2.   Sucrose density gradient analysis of RNA synthesized
           in vitro.
One hundred μg $\phi80psu_3^+$ DNA were transcribed in vitro by RNA polymerase in the presence (●——●) or absence (o——o) of the ρ termination factor in the reaction mixture.   Each preparation of
synthesized RNA was dissolved in 0.1 ml of 1 x SSC, layered on to
a 5 ml of 5-20 percent sucrose gradient in 1 x SSC, and centrifuged
for 4 hr at 50,000 rpm and 4°C in the SW 50.1 rotor of a Spinco
model L centrifuge.   Fractions of six drops each were collected.
Sedimentation constants were estimated by centrifuging 16S E.coli
ribosomal RNA and 4S E.coli tRNA in a separate sucrose gradient in
the same rotor.   Aliquots of 10 μl of each fraction were precipitated with trichloroacetic acid and passed through nitrocellulose
filters.   Distribution of the ^{14}C-labeled-synthesized RNA was
determined by counting the filters in a scintillation spectrophoto-
meter.   For the competition-hybridization studies, the individual
fractions were combined into four samples (I-IV) representing
different S regions of the sucrose gradient as indicated by the
brackets.

ISOLATION OF THE E.COLI DNA FRAGMENT CARRYING THE tRNA^{TYR} GENE

The method for the isolation of the DNA fragment was the same
as that used by Shapiro et al. (6) for the isolation of the lac
operon. The purification procedure took advantage of the fact
that the two phages $\phi 80psu_3^+$ (0) (1) and $\phi 80psu_3^+$ (S) (2) carry the
E.coli DNA fragment containing the su_3^+ gene inserted into the phage
DNA in opposite orientations, i.e. the sense strand for su_3^+ gene
transcription on opposite phage DNA strands. In order to determine the DNA strand on which the tRNA^{Tyr} is transcribed, the complementary strands of the two $\phi 80psu_3^+$ phage DNAs were separated
and purified in CsCl gradients. The transcribed strand of each of
the phage DNAs was identified by hybridization with ^{32}P-labeled
E.coli tRNA (Table 1). In the case of $\phi 80psu_3^+$ (0) (1), the tRNA^{Tyr}
chains are transcribed from the light strand while in the case of
$\phi 80psu_3^+$ DNA (2) there is an inversion of the E.coli DNA fragment
carrying the su_3 gene and transcription of the tRNA^{Tyr} chains
takes place on the heavy strand. When the separated heavy strands
of both phages are hybridized, only the inserted E.coli sequences
including the tRNA^{Tyr} gene are complementary and will anneal to
form a duplex DNA (Fig. 3). The other phage sequences are identical and non-complementary and therefore remain single stranded.
The single stranded tails of the heteroduplex were removed by
digestion with the specific Neurospora endonuclease and the E.coli
DNA fragment was isolated.

These studies were complemented by electron microscopic
observations. Hybridization of the two heavy DNA strands resulted
in the formation of a duplex showing short, double stranded structures with single-stranded bush-like tails. After digesting the
single-stranded tails with Neurospora endonuclease, a pure population of short, duplex molecules was seen. The length of the
endonuclease-resistant duplex molecules was about 0.57 μm. Thus,
the mass of the isolated E.coli DNA fragment carrying the tRNA^{Tyr}
gene is about 1.08×10^6 daltons, which represents a purification of
about 2000-fold, compared to the E.coli genome. The isolated
duplex molecules were shown to serve as templates for in vitro
tRNA^{Tyr} transcription (25-80 percent of the total RNA are tRNA^{Tyr}-
like molecules)thus establishing their identity as E.coli DNA
fragments containing the su_3 gene.

TABLE   1

HYBRIDIZATION OF ^{32}P-LABELED E.COLI tRNA WITH THE
SEPARATED STRANDS OF $\phi80psu_3^+(0)$ AND $\phi80psu_3^{+,-}(S)$ DNA

DNA	Strand	Hybridized E. coli $[^{32}P]$tRNA(cpm)
$\phi80psu_3^+(0)$	Light	1,970
$\phi80psu_3^+(0)$	Heavy	50
$\phi80psu_3^{+,-}(S)$	Light	40
$\phi80psu_3^{+,-}(S)$	Heavy	2,180

The hybridization mixture contained in a total volume
of 0.3 ml: 0.3 M NaCl, 0.03 M sodium citrate (2 x SSC),
2 µg of the separated single-stranded DNA and 0.22 µg
of E.coli $[^{32}P]$tRNA. The mixtures were incubated at
68°C for 120 min, diluted with 2 ml of 2 x SSC, loaded
on nitrocellulose filters (Schleicher and Schuell B6,
27 mm), and washed with 50 ml of 2 x SSC on each side.
The filters were treated with pancreatic RNase (25
µg/ml in 2 x SSC) for 60 min at room temperature,
washed again with 50 ml of 2 x SSC on each side, dried,
and counted.

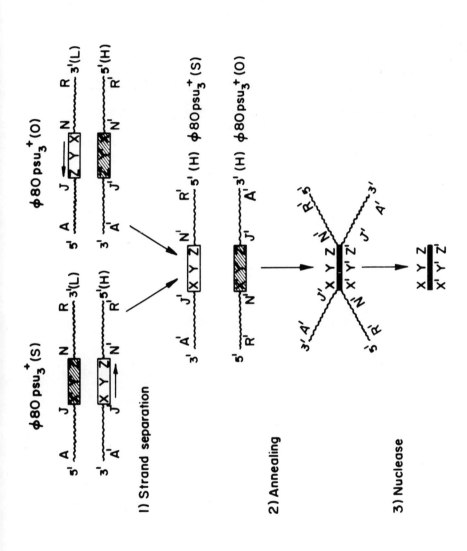

Fig. 3. Purification of the E.coli DNA fragment carrying the tRNA^Tyr gene.

REFERENCES

1. T. ANDOH & H. OZEKI.(1968) *Proc.Natl.Acad.Sci. USA*, 59, 792.
2. S. KAPLAN, A.O.W. STRETTON & S. J. BRENNER (1965).
    J.Mol.Biol. 14, 528.
3. M.G. WEIGERT, E. LANKA & A. GAREN. (1965) *J.Mol.Biol.* 14, 522.
4. V. DANIEL, S. SARID, J.S. BECKMANN & U.Z. LITTAUER. (1970)
    Proc.Natl.Acad.Science USA, 66, 1260.
5. H.D. ROBERTSON, S. ALTMAN & J.D. SMITH. (1972) *J.Biol.Chem.*
    247, 5243.
6. F. SHAPIRO, L. MacHATTIE, L. ERON, G. IHLER, K. IPPEN &
    J. BECKWITH.(1969) *Nature, 224*, 768.
7. V. DANIEL, J.S. BECKMANN, S. SARID, J. GRIMBERG, M. HERZBERG
    & U.Z. LITTAUER. (1971) *Proc.Natl.Acad.Sci. USA, 68*, 2268.

SYMMETRICAL TRANSCRIPTION IN ANIMAL CELLS AND VIRUSES

Yosef Aloni

Department of Genetics, Weizmann Institute of Science
Rehovot, Israel

INTRODUCTION

I would like to discuss the first step of genetic transfer, that from DNA to RNA, namely the transcription process. It is assumed that there is a selectivity in transcription; thus, not all the genetic information of the DNA is transcribed to RNA; there is transcription of only portions of certain DNA templates and non-transcription of others. In other words, in vivo transcription proceeds from defined initiation points to defined stopping points. There is another type of selectivity in the transcription process: It has been generally accepted that transcription is asymmetric, in the sense that only one strand of a given gene is transcribed. The idea of asymmetric transcription is based on the assumption that if each of the two DNA strands of a given gene serves as an RNA template, each gene would produce two RNA products with complementary sequences, which should code for two different proteins. Since, from genetic evidence we know that each gene controls only one protein, we must assume that either only one of the two possible RNA strands is made, or if both are synthesized, for some specific reason, only one is functional. Using bacteriophages as model systems, it appeared that the former possibility is correct and since then the dogma is that in vivo transcription is asymmetric.

Figure 1 illustrates some of the differences between asymmetric and symmetric transcription: It can be seen that there are two types of asymmetric transcription; in the first, only one

45

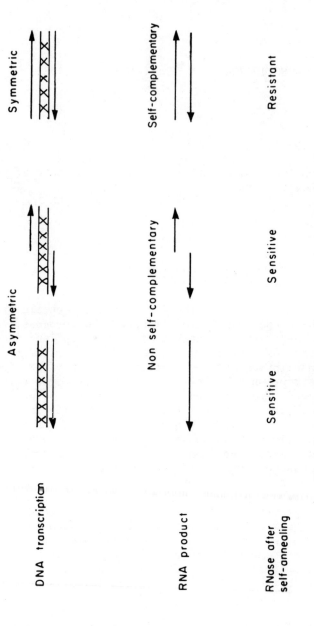

Fig. 1. Symmetric and asymmetric transcription.

DNA strand is transcribed while in the second there is a switch from one DNA strand to its complement. In both cases, there is no transcription of overlapping sequences. However, in symmetric transcription overlapping sequences are transcribed.

The RNA products of asymmetric transcription are non self-complementary, unlike those of symmetric transcription. Consequently, upon self-annealing and RNase treatment, the products of asymmetric transcription would be RNase-sensitive while those of symmetric transcription would form double-stranded (ds) RNA and would be RNase-resistant.

Based on these differences the two main tests to distinguish between asymmetric and symmetric transcription are: (i) complementarity of the RNA products to the separated strands of the DNA template (ii) self-complementarity of the RNA products and consequently their ability to form ds RNA upon self-annealing. It should be mentioned that in each case the newly synthesized RNA must be analyzed, in order to avoid the possibility of RNA processing from symmetry to asymmetry.

The purpose of this communication is to describe experiments which demonstrate that, at least in two different genetic systems, the concept of asymmetric transcription is incorrect; and that the alternative symmetric type of transcription is taking place. The first system is the mitochondrial DNA in HeLa cells and the second is the DNA tumor viruses, polyoma and SV_{40} in lytically infected cells. Part of the work summarised in the present communication has been published (1-6).

SYMMETRICAL IN VIVO TRANSCRIPTION OF MITOCHONDRIAL
DNA IN HELA CELLS

The reason for first studying asymmetry vs. symmetry of transcription in the mitochondrial genetic system in HeLa cells is because of the relative simplicity and compartmentalized character of this system, which offers unique advantages for the study of gene expression in eukaryotes. Furthermore, the mitochondrial DNA is relatively simple, it has a circular configuration of about 5 μm equivalent to a M.W. of $1x10^7$ and the two strands of the mitochondrial DNA can easily be separated.

a.   Separation of the Mitochondrial DNA Strands

Figure 2 shows the quality of strand separation obtained by centrifuging [14C] thymidine-labeled mit-DNA in an alkaline CsCl density gradient. The ratio of radioactivities associated with the two bands in this experiment was 1.4. This difference in [14C] thymidine radioactivity associated with the two strands presumably reflects the difference in their thymidine content. Therefore, one would expect that after short pulses of [3H] uridine, when essentially all label incorporated is in UMP, the potential transcripts of the L strands would have, on the average, a specific activity 1.4 times higher than the transcripts of the H strand. Having the separated mit-DNA strands, one can analyze the mit-RNA with respect to its complementarity to each of the DNA strands. In order to avoid the possibility of RNA processing from symmetry to asymmetry, the newly synthesized RNA of the nascent chains present in the transcription complexes of the mitochondrial DNA was investigated.

b.   Isolation and Characterization of Transcription Complexes of
Mitochondrial DNA

Isolation of transcription complexes of mitochondrial DNA was based on the expectation that these complexes, due to the presence of attached RNA chains, would band in a CsCl/ethidium bromide density-gradient at a position of higher density than closed circular mit-DNA. In Fig. 3a, it can be seen that a whole spectrum of components containing RNA labeled in a 5 min [3H] uridine pulse was found in the density region $\sim$1.60 g/cm^3 to $\sim$1.80 g/cm^3. DNA long-term labeled with [14C] thymidine was also found in this region of the gradient.

Electron microscopic analysis of the heaviest 14C-thymidine-labeled components in the gradient ($\sim$1.78 g/cm^3) showed that these consisted primarily of complexes of open or closed circular mit-DNA with collapsed molecules. A few typical mitochondrial DNA molecules with RNA bushes attached are shown in Plate 1. The 5 μm open circular mit-DNA molecule is recognizable by its uniform extended appearance, typical of duplex DNA. At least 25 bushes of various sizes can be seen attached to the circular DNA. In Plate 2, two loosely twisted circular mit-DNA molecules, possibly concatenated, with very large RNA bushes are seen. Plates 3a, b and c show some highly twisted circular mit-DNA molecules with a few relatively large RNA bushes attached to them. On the basis of the fine structural features of the attachment of the RNA molecules to DNA, and of the failure to observe such a type of association by mixing 45S rRNA precursor molecules and mit-DNA, (Plate 3d) one

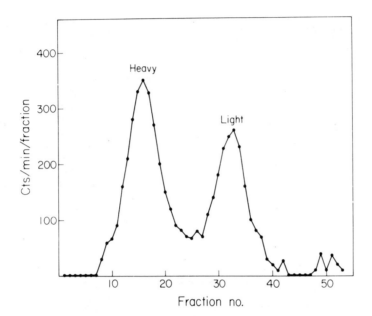

Fig. 2. Separation of the complementary strands of ^{14}C-labeled HeLa mit-DNA in an alkaline CsCl density gradient.
A solution containing 13 µg closed circular mit-DNA in 4.0 ml of 0.055 M K_3PO_4 and 0.01 percent SDS was brought to a refraction index of about 1.405 with solid CsCl and to pH 12.4 with KOH. The mixture was centrifuged in a polyallomer tube in the Spinco 65 angle rotor at 42,000 rpm for 42 h at 20°.

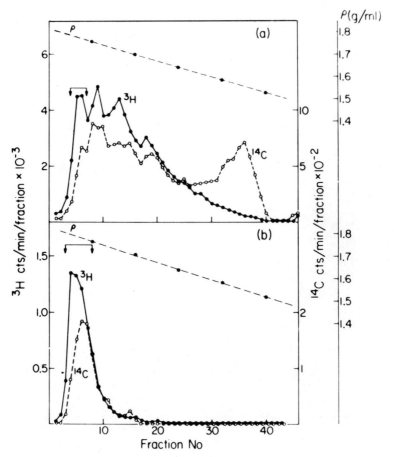

Fig. 3.   Fractionation of ^{3}H-labeled RNA and ^{14}C-labeled DNA
by CsCl/EB density-gradient centrifugation.
(a) The mitochondrial fraction was prepared by differential centrifugation as previously described (2) from cells pulse-labeled
for 5 min with ^{3}H-uridine and long term labeled with ^{14}C-thymi-
dine.   The mitochondrial fraction was dissolved in SDS buffer and
passed through a sucrose gradient (3).   The fast sedimenting
structures of the sucrose gradient were collected by ethanol precipitation, dissolved in 3.7 ml   Tris/Na/EDTA and, after addition
of ethidium bromide (EB) to a final concentration of 100 µg and
CsCl to a density of 1.63 g/cm^3, centrifuged in the Spinco SW65
rotor at 48,000 rpm for 27 h at 4°.   Fractions were collected
from the bottom of the tube, and assayed for radioactivity and
refractive index as described (2).
(b) The fractions corresponding to the peaks of ^{3}H and ^{14}C radioactivity with the highest density (indicated by arrows in (a))
were pooled, and the sample was recentrifuged in a CsCl/ED density
gradient under the same conditions as in (a).

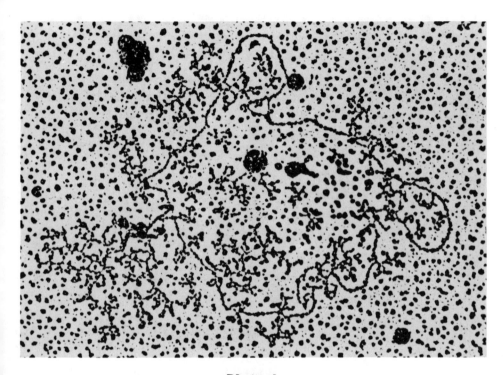

Plate 1

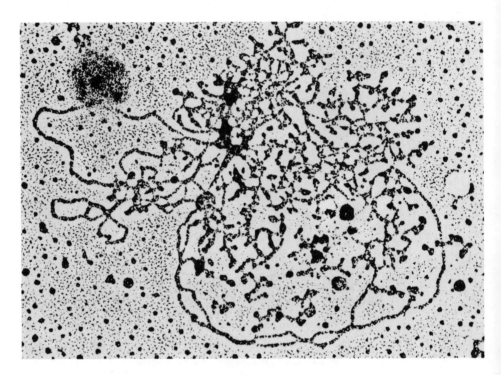

Plate 2

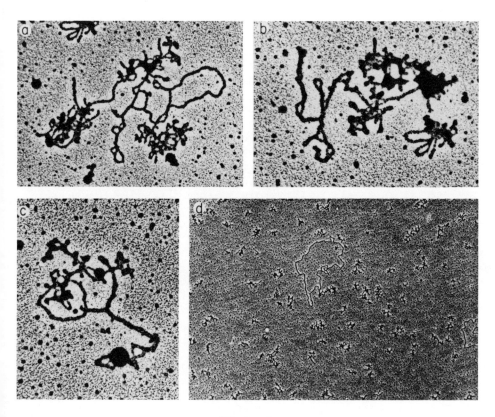

Plate 3

may conclude that the complexes observed here occur in vivo. The
most plausible interpretation of these structures is that they are
transcription complexes with growing RNA chains which have been
labeled during the [^{3}H] uridine pulse. The observation that the
closed transcription complexes detected here carried only a few
nascent chains, and that in intermediate forms, i.e. in partially
relaxed transcription complexes, the nascent chains were preferentially associated with the relaxed portion of the circle, suggests
that the physiological process goes from the twisted to the relaxed
form. Each local unwinding of the DNA duplex, necessary for initiation and propagation of transcription, would produce a partial
relaxation of the original supercoiled structure, until, for a
sufficient number of initiation points, the superhelical density
would become zero. The occurrence, in some of the transcription
complexes we have analyzed, of growing RNA chains attached at
fairly regular intervals to many points along the whole length of
mitochondrial DNA, is in agreement with the conclusion previously
reached that mitochondrial DNA in HeLa cells is completely or
almost completely transcribed. The largest RNA bushes found to be
attached to mitochondrial DNA were at least as large as collapsed
45S rRNA precursor molecules (M.W. 4.5x10^6), indicating that at
least one of the two mit-DNA strands is transcribed as a continuous chain over its entire, or almost entire, length. On the other
hand, the fact that no obvious size pattern of the nascent RNA
chains along the mit-DNA molecules, such as one of progressive increase, was observed in the transcription complexes, suggests the
occurrence of multiple initiation points for transcription. These
two conclusions are not mutually exclusive. In fact, if the two
strands of the same mit-DNA molecule are transcribed concurrently
in opposite directions, the presence of intermixed small and large
RNA bushes in more than one area of the contour of the mit-DNA
molecule would be compatible with a single initiation point for
the transcript of at least one of the two strands, provided that
transcription of the other strand were to start at different posi-
tion(s) on the mit-DNA molecule.

c. Sequence Homology of Nascent RNA Recovered from Transcription
Complexes to Heavy and Light Mitochondrial DNA Strands

The transcription complexes banded at the density of
1.78 g/cm^3 in CsCl/ethidium bromide (Fig. 3b) were digested with
DNase extracted with SDS/phenol and a constant amount of the
purified RNA was subjected to hybridization tests with increasing
amounts of the separated strands of mit-DNA. From Fig. 4, it
appears that about 1.5 times as much labeled RNA hybridized with
the L as with the H strands. This ratio, which reflects the relative proportion of labeled RNA complementary to the two mit-DNA

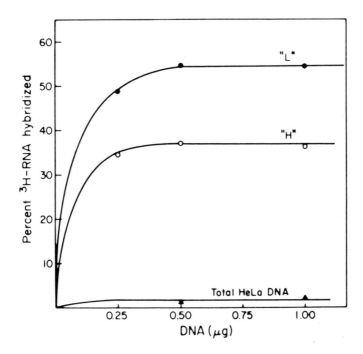

Fig. 4. Hybridization tests between ^{3}H-RNA isolated from transcription complexes and varying amounts of L and H mit-DNA strands.
The material banding at a density of 1.78 g/cm^3 in the test
shown in Fig. 3b was dialyzed against Tris/K/Mg buffer (2), and
subjected to digestion with DNase, SDS/phenol extraction and
chromatographed-through Sephadex G100 (2). Portions of the eluate
containing 100 cpm were used for hybridization tests with varying
amounts of L or H mit-DNA strands (3).

strands, strongly suggests that the two mit-DNA strands are transcribed at a similar rate. In view of the evidence of complete
transcription of the H strands, this is in accord with the idea
that the symmetric transcription of mit-DNA in HeLa cells involves
a considerable portion, if not all, of the mit-DNA molecule. The
observation that RNA molecules complementary to both mit-DNA
strands are associated with transcription complexes would exclude
the possibility that transcription of mit-DNA is asymmetrical, and
the apparent symmetry of transcription results from copying of the
asymmetric transcription product by an enzyme of the RNA replicase
type.

d. RNase-Resistance of Self-Annealed Mit-RNA

Symmetrical transcription predicts the formation of RNA products capable of extensive self-pairing. The amount of double-
helical structures in the labeled mit-RNA after a 20-min pulse is
shown in Table 1. The RNase resistance was 15 percent; however,
after self-annealing, it increased considerably, to about 60 percent, and disappeared after heating at low ionic strength. The
incomplete RNase resistance of the self-annealed preparations
implies that the amount of sequences complementary to one of the
two mit-DNA strands was in excess.

TABLE 1

RIBONUCLEASE RESISTANCE OF NEWLY SYNTHESIZED MITOCHONDRIAL RNA

Original preparation	After self-annealing	After denaturation
15	60	0

[3]H-RNA sample (about 1000 cpm) from the mitochondrial fraction of
HeLa cells labeled with ^{3}H-uridine for 20 min, tested for RNase
resistance as detailed in Table 3.

e. Relationship Between Labeling Time and the Proportion of Radioactive RNA Hybridized with the H and L mit-DNA Strands

   Table 2 shows the ratio of ^{3}H mit-RNA hybridized with the L
and H mit-DNA strands in hybridization-exhaustion experiments
utilizing mit-RNA extracted with phenol and SDS from cells labeled
with ^{3}H uridine for different periods of time. Almost equal
amounts of ^{3}H RNA (in cpm) extracted from cells labeled for 1 min
hybridized with the two strands; the proportion of labeled RNA hybridized with the H strand increased with increasing pulse length,
which suggests a greater accumulation of the transcripts of this
strand

TABLE   2

HYBRIDIZATION OF 5-^{3}H URIDINE PULSE LABELED mit-RNA WITH
SEPARATED mit-DNA STRANDS

RNA Extraction Procedure	Labeling Time (min)	$\dfrac{[^3\text{H}]\text{RNA Hybridized with "L"}}{[^3\text{H}]\text{RNA Hybridized with "H"}}$
SDS-phenol	1	0.98
	5	0.74
	20	0.58
	45	0.25
SDS-pronase-phenol	5	1.43

The data were obtained from the results of hybridization
experiments as presented in Fig. 4.

   A symmetric transcription has previously been reported for
portions of the genome of bacteriophages lambda (7) and T$_4$ (8)
and the presence of virus-specific double-stranded RNA has been

described in vaccinia-infected chick cells (9). The present observation constitutes the first known instance of symmetric in
vivo transcription of the entire, or almost the entire, genome.
Whether this represents a peculiar property of mit-DNA or whether
the same mode of transcription operates in other DNAs remained to
be established.

SYMMETRICAL TRANSCRIPTION OF SV_{40} DNA AND POLYOMA DNA IN LYTICALLY INFECTED CELLS

SV_{40} and polyoma DNA have circular configurations similar to
that of mit-DNA in HeLa cells: Early after infection, and in
transformed cells, the viral genome is only partially transcribed,
while at later stages in the infection process, most or all of
the genetic information contained in the viral DNA's is transcribed
(10). Two contradictory mechanisms concerning the transcription
and ultimate regulation of expression of SV_{40} DNA late during
infection have recently been reported; one claims asymmetrical
and the other symmetrical transcription. Asymmetrical transcription is based upon the observations that in a late stage in the
infection, RNA equivalent of 100 percent of one SV_{40} DNA strand
is found, with 30-40 percent complementary to the minus strand
and 60-70 percent complementary to the plus strand (11-13). These
results at first glance imply a mechanism of asymmetric transcription in the sense that only one of the two DNA strands of a
given gene serves as a template for RNA. Consequently, it has
been concluded that the regulation of genetic expression of SV_{40}
operates on the transcriptional level. The RNA species in these
studies were stable and non-complementary viral RNA transcripts
that accumulate in lytically infected cells. The possibility
cannot be excluded, however, that SV_{40} DNA is first transcribed
symmetrically, and afterwards certain RNA sequences are degraded,
leaving the stable products.

We now describe experiments that show that when newly synthesized viral RNA is analyzed, symmetrical transcription of the
complete viral DNA is revealed.

a. Isolation of RNase-Resistant Viral RNA

BSC-1-cells were exposed to [^{3}H]uridine for 20 min,
48 h after infection with SV_{40}, in order to identify self-complementary viral RNA in the infected cells. Mock-infected cells
were similarly treated. The [^{3}H] labeled RNA extracted from these
cells was incubated in 0.2 ml of 4xSSC at 70° for 20 h, treated

with pancreatic and T_1 RNase extracted with SDS-phenol, collected by ethanol precipitation, dissolved in 0.25 M NaCl and passed through columns of Sephadex G-100. Figure 5 shows that only a small amount of the labeled RNA from mock-infected cells treated in this way is found in the excluded peak, as compared with the RNA from infected cells. The RNA from infected cells found in the excluded peak of the Sephadex column was used in all further experiments.

b. Nuclease Sensitivity

TABLE 3

NUCLEASE RESISTANCE OF SELF-ANNEALED RNA

Enzyme Treatment	TCA Precipitability (percent)
(a) None	100
(b) Pancreatic RNase and T_1 RNase	98
(c) As (b) with the addition of pancreatic DNase	96
(d) Thermal denaturation and treatment as in (b)	0

[3]H-RNA was taken from the excluded peak of a Sephadex G-100 column as in Fig. 5. Equal amounts of radioactivity (about 2000 cpm) were used in each of the four treatments. Nuclease treatment: pancreatic RNase, 25 µg/ml; T_1 RNase 5 units/ml; pancreatic DNase, 50 µg/ml were incubated for 45 min at 37° in 0.23 M NaCl and 0.01 M Tris-HCl (pH 7.4 at 25°). For the simultaneous incubation of RNase and DNase, 0.0025 M $MgCl_2$ was added. Thermal denaturation was carried out in 0.01 M NaCl Tris-HCl, (pH 7.4 at 25°) at 100° for 4 min, after which the samples were quickly cooled. After each treatment, the TCA precipitable material on Millipore filters was counted.

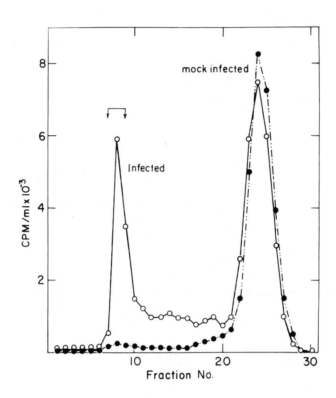

Fig. 5. Exclusion chromatography of self-annealed, RNase treated RNA on a column of Sephadex G-100.
RNA samples from infected and mock-infected cells were dissolved in 0.5 ml of 0.25 M NaCl and layered on separate 1.1x55 cm Sephadex G-100 columns equilibrated with 0.25 M NaCl. Two ml fractions were collected and 0.1 ml portions were counted. The first peak is excluded with the void volume, while the second peak contains lower molecular weight products.
0 —— 0, infected; o — .. — o mock-infected.

Table 3 shows self-annealed RNA to be 98 percent resistant to the action of RNase and 96 percent resistant to the combined effects of RNase and DNase. However, it is completely degraded by RNase after first undergoing thermal denaturation. Consequently, all the [^{3}H] label must be in the RNA. Moreover, it should be noted that under the conditions of the experiment, RNA-DNA hybrids are known to be sensitive to the combined effects of DNase and RNase.

c. RNase Susceptibility as a Function of Salt Concentration and Temperature

The material eluted in the excluded peak of the Sephadex column was tested for susceptibility to RNase as a function of salt concentration and temperature. The RNase susceptibility decreased with increasing ionic strength (Fig. 6a). This was also true of single-stranded 28S ribosomal RNA, which at a salt concentration greater than 2xSSC (about 0.4 M) showed significant resistance to the enzyme. The most pronounced difference between the 28S rRNA and RNA present in the excluded peak of the Sephadex column is in the steepness of the transition from RNase-resistance to sensitivity. In addition, at 2xSSC the RNA from the excluded peak is almost completely resistant to the enzyme.

To determine the T_m of the transition from RNase-resistance to RNase-sensitivity, samples were heated to different temperatures, cooled rapidly and the RNase resistance in 2xSSC measured. Figure 6b shows the results obtained when samples were heated at two different salt concentrations. Sharp transitions, with midpoints at 95° in 1xSSC and 81° in 0.1xSSC, were observed. Such transitions and temperatures are indicative of double-stranded molecules.

d. Buoyant Density of the Self-Annealed RNA

Single-stranded and double-stranded viral RNA's exhibit characteristic and distinguishable buoyant densities in Cs_2SO_4 of 1.63 and 1.61 g/cm^3, respectively (14). Single-stranded and double-stranded DNA's are less dense (2) and have densities of about 1.44 g/cm^3. As expected, RNA-DNA hybrids have intermediate densities (2) of about 1.50 g/cm^3. Figure 7a shows the buoyant density of self-annealed RNA in Cs_2SO_4. The value obtained (1.61 g/cm^3) is in full accord with the identification of the material as a double-stranded RNA. In addition, when the self-annealed RNA was first denatured and then centrifuged to equilibrium in Cs_2SO_4, the density increased by 0.02 g/cm^3 to become

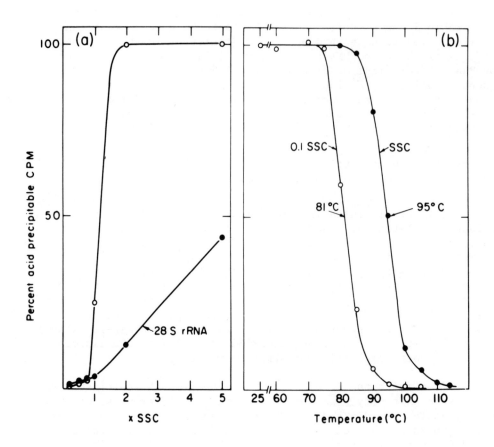

Fig. 6. Degradation of the material present in the excluded peak
of the Sephadex column by RNase at different salt concentrations
and at different temperatures.
(a) Each sample in 2 ml contained the indicated concentrations
of SSC, ^{32}P-labeled 28S rRNA (800 cpm), and ^{3}H-labeled RNA
(800 cpm) from the excluded peak of the Sephadex column. RNase-
resistance was tested with 50 μg/ml of enzyme for 30 min at 25°.
The samples were then precipitated with TCA and counted. The
amount of acid-precipitable material before treatment with RNase
was assigned a value of 100 percent.
(b) Samples 0.6 ml of ^{3}H-labeled RNA (700 cpm) from the excluded
peak of the Sephadex column were brought to SSC or 0.1xSSC,
heated for 4 min at the indicated temperatures, and rapidly cooled.
The samples were then brought to 2xSSC, and the RNase-resistance
tests were performed as in (a).

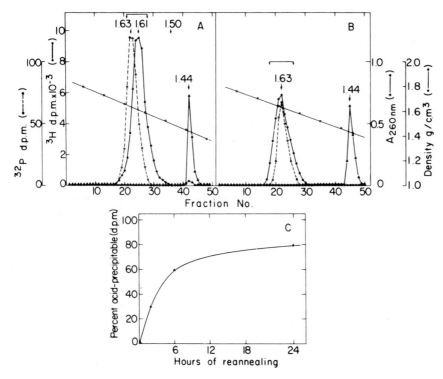

Fig. 7.   Buoyant density of self-complementary RNA in Cs_2SO_4.
(a) Four ml of Cs_2SO_4 solution (final ρ = 1.605) containing
0.05 M Tris-HCl (pH 7.4 at 25°), 0.005 M EDTA, E.coli DNA (40 µg),
(^{32}P) single-stranded viral RNA (see below) and (^{3}H)-self-com-
plementary RNA from the excluded peak of the Sephadex column
(Fig.5) were centrifuged at 35,000 rpm for 60 h at 22° in the
Spinco SW50 rotor. Fractions were collected from the bottom of
the tube and the refractive index determined. After addition of
0.5 ml H_2O to each fraction, the absorbance at 260 nm was recorded and 0.1 ml aliquots were taken for measurement of radioactivity. To prepare the single-stranded viral RNA, standard infected cells were labeled 42 h post-infection for 6 h with 0.1 mC
^{32}P/ml and the RNA was extracted. Viral RNA was selected by
hybridizing to, and eluting from, SV_{40} DNA filters.
(b) The fractions between the arrows in (a) were pooled, brought
to a concentration of 0.01 M NaCl, 0.01 M Tris-HCl (pH 7.4 at
25°), heated to 100° for 5 min and rapidly cooled. The denatured
RNA was then recentrifuged and assayed as in (a).
(c) The denatured RNA from (b) was collected, dialyzed against
0.1 M NaCl precipitated with ethanol, dissolved in 0.15 ml of
4xSSC and reannealed at 70°. Aliquots containing 2,500 dpm (H^3)-
RNA(and 20 dpm (^{32}P)-RNA) were removed at the times indicated
and tested for resistance to RNase (50 µg/ml pancreatic RNase,
5 units/ml T_1 RNase in 2xSSC at 25° for 60 min).

coincident with the density of the single-stranded viral RNA
marker (Fig. 7b). Both before and after this treatment, no
radioactivity was found at the density characteristic for RNA-
DNA hybrid molecules. The denatured RNA shown in Fig. 7b was
collected from the Cs_2SO_4 gradient and incubated at 70° in
4xSSC. Figure 7c shows the ability of the denatured material to
re-anneal, with almost 80 percent renaturation occurring within
24 h.

Thus, multiple evidence shows self-annealed RNA to be composed of double-stranded RNA molecules. Since symmetrical transcription of DNA predicts the formation of RNA products capable of
extensive self-pairing, the most likely interpretation of the
data is that the self-complementary RNA was produced during symmetrical transcription of SV_{40} DNA late in infection.

e. Relation of the Annealed Self-Complementary RNA to SV_{40}

The relation of the double-stranded RNA to SV_{40} was suggested
by its occurrence in infected cells and not in mock-infected
cells, and was clearly established by RNA-DNA hybridization experiments. "Native" and denatured RNA samples were incubated with
filters containing excess amounts of component I SV_{40} DNA from
plaque-purified virus or with filters containing BS-C-1 DNA.
Almost 50 percent (> 90 percent if corrected for efficiency of
hybridization) of the denatured RNA hybridized with SV_{40} DNA, and
about 8 percent hybridized with BS-C-1 DNA (Table 4). No hybridization was registered with either SV_{40} DNA or BS-C-1 DNA when
"native" RNA was used. These results again indicate the duplex
nature of the RNA, as well as its high specificity toward SV_{40}
DNA.

f. The Fraction of the Newly Synthesized Viral RNA That
Can Become ds RNA

The fraction of the newly synthesized viral RNA that can
become ds RNA was estimated by separation in a sucrose gradient,
as shown in Fig. 8. To minimize thermal and enzymatic degradation, self-annealing was carried out at 37° in 60 percent formamide, and the RNase digestion was performed with a low concentration of the enzyme. Figure 8a shows a main peak of RNase-
resistant [3H] labeled RNA at about 4S. There was also some
faster sedimenting RNA, which was pooled as indicated. A portion
of this RNA was centrifuged to equilibrium in Cs_2SO_4 and banded

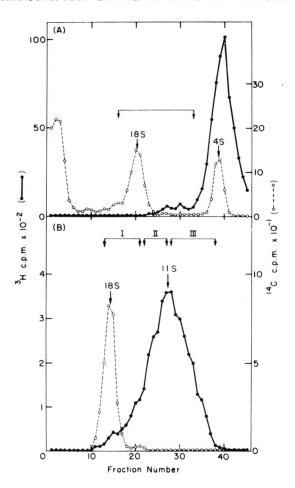

Fig. 8. Sedimentation of RNase-resistant RNA through sucrose
gradients.
Polyoma infected cells (3×10^7) were labeled for 20 min with ^{3}H-
uridine. Labeled RNA was extracted from whole cells, self-
annealed for 20 h in 0.2 ml 60 percent (v/v) formamide, 0.75 M
NaCl, 0.5 percent (w/v) SDS, 0.01 M Tris (pH 7.9 at 25°), digested
with 5 µg/ml pancreatic RNase and 1 unit/ml T_1 RNase in 2xSSC for
1 h at 25°, extracted with SDS-phenol and collected by ethanol
precipitation. (a) RNA was sedimented through a linear 15-30 percent (w/w) sucrose gradient in SDS buffer in a Spinco SW41 rotor
for 16 h, at 33,000 rpm at 20°. ^{14}C-18S rRNA and 4S RNA served as
sedimentation markers. Twenty µl fractions were collected, precipitated in 10 percent TCA and counted. (b) The material for the
region between the arrows in(a)was pooled,collected by ethanol precipitation and rerun as in (a) in a Spinco SW 41 rotor for 17 h at
33,000 rpm at 20°. Fractions (20 µl) were collected, precipitated
in 10 percent TCA on glass fiber filters and counted.

TABLE   4

HYBRIDIZATION OF SV$_{40}$ WITH "NATIVE" AND DENATURED RNA

RNA	DNA on Filter	μg/DNA Filter	cpm Bound to Filter[*]
"Native"	SV$_{40}$	10	15 (0.5)
	BS-C-1	50	12 (0.4)
	None	0	8 (0.3)
Denatured	SV$_{40}$	10	1360 (47.5)
	BS-C-1	50	233 (8.2)
	None	0	14 (0.5)

Labeled RNA used in the hybridization assay was obtained from the
excluded peak of a Sephadex G-100 column (see Fig.5). SV$_{40}$ DNA
was extracted from plaque-purified virus. Each hybridization
mixture contained DNA immobilized on Millipore filters, as indicated, and 2850 cpm of "native" or denatured RNA.

[*] The numbers in parentheses give cpm bound as percent of input,
not corrected for efficiency of hybridization, which was 50-60
percent.

(Fig. 7a) at 1.62 g/cm^3, the density of double-stranded RNA (14).
A second portion was denatured and hybridized with an excess
amount of viral DNA; 60 percent of the RNA hybridized, thus showing a high specificity towards viral DNA. The remainder was
centrifuged through a second sucrose gradient. A broad peak with
a median at about 11S was obtained (Fig.8b) with faster and slower
sedimenting RNA components. This peak represents between 0.6-1.0
percent of the total labeled RNA extracted from whole infected
cells and it corresponds to ds RNA of molecular weight $\sim 10^6$.

As mentioned above, the RNA of the 11S peak represents 0.6-1
percent of the total labeled RNA of infected cells and 60 percent
of it hybridized with excess amounts of viral DNA. Therefore,
0.36-0.60 percent of the total labeled RNA of infected cells (in
a 20 min pulse with [^{3}H] uridine) is viral ds RNA. As 2 percent

of the $[^3H]$ labeled RNA hybridized with excess amounts of viral DNA prior to self-annealing, it can be calculated that between 18-30 percent of the viral $[^3H]$ RNA of infected cells, labeled for 20 min, is self-complementary and can form ds RNA upon self-annealing.

g. Proportion of the Viral DNA Transcribed Symmetrically

The strategy for testing the proportion of the viral DNA transcribed symmetrically is illustrated in Fig. 9. RNA extracted from infected cells, labeled with ^{32}P between 35-52 h post infection, was hybridized to and eluted from SV_{40} DNA filters. This procedure yielded asymmetric ^{32}P labeled viral RNA representing 60 and 40 percent of each of the two viral DNA strands (11-13).

RNA extracted from infected cells, labeled with $[^3H]$ uridine for 20 min at 48 h post infection, was self-annealed, RNase treated and the viral ds RNA was isolated by Sephadex G-100 chromatography, as in Fig. 5. The labeled viral ds RNA was further purified by centrifuging in a Cs_2SO_4 density gradient (see Fig. 7a). Only the material that banded at a density of 1.61 g/cm^3 was collected.

The proportion of the viral DNA transcribed symmetrically was then determined from the amount of ^{32}P labeled asymmetric viral RNA that anneals with excess denatured viral ds RNA. Figure 10 shows that with increasing amounts of denatured ds RNA, almost 100 percent of the ^{32}P labeled viral RNA became RNase resistant, indicating that the complete SV_{40} DNA molecule is transcribed symmetrically.

CONCLUSION

The question of symmetric versus asymmetric transcription seems to be extremely important. As a consequence of the data presented here, much work in the field of genetic expression of mitochondrial DNA in higher cells and of the DNA tumor viruses SV_{40} and polyoma in lytically infected cells needs to be reassessed. Moreover, apart from raising new questions as how selective degradation is achieved, and what is the relation of symmetric transcription to the occurrence of ds RNA in normal and cancer cells, our data raise the possibility that post-transcriptional regulation of gene expression may be a more widespread phenomenon than has previously been considered.

TEST FOR THE PROPORTION OF THE VIRAL DNA
TRANSCRIBED SYMMETRICALLY

Asymmetric RNA transcripts equivalent to a
complete viral DNA strand accumulate late in
infection.

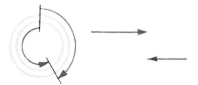

RNase digestion of self-annealed RNA from
infected cells yields *ds* viral RNA.

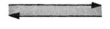

The amount of labeled asymmetric RNA that
anneals with excess denatured *ds* RNA, determines the proportion of the viral DNA transcribed symmetrically.

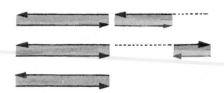

Fig. 9. Test for the proportion of the viral DNA transcribed
symmetrically.

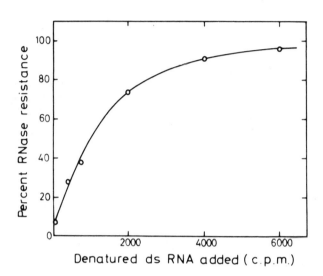

Fig. 10.   The proportion of the viral DNA transcribed symmetrically.
To prepare single-stranded viral RNA standard infected cells were
labeled between 35-52 h post-infection with 0.5 mC ^{32}P/plate and
the RNA was extracted.   Viral RNA was selected by hybridizing to,
and eluting from, SV$_{40}$ DNA filters.   The ^{32}P viral RNA was further
purified by DNase treatment and Sephadex chromatography.   To
prepare ds RNA, standard infected cells were labeled for 20 min
with ^{3}H-uridine at 48 h post-infection.   The ^{3}H ds RNA was prepared as described in Fig. 5 and was further purified by passage
through a Cs$_2$SO$_4$ density gradient as in Fig. 7a.   The material
banded at a density of 1.61 g/cm^3 was collected.   A constant
amount of ^{32}P viral RNA (500 cpm) was incubated with increasing
amounts of denatured ^{3}H ds RNA, in 0.1 ml of 4xSSC at 70° for
20 h.   The sample was then brought to 10 ml of 2xSSC and the RNase
resistant material was determined as in Table 3.

ACKNOWLEDGEMENT

This work was supported in part by grants from the Israel Cancer Association and the Israel Academy of Sciences and Humanities.

REFERENCES

1. ALONI, Y. & ATTARDI, G. (1971a). Proc.Nat.Acad.Sci. US. 68, 1757.
2. ALONI, Y. & ATTARDI, G. (1971b). J.Mol.Biol. 55, 251.
3. ALONI, Y. & ATTARDI, G. (1972). J.Mol.Biol. 70, 363.
4. ALONI, Y. (1972). Proc.Nat.Acad.Sci.U.S. 69, 2404.
5. ALONI, Y. (1973). Nature, In press.
6. ALONI, Y. & LOCKER, H. (1973). Virology, In press.
7. BØVRE, K. & SZYBALSKI, W. (1969). Virology, 38, 614.
8. GEIDUSCHEK, E.P. & GRAU, O. (1970). Le petit Colloq. Ed. Silverstri (North Holland Publ.Co. Amsterdam) p.190.
9. COLBY, C. & DUESBERG, P.H. (1969). Nature, 222, 940.
10. ALONI, Y., WINOCOUR, E. & SACHS, L. (1968). J.Mol.Biol. 31, 415.
11. LINDSTROM, D.M. & DULBECCO, R. (1972). Proc.Nat.Acad.Sci. U.S. 69, 1517.
12. KHOURY, G., BYRNE, J.C. & MARTIN, M.A. (1972). Proc.Nat. Acad.Sci.U.S. 69, 1925.
13. SAMBROOK, J., SHARP, P. & KELLER, W. (1972). J.Mol.Biol. 70, 57.
14. SZYBALSKI, W. (1968). Methods in Enzymology. 12B, 330.

CHROMATIN STRUCTURE AND GENE EXPRESSION IN EUKARYOTES

Brian J. McCarthy, James T. Nishiura[*], Margaret
N. Farquhar[+]

Department of Biochemistry and Biophysics, University
of California, San Francisco, San Francisco, Calif. 94143

INTRODUCTION

Control of gene expression in eukaryotes appears to be
exerted, at least in part, through selective transcription.
Cytological and biochemical evidence indicates that the synthesis
of RNA occurs at selected loci in interphase chromosomes. Thus
RNA synthesis occurs in extended euchromatic fibrils and not in
condensed, heterochromatic masses. Similar cytological observations tend to correlate RNA synthesis with loops of amphibian lampbrush chromosomes and with puffs in insect polytene chromosomes. The
concept that active and inactive portions of the genome may differ
in chemical and physical terms has provided an impetus for the
development of biochemical procedures for fractionating interphase
upon two overriding considerations. First, it is probable that in
many ukaryotic cells, the genome is repressed at any one time.
Therefore, biochemical or physical studies of total chromatin

[*]Present Address: Department of Genetics, University of California
                   Berkeley, California

[+]Present Address: Department of Zoology, University of Washington
                   Seattle, Washington 98195

refer primarily to the genome in its inactive state so that
features characteristic of active chromatin may be obscured.
Furthermore, the quite distinct appearance of condensed and extended
chromatin on microscopic examination must have a chemical basis.
Thus a separation of active from inactive chromatin should allow
determination of the chemical elements responsible for both
transcriptional activity and distinctive morphological features.

Since the size of mammalian and many other eukaryotic
genomes is so large compared to that of bacteria, it might be
supposed that the fraction of transcribed DNA in any cell is quite
small. Certainly, a few percent of the mammalian genome would
suffice to specify all known enzymes and structural proteins.
However, this argument is complicated by the existence of giant
heterogeneous nuclear RNA assumed to be the precursor to messenger
RNA. If only a minor part of each HnRNA molecule survives to
become mRNA (1) it is conceivable that the fraction of the genome
transcribed is large even in specialized cells where only few
messenger RNA molecules are evident. This possibility implies
that transcriptional activity need not be closely correlated
with translational capabilities. Measurement of the percent of
the genome transcribed may not therefore be useful in distinguishing
spacer from informational DNA. Nevertheless, to effect an efficient
fractionation of chromatin, it is important to know what fraction
of the genome is transcribed. In the most general terms, the
fraction of the genome transcribed in a single cell is equivalent
to the fraction of active chromatin. In practice, this equation
may not be exact, since the cell population may be heterogeneous
and different sites in the genome may be transcribed at different
rates. Nevertheless, a consideration of the fraction of the genome
transcribed is relevant to undertaking chromatin fractionation
since the isolation of active chromatin is inherently more difficult
in cases where genome expression is quite limited.

HOW MUCH OF THE GENOME IS TRANSCRIBED IN EUKARYOTES?

Estimates of the fraction of various eukaryotic genomes
transcribed are of interest for several reasons. In principle they
bear on the issue of non-transcribed spacer DNA which may represent
a substantial portion of some genomes. However such estimates do
not necessarily contribute to the solution of the problem of
how much of the genome represents genes in the sense of DNA coding
for the amino acid sequence of proteins. In some cells or some
genomes transcripts of HnRNA representing single mRNA species may
be much larger than in other cases.

The transcriptional diversity of a population of RNA
molecules may be measured by an excess RNA hybridization reaction.
In eukaryotes, where the existence of operationally redundant DNA

sequences complicates the interpretation of such experiments (2,3), quantitative estimates can be made only with reference to the unique part of the genome. In general, labeled single-stranded fragments of unique DNA are prepared by annealing and hydroxyapatite fractionation and hybridized with RNA in gross excess for extended periods of time (4,5,6,7,8).

This kind of experiment has been conducted by several groups with a variety of eukaryotic cells. Many of these results are tabulated for comparative purposes (Table 1).

TABLE   I

The Extent of Transcription of Various Genomes

	Genome Size Daltons	Percent Transcribed	Reference
1. Bacteria			
E. Coli	2.8×10^9	40-50	(32)
B. subtilis	2×10^9	40	(33)
			(8)
11. Eukaryotes			
Dictyostelium discoideum	30×10^9		
amoebae		15	(34)
Total		28	
Drosophila melanogaster	120×10^9		
cultured cells		15	(35) (19)
embryos		15	
adults		10	
Xenopus laevis	2×10^{12}		
oocytes		0.6	(5)
Chicken	1×10^{12}		
red blood cells		2	(16)
liver		15	
Mouse	3×10^{12}		
hepatoma cells		2	(4)
liver, kidney, spleen		4-5	(6)
embryo		8	(7)
brain		11	(8)
Bovine			
brain	3×10^{12}	4.2	(36)
Human	3×10^{12}		
HeLa cells		4	(37)
Liver, kidney, spleen etc.		4-5	(9)
Brain		22	

Included are estimates for two species of bacteria, from which it
appears that the majority of the genome (80-100%) is expressed,
assuming that only one DNA strand is transcribed in every region.
In eukaryotes, it is apparent that, especially for organisms
with relatively small genomes, such as the cellular slime mold and
Drosophila melanogaster, the fraction of the genome transcribed
may be a sizeable fraction of the total. It should be emphasized
that all these estimates are necessarily minimal for obvious
technical reasons involving the concentration of rarer RNA
species and the long incubation times employed (8).

     In the case of vertebrates, a pattern is apparent in the
sense that the more specialized cell types or the more limited mixtures of cells found in tissues, yield the lowest values.
Seemingly paradoxical is the low transcriptional representation
of Xenopus laevis oocytes, considering the apparent diversity
of maternal messengers. However, it should be noted that in
all these tests (Table 1) total RNA was used. Although mostly
the titration value is dominated by the base sequences of HnRNA,
in the case of maternal messenger in eggs, such RNA may already
be processed to mRNA. An obvious interpretation of the high
values for brain RNA may be made in terms of a large amount of
the genome devoted to nervous function, but it is equally likely
that this simply represents cumulative contributions from a
diverse admixture of cells (9).

     In terms of implications for chromatin fractionation, it
is immediately obvious that Drosophila cells, where about 30%
of the chromatin appears to be active, is a most promising
system. In vertebrates the problem is seemingly more difficult,
since RNA from single cell types leads to values of percent
transcription of only a few percent. In the case of tissues
such as mammalian liver, it is likely that each cell type
contributes a different population of RNA molecules so that
the percent of active genome in any one cell is less than the
value obtained for RNA isolated from the whole tissue.

     By virtue of the favorable situation presented by the
expression of the Drosophila genome, we will present data
concerned with chromatin of such cells. Other studies with
sea urchin or vertebrate chromatin will also be discussed.

FRACTIONATION OF DROSOPHILA CHROMATIN

     The earliest successful chromatin fractionation was reported
by Frenster et al (10), who separated thymocyte chromatin into
two fractions by sonication and differential centrifugation.

The same approach was refined and developed by Chalkley and
Jensen (11). Yunis and Yasmineh (12) and Duerksen and McCarthy
(13). These studies demonstrated that satellite DNA's reside exclusively in condensed portions of chromatin. Several other fractionation approaches have proved successful, including enzymatic
digestion (14), chromatography on ECTHAM cellulose (15), thermal
chromatography on hydroxyapatite (16) and agarose gel filtration
(17).

We now consider the efficacy of some of these procedures
and the implications of some of the results obtained.

Attempts have been made to fractionate Drosophila chromatin isolated from embryos or cultural cells (Schneider's line 2).
First the chromatin must be fragmented, and ideally, such breaks
should be made at the boundaries between active and inactive segments. Since there is no obvious way to attain this ideal, random
breaks are introduced by the use of a sonicator, a Virtis high-
speed homogenizer, or a French pressure cell. Each method may be
adapted to yield larger or smaller fragments. However, fractionation has been reproducibly obtained to date only with fragments
containing DNA with a double-stranded molecular weight of less
than 3×10^6 daltons. Such pieces represent only a portion of a
transcription unit or chromomere, containing perhaps $1\text{-}2 \times 10^7$
daltons of DNA (18). Larger fragments have been obtained by these
methods and treatment with restriction endonucleases, but they
have not yet been separated into active and inactive moieties.

In the case of Drosophila, chromatin separation can be
obtained by sedimentation through a steep sucrose gradient
$(0.17\text{M} \to 1.7\text{M})$ (19). The degree of separation depends upon the
shear regimen and the centrifugation time but under optimal conditions two well-separated peaks are obtained with embryo chromatin
(Figure 1).

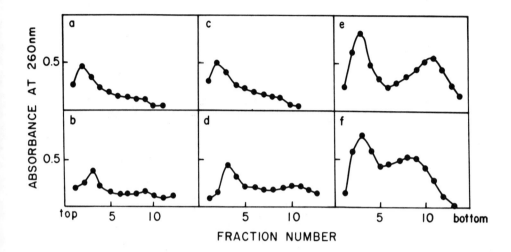

FIGURE 1.   Sucrose Gradient Profiles of Sheared Chromatin

D. melanogaster embryo chromatin, purified by sedimentation
through sucrose, was sheared in a refrigerated Virtis homogenizer
for various times at either of two voltage settings and centrifuged
at 12,000 xg for 10 min. The supernatant fraction was layered
over linear 0.17 → 1.7M sucrose gradients and centrifuged for
various periods at 113,000 xg at 4°.

(a) Sheared for 100 sec at 40 volts, centrifuged for 2 h.
(b) Sheared for 100 sec at 40 volts, centrifuged for 4 h.
(c) Sheared for 200 sec at 40 volts, centrifuged for 2 h..
(d) Sheared for 200 sec at 40 volts, centrifuged for 4 h.
(e) Sheared for 300 sec at 40 volts, centrifuged for 6 h.
(f) Sheared for 300 sec at 80 volts, centrifuged for 6 h.

A similar distribution may be obtained with Schneider's line 2
chromatin either by shearing in the Virtis homogenizer or in a
French pressure cell (Figure 2).

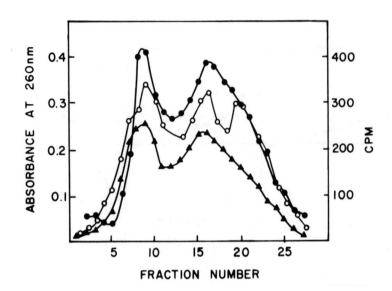

FIGURE 2.   Sucrose Gradient Profile of D. melanogaster Chromatin
             labeled with 3H-tryptophan and 14C-lysine.

        Cells (Schneider's line 2) were grown in Schneider's medium
lacking unlabeled lysine and tryptophan but containing 1 μCi/ml
3H-tryptophan and 0.2 mCi 14C-lysine for 48 h at 26°. Chromatin
was extracted from washed nuclei, purified by centrifuging through
1.7M sucrose and sheared at 3000 lbs/sq inch in a French pressure
cell in 0.01M Tris, pH 8.0. After centrifuging at 12,000 g for
10 min, the supernatant was layered over a linear 0.17M → 1.7M
sucrose gradient and centrifuged at 113,000 g for 14 hrs. at 4°
in the SW41 rotor. Fractions were collected and analyzed for
optical density at 260 nm ●---●,14C cpm ▲---▲ and 3H cpm O---O.

In this case, the cells were labeled with both 3H-tryptophan and
14C-lysine. No consistent differences in the 3H/14C ratio
or the radioactivity/Abs. 260 nm ratio is apparent. Since the
14C-lysine represents mostly histones and the 3H-tryptophan non-

histone proteins, this experiment implies that both classes of
chromosomal proteins are approximately equally distributed between
the two peaks.

With both embryo and cultured cell chromatin, two peaks
were consistently observed: a slowly sedimenting peak representing
about one-third of the material and the remainder in a rapidly
sedimenting peak. The explanation of the data in Table 1 is that
in both cases approximately 30% of one strand of the DNA is
transcribed. The sucrose gradient results can be reconciled with
this by assuming that the slowly sedimenting peak represents
active chromatin. That these two peaks represent independent
separable entities is shown by their behavior after a second
sucrose gradient centrifugation (19). Each peak re-runs at its
original position.

Several observations are consistent with the assignment of
active chromatin to the slowly sedimenting peak. When cells are
briefly pulse-labeled with ^{3}H-uridine, most of the nascent RNA
chains are associated with the slowly sedimenting peak. Similarly,
the endogenous RNA polymerase activity is found in the same
region of the gradient (Nishiura and McCarthy, unpublished results).
The difference in template activity also reveals itself in
in vitro assays. When each sucrose gradient fraction was tested
for its ability to support RNA synthesis with added excess E. coli
RNA polymerase, all the activity was associated with slowly
sedimenting chromatin. Presumably this is simply a reflection of
the availability of binding sites for RNA polymerase. We make
no claims f   fidelity of transcription and have yet to carry
out the corresponding test with homologous enzyme

A well established index of inactive, heterochromatin is its
content of satellite or very rapidly renaturing DNA (12,13). The
association of satellite DNA's with heterochromatin has been
established for several species of vertebrates and invertebrates.
Thus the validity of the sucrose gradient fractionation may be
tested by demonstrating the absence of very rapidly renaturing DNA
from the putatively active peak. This was accomplished by
fractionating ^{3}H-thymidine - and ^{14}C-thymidine - labeled chromatin,
recovering the DNA from various pooled fractions, fragmenting
and denaturing the DNA and mixing it with an excess of unlabeled
adult DNA. The renaturation kinetics (Figure 3) demonstrate the
essential absence of extremely rapidly renaturing DNA from the
slowly sedimenting peak and enrichment of the rapidly sedimenting
chromatin.

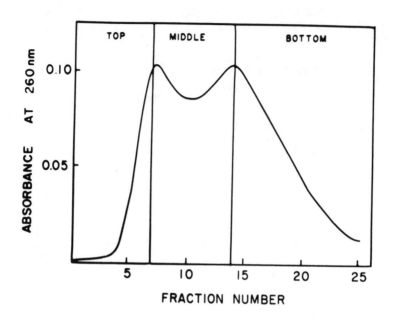

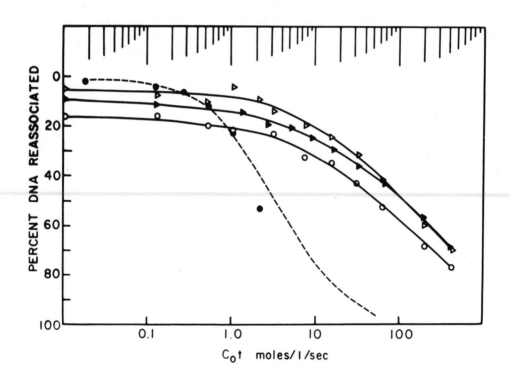

FIGURE 3.   Renaturation of DNA extracted from Fractionated Chromatin

Schneider's cells were labeled with either ^{3}H-thymidine (2 µCi/ml) or ^{14}C-thymidine.   Chromatin was extracted and fractionated as described in the legend to Figure 2.

The optical density profile is illustrated.   Chromatin fractions 5-7, 8-14, and 15-25 were combined, dialyzed overnight against 0.01M Tris, and the labeled DNA was isolated. ^{3}H-labeled DNA (0.3 µg, specific activity: 46,000 cpm/µg) from fractions 5-7 and 1.0 µg of ^{14}C-labeled DNA (specific activity: 3900 cpm/µg) from fractions 15-25 were added to 150 µg of unlabeled adult DNA and the mixture sheared at 12,000 psi in a French press.   In a separate tube 0.3 µg of ^{3}H-labeled DNA from fractions 8-14 was mixed with 150 µg of unlabeled adult DNA and the mixture sheared in the same way.   Each sample was denatured and the kinetics of renaturation measured by hydroxyapatite chromatography (8).

O---O : ^{14}C-labeled DNA from fractions 15-25
Δ---Δ : ^{3}H-labeled DNA from fractions 5-7
▲---▲ : ^{3}H-labeled DNA from fractions 8-14
●---● : ^{3}H-labeled B. subtilis DNA.

The experiment illustrated in Figure 2 demonstrates that no large differences in protein content exist between the two peaks.   Furthermore, when total chromosomal protein isolated from three regions of the gradient was analyzed on SDS polyacrylamide gels, no substantial difference was observable either in the pattern of stained bands or in the distribution of ^{3}H-leucine (19) Histones, though not well-resolved in this system, appear similar, at the front of the gel, while the only obvious difference in non-histone proteins appeared in the apparently very high molecular weight species which are enriched in rapidly sedimenting chromatin.

More direct assays of histone content were made by isolating histones from the two chromatin peaks and resolving the various species according to the urea acrylamide gel method of Panyim and Chalkley (20) Again it appears that all the histones are present in both peaks and in approximately the same relative proportion (Figure 4).

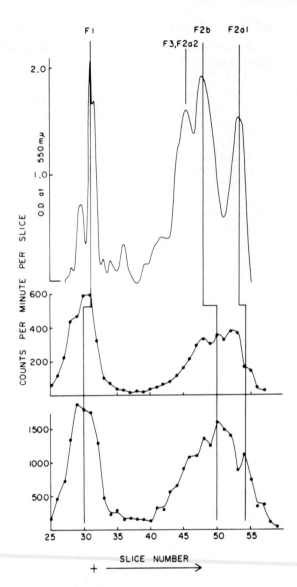

FIGURE 4.   Electrophoretic Comparison of Histones Isolated from
             Fractionated Chromatin.

^{3}H-lysine labeled chromatin was fractionated on a sucrose
gradient as in Figure 1. Histones were isolated from fractions
corresponding to the two peaks and placed on 4M urea, 15%
acrylamide gels according to Panyim and Chalkley (20).   A
densitometer trace of total histones is shown at the top.   Second
and third frames: ^{3}H cpm of 1.5 mm slices from histone gels of
slowly and rapidly sedimenting chromatin respectively

   Structural differences between the chromatin of the peaks
are most evident from their thermal denaturation behavior. Thermal
denaturation of total Drosophila chromatin takes place over a
broad range of temperature with a profile suggesting two peaks
(Figure 5). However, when fractionated chromatin is thermally
denatured, the slowly sedimenting chromatin denatures over a
lower temperature range than does the main peak. This result is
consistent with other evidence suggesting that thermal denaturation
at lower temperatures is indicative of active chromatin (16,21,22).
Perhaps the same alterations in chromosomal protein association with
DNA which diminish stabilization against thermal denaturation are
responsible for the increased availability to RNA polymerase.

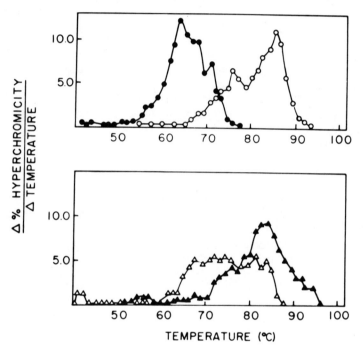

FIGURE 5.   Thermal Denaturation of Fractionated Chromatin.

     Chromatin prepared from D. melanogaster chromatin was sheared
in a Virtis homogenizer at 40 volts for 5 min and centrifuged on
a sucrose gradient as in Figure 1. Two clearly separated peaks were
obtained : the profile is illustrated in Figure 1 (e). Fractions
1-5 and 6-13 were combined, dialyzed and subjected to thermal
denaturation in 0.01M Tris, pH 8.0. The hyperchromicity was
recorded and the data transformed and plotted in differential
form (38).

●---● : D. melanogaster DNA; O---O : D. melanogaster chromatin;
Δ---Δ : chromatin fractions 1-5; ▲---▲ : chromatin fractions 6-13.

FRACTIONATION OF CHROMATIN BY THERMAL CHROMATOGRAPHY

Differences in thermal denaturation profiles of extended and condensed fractions of chromatin (13,21) suggest a relationship between the denaturation temperature and transcriptional activity of chromatin. This has been shown to be the case in chick erythrocyte chromatin, where only the DNA from the lowest melting chromatin fractions forms hybrids with homologous RNA (16). This demonstration was made possible through the use of thermal chromatography on hydroxyapatite. ^{3}H-thymidine labeled chromatin is eluted from the column as it reaches its thermal denaturation temperature. The general applicability of this method was tested in studies of sea urchin embryo chromatin.

Chromatin was isolated from S. droebachiensis and S. purpuratus embryos at various developmental stages. Optical properties, such as UV absorbance spectra and hyperchromicity during thermal denaturation, were used to monitor the effects of various physical treatments and to assay for possible species and/or developmental stage differences. Figure 6 shows the thermal denaturation profiles of S. purpuratus sperm, early and hatched blastula chromatin. The proportion of low melting chromatin increases as embryogenesis proceeds.

Sea urchin chromatin fragments were fractionated by thermal elution from HAP as described by McConaughy and McCarthy (16). Elution patterns of chromatin from morulae and hatched blastulae are shown in Figure 7. Hatched blastula chromatin is eluted from HAP at somewhat lower temperatures than chromatin from morulae; at 95°, 46% of the hatched blastula chromatin has been eluted, as compared to 37% of the morula chromatin.

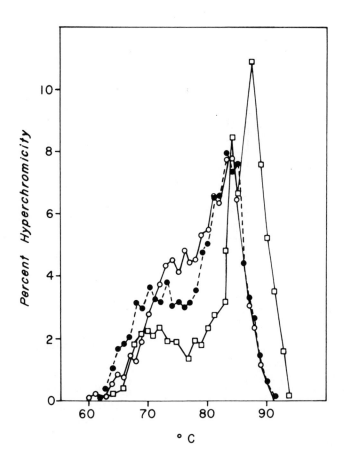

FIGURE 6.   Thermal Denaturation Profiles of Chromatin Isolated
            From Sea Urchins at Different Stages of Development

        Denaturation in 10mM phosphate buffer, pH 6.8.   Differential
denaturation profiles are shown for sperm chromatin (□)
(Tm = 83.5, hyperchromicity = 40%), early blastula chromatin (O)
(Tm = 79.0, hyperchromicity = 32%) and hatched blastula chromatin
(●) (Tm = 79.5, hyperchromicity = 36%).

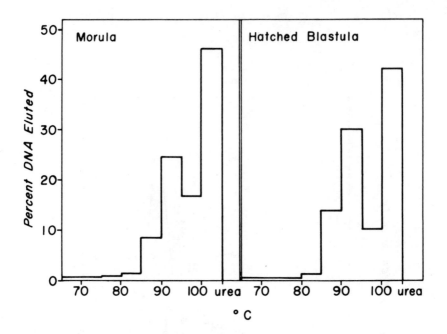

FIGURE 7.   Thermal Elution Patterns of Sea Urchin Chromatin From
             HAP Columns.

        Unlabeled morula chromatin (4.2 mg) and ^{3}H-thymidine labeled
hatched blastula chromatin (3.3 mg, 3700 cpm/µg) were fractionated
by thermal elution from HAP columns (each containing 6 ml packed
Clarkson HAP) in 0.12$\underline{M}$ phosphate buffer pH 6.8 as described by
McConaughy and McCarthy (16).   Material remaining on the columns
at 100° was eluted with MUP (8$\underline{M}$ urea, 0.24$\underline{M}$ phosphate buffer,
pH 6.8, 0.01$\underline{M}$ EDTA).

        DNA renaturation was used to assay for possible differences
in amounts of repeated and unique sequences in thermally fractionated chromatin. ^{3}H-thymidine DNA from each fraction of hatched
blastula chromatin was combined with excess total sperm DNA;
renaturation kinetics of these fractions are plotted as "C_0t curves"
(2) in Figure 8.   The lowest melting fractions are enriched in
unique sequences.   Fractions eluted at 95° and 100° display

renaturation kinetics similar to total DNA, while there is an
increase in the proportion of rapidly renaturing sequences in
DNA isolated from chromatin which is eluted from hydroxyapatite
by the urea buffer. A comparison of the $C_o t_{\frac{1}{2}}$ values of these
fractions shows an approximate four-fold difference in the
renaturation rates of the 90° fraction and the urea fraction.
This is undoubtedly a minimum estimate of the renaturation rate
differences since the imperfectly repeated sequences renature
more slowly than the well-matched unique sequences.

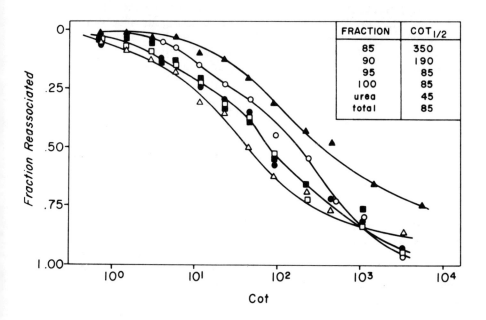

FRACTION	$COT_{1/2}$
85	350
90	190
95	85
100	85
urea	45
total	85

FIGURE 8.   Renaturation Kinetics of DNA from Hatched Blastula
            Chromatin Fractions.

        Purified ^{3}H-DNA sequences from thermal elution fractions
(Figure 7) were mixed with 1000-fold excess of total sheared sea
urchin sperm DNA. Reaction mixtures contained 3.3 µg/ml ^{3}H-labeled
DNA (3,700 cpm) from the indicated fractions and 3.3 mg/ml
total DNA in 48% formamide and 5 x SSC. Early points $(C_o t = 6)$
were determined from reaction mixtures which were diluted 1:20.
After heat denaturation at 75° for 10 min., samples were incubated
at 37° as indicated by the $C_o t$ values. Single and double strand
duplexes were assayed on HAP columns. Kinetics for DNA isolated
from chromatin eluted from the column at 85° (▲), 90° (O), 95°
(■), 100° (●), or by MUP (Δ) are compared with total DNA (□).

RNA-DNA hybridization was used to determine if these
fractionated segments which differed in sequence composition were
also differentially transcribed. Unlabeled DNA fractions were
allowed to react with pulse-labeled polysomal RNA under conditions
of excess DNA. Renaturation of trace amounts of labeled RNA and
excess DNA can be used to approximate the repeat frequencies of
the RNA species (23,24). Since the concentration of RNA is
small compared to that of the DNA, reaction kinetics are determined
by the concentration of DNA. In an ideal situation,RNA hybrids
would form at a rate equal to that of the DNA sequences from
which they were transcribed. However, the rates of RNA-DNA
hybridization are different from those of DNA-DNA duplex
formation (25) and the relative rates change, depending on the
renaturation conditions (26). In addition, the amount of hybrid
formation depends on the ratio of RNA to homologous DNA sequences.
In other words, for complete reaction one must have not just
excess total DNA, but an excess of those DNA sequences which
hybridize to the labeled RNA. If the labeled RNA represents
only a small fraction of the genome, then true DNA excess is
often difficult to obtain. For example, if histone genes
represent 0.5% of the sea urchin genome (23,27), a ten-fold DNA
excess of histone genes would require 2 mg of total DNA per μg
of histone mRNA. DNA to RNA ratios of approximately 2×10^6
are necessary for a similar DNA excess in the case of unique genes.

Pulse-labeled polysomal RNA from morulae was reacted with
unlabeled DNA from chromatin which had been isolated from embryos
at the same stage of development and fractionated as shown in
Figure 7. Reaction kinetics are shown in Figure 9. The RNA reacts
most rapidly with DNA sequences which are eluted from HAP at the
lowest temperature. Little or no hybrid formation occurs with
DNA sequences which are eluted with the urea buffer. The 25% to
30% reactions of the various fractions and total DNA indicate
that excess DNA sequences were not available for all RNA molecules.
Because of this, the relative amounts of repeated and unique RNA
transcripts cannot be determined quantitatively. However, it is
apparent from the renaturation profiles that both repeated and
unique RNA transcripts are represented in morula pulse labeled RNA.
The "C_0t curves" suggest a biphasic renaturation pattern in
all the fractions. In some cases, the more rapidly renaturing
component appears as double-stranded hybrid by the time the
earliest points are recorded. This biphasic pattern is more
evident in the lower frame of Figure 9, where the kinetics are
plotted in reciprocal form (28). Rate constants of the two
components are consistent with those expected for repeated and
unique transcripts (24). These results suggest that the thermal
chromatography method for chromatin fractionation may be of
general value. Clearly, DNA sequences complementary to RNA

synthesized in sea urchin embryos are specifically localized in
low melting chromatin. Much of the pulse-labeled morula RNA
has been shown to be histone mRNA (23,29,30,31). Thus we
tentatively conclude that histone genes are represented in the
low melting fraction of sea urchin chromatin. Further experiments
are needed to obtain definitive proof and to determine the state
and localization of histone genes in cells without mitotic activity.

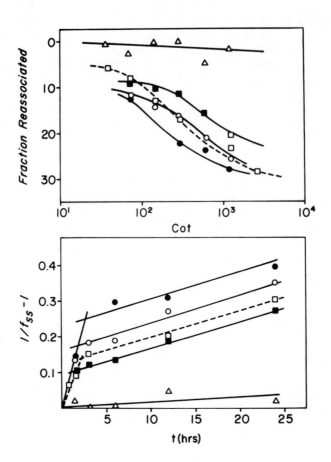

FIGURE 9.   Hybridization of DNA from Morula Chromatin Fractions
            with pulse labeled Polysomal RNA.

        Purified DNA sequences from thermal elution fractions
(Figure 7) were mixed with ^{3}H-uridine pulse-labeled polysomal
RNA and 20 µl aliquots were sealed in capillary tubes.   Each
sample contained 200 µg DNA (4 mg/ml) and 300 cpm ^{3}H-RNA in 48%
formamide and 5xSSC and was incubated at 45°.   At times indicated
by the C_ot values samples were diluted to 1 ml 2xSSC and incubated
at 37° with 5g carrier E. coli RNA, 5 units T1 RNase and 40 µg/ml
pancreatic RNAse. RNAse resistant hybrids were precipitated
with 10% TCA, and measured for radioactivity.   Reaction kinetics
are shown for the 85-90° fraction (●), 95° fraction (O), 100°
fraction (■), MUP fraction (Δ) and total DNA (□).   Data are
plotted as C_ot curves (2) in the upper figure and in reciprocal form
(28) in the lower figure.

CONCLUSIONS

It is clear that considerable technical problems remain to
be solved before chromatin fractionation can be considered a
complete success. At the present time a major weakness of this
approach to gene regulation derives from the lack of precise
methods for fragmenting interphase chromosomes. Even with
gentle enzymatic treatment with restriction endonucleases, there
is no obvious way to cut out single transcription units from the
body of the chromosome.

Despite these difficulties, it is possible to isolate a
fraction of chromatin having many of the expected attributes of
active regions. Such a fraction contains the endogenous RNA
polymerase and the nascent RNA chains and displays in vitro
template activity. (19) Though differences in physical properties
are readily apparent, the overall chemical composition of active
and inactive chromatin is, to a first approximation, quite similar.
Since differences in histone content are not readily apparent, it
seems that histones are equally present in transcribed and non-
transcribed regions. This is consistent with a role as structural
components of chromosomes rather than regulators of gene expression.
Nevertheless, it is possible that histone modifications contribute
to the differences in physical properties revealed by thermal
denaturation.

ACKNOWLEDGEMENT

The research described above was supported by grants from
the USPHS (GM20287) and the National Science Foundation (GB6099).

REFERENCES

1. IMAIZUMI,T., DIGGELMAN,H. and SCHERRER, K.(1973). Proc. Nat.
    Acad. Sci. USA 70:1122
2. BRITTEN, R.J. AND KOHNE,D.E. (1968). Science 161:529.
3. McCARTHY,B.J. and CHURCH, R.B. (1970). Ann. Rev. Biochem.
    39:131.
4. GELDERMAN, A.H., RAKE, A.V. and BRITTEN, R.J. (1971). Proc.
    Nat. Acad. Sci. USA 68:172.
5. DAVIDSON, E.H. and HOUGH, B.R. (1971). J. Mol. Biol. 56:491.
6. HAHN, W.E. and LAIRD,C.D. (1971). Science 173.:158.
7. BROWN, I.R. and CHURCH, R.B. (1971). Biochem. Biophys. Res.
    Commun. 42:850.
8. GROUSE, L., CHILTON, M.D. and McCARTHY,B.J. (1972).
    Biochemistry 11:798.
9. GROUSE,L., OMENN, G.A. and McCARTHY, B.J. (1973). J.
    Neurochem. 20:1063.
10. FRENSTER, J.H., ALLFREY, V.G. and MIRSKY, A.E. (1963). Proc
    Nat. Acad. Sci. USA 50:1026.
11. CHALKLEY, R. and JENSEN, R.H. (1968). Biochemistry 7:4380.
12. YUNIS, J.J., and YASMINEH, W.G. (1971). Science 174:1200.
13. DUERKSEN, J.D. and McCARTHY, B.J. (1971). Biochemistry 10:1471.
14. BILLING, R.J. and BONNER, J. (1972). Biochim. Biophys.
    Acta 281:453.
15. REECK, G.R., SIMPSON, R.T. and SOBER, H.A. (1972). Proc.
    Nat. Acad. Sci. USA 69:2317.
16. McCONAUGHY, B.L. and McCARTHY, B.J. (1972). Biochemistry 11:998.
17. JANOWSKI,M., NASSER,D.S. and McCARTHY, B.J. (1972). In: 5th
    Karolinska Symposium on Research Methods in Reproductive
    Endocrinology (E. Diczfalusy, ed), p. 112.
18. BEERMAN, W. (1972). In: Developmental Studies on Giant
    Chromosomes. Results and Problems in Cellular Differentiation
    Vol. 4, (W. Beerman, ed).
19. McCARTHY, B.J., NISHIURA, J.T., DOENECKE, D., NASSER, D.S.
    and JOHNSON C.B. (1973). Cold Spring Harbor Symp. Quant. Biol.
    38, in press
20. PANYIM, S. and CHALKLEY, R. (1969). Arch. Biochem. Biophys.
    130:337.
21. FRENSTER, J.H. (1969). In: Handbook of Molecular Cytology
    (A. Lima-de-Faria, ed), North Holland Press, p. 251.
22. HUANG, R.C., BONNER, J. AND MURRAY, K. (1964). J. Mol. Biol.
    8:54.
23. KEDES, L.H. and BIRNSTIEL,M.L. (1971). Nature New Biol. 230:165.
24. MELLI, M., WHITFIELD, C., RAO, K.V., RICHARDSON, M. and BISHOP,
    J.O. (1971). Nature New Biol. 231, 8.
25. BISHOP, J.O. (1972). Biochem. J. 126, 171.
26. STRAUS, N.A. and BONNER, T.I. (1972). Biochim. Biophys. Acta.
    277:87.

27. McCARTHY, B.J. and FARQUHAR, M.N. (1972). Brookhaven Symp.
    31,1.
28. WETMUR, J.G. and DAVIDSON, N. (1968). J. Mol. Biol.
    31:349.
29. WEINBERG, E.S., BIRNSTIEL, M.L., PURDOM, I.F. and WILLIAMSON,
    R. (1972). Nature 240:225.
30. FARQUHAR, M.N. and McCARTHY, B.J. (1973a). Biochem. Biophys.
    Res. Commun. 53:515.
31. FARQUHAR, M.N. and McCARTHY, B.J. (1973b). Biochemistry, in
    press.
32. McCARTHY, B.J. and BOLTON, E.T. (1964). J. Mol. Biol. 8:184.
33. KENNELL, D. (1968). J. Mol. Biol. 34:85.
34. FIRTEL, R.A. (1972). J. Mol. Biol. 66:363.
35. TURNER, S.H. and LAIRD, C.D. (1973). Biochem. Genet. in press.
36. KOHNE, D.E. and BYERS, M.J. (1973). Biochemistry 12:2373.
37. SCHERRER, K., SPOHR, G., GRANBOULAN, N., MOREL, C.,
    GROSCLAUDE, J. and CHEZZI, C. (1970). Cold Spring Harbor
    Symp. Quant. Biol. 35:539.
38. LI, H.J. and BONNER, J. (1971). Biochemistry 10:1461.

NEW DEVELOPMENTS IN PROTEIN SYNTHESIS.   A SURVEY

P. Lengyel

Yale University, New Haven, Connecticut

In the framework of an outline of the mechanism of protein
synthesis the following topics were discussed more exten;ively:
1) Specificity in peptide chain initiation and the problem of
translational control. 2) GTP cleavage as promoted by elongation
factors Tu and G and the role of particular ribosomal proteins.
3) Protein synthesis and the stringent control of RNA synthesis
and other processes by amino acids. 4) The interferon defense
mechanism.

REFERENCES

No references are provided for topic (1) since this was discussed by M. Revel et al. in this symposium, and a list of references can be found after their contribution.

for topic (2)

1. LENGYEL, P. & SOLL, D. (1969). Bact.Rev. 33, 264.
2. LUCAS-LENARD, J. & LIPMANN, F. (1971). Ann.Rev.Biochem.
       40, 409.
3. LENGYEL, P., SOPORI, M.L., GUPTA, S.L. & WATERSON, J. (1972).
       In RNA/Viruses/Ribosomes, p.291, North Holland, Amsterdam.
4. HASELKORN, R. & ROTHMAN-DENES, L.B. (1973). Ann.Rev.Biochem.
       42, in the press.
5. KURLAND, C. (1972). Ann.Rev.Biochem. 41, 377.
6. NOMURA,, M. (1973). Science, 179, 864.

7. KISCHA, K., MOLLER, W. & STOFFLER, J. (1971). Nature,New
    Biology, 233, 62.
8. HAMEL, E., KOKA, M. & NAKAMOTO, T. (1972). J.Biol.Chem.
    247, 805.
9. SOPORI, M. & LENGYEL, P. (1972). Biochem.Biophys.Res.Comm.
    46, 238.
10. WEISSBACH, H., REDFIELD, B., YAMASAKI, E., DAVIS, R., PESTKA,
    S. & BROT, N. (1972). Arch.Biochem.Biophys. 149, 110.
11. CABRER, B., VAZQUEZ, D. & MODOLLEL, J. (1972). Proc.Nat.Acad.
    Sci. USA, 69, 733.
12. MILLER, D.L. (1972). Proc.Nat.Acad.Sci. USA, 69, 752.
13. RICHTER, D. (1972). Biochem.Biophys.Res.Comm. 46, 1850.
14. COX, T., MOLLER, W., LAURSEN, R. & WITTMAN-LIEBOLD, B. (1973).
    Eur.J.Biochem. 34, 138.
15. HIGHLAND, J.H., BODLEY, J.W., GORDON, J., HASERNBANK, R. &
    STOFFLER, J. (1973). Proc.Nat.Acad.Sci. USA, 70, 147.
16. THAMMANA, P., KURLAND, C.G., DEUSSER, E., WEBER, J.,
    MASCHLER, R., STOFFLER, J. & WITTMAN, H.G. (1973). Nature,
    New Biology, 242, 47.

for topic (3)

1. EDLIN, G. & BRODA, P. (1968). Bact.Rev. 32, 206.
2. CASHEL, M. & GALLANT, J. (1969). Nature, 221, 838.
3. CASHEL, M. (1969). J.Biol.Chem. 244, 3133.
4. SOKAWA, L.J., SOKAWA, Y. & KAZIRO, Y. (1972). Nature, New
    Biology, 240, 242.
5. HALL, B. & GALLANT, J. (1972). Nature, New Biology, 237, 131.
6. HOCHSTADT-OZER, J. & CASHEL, M. (1972). J.Biol.Chem. 247,
    7067.
7. HASELTINE, W.A., BLOCK, R., GILBERT, W. & WEBER, K. (1972).
    Nature, 238, 381.
8. LUND, E. & KJELDGAARD, N.O. (1972). Eur.J.Biochem. 28, 316.
9. SLY, J. & LIPMANN, F. (1973). Proc.Nat.Acad.Sci. USA, 70,
    306.
10. HASELTINE, W.A. & BLOCK, R. (1973). Proc.Nat.Acad.Sci. USA,
    70, 1564.
11. PEDERSEN, F.S., LUND, E. & KJELDGAARD, N.O. (1973). Nature,
    New Biology, 243, 13.

for topic (4)

1. NG, M.H. & VILCEK, J. (1972). Adv.Prot.Chem. 26, 173.
2. LAI, M.T. & JOKLIK, W.K. (1973). Virol. 51, 191.
3. STEWART, W.E., deCLERCQ, E. & DeSOMER, P. (1972). J.Virol.
    10, 707.

4. OXMAN, M.N. & LEVIN, M.J. (1971). Proc.Nat.Acad.Sci. USA,
    68, 299.
5. MARCUS, P.L., ENGELHARDT, D.L., HUNT, J.M. & SEKELLICK, M.J.
    (1971). Science, 174, 593.
6. BIALY, H.S. & COLBY, C. (1972). J.Virol. 9, 286.
7. MANDERS, E.K., TILLES, J.G. & HUANG, A.S. (1972). Virol.
    49, 573.
8. GRAVELL, M. & CROMEANS, T.L. (1972). Virol. 50, 916.
9. METZ, D.H. & ESTEBAN, M. (1972). Nature, 238, 385.
10. FALCOFF, E., FALCOFF, R., LEBLEU, B. & REVEL, M. (1972).
    Nature, New Biology, 240, 145.
11. FRIEDMAN, R.M., METZ, D.H., ESTEBAN, R.M., TOVELL, D.R.,
    BALL, L.A. & KERR, I.M. (1972). J.Virol. 10, 1184.
12. STEWART II, W.E., GOSSER, L.B. & LOCKART, R.Z. (1973).
    J.Gen.Virol. 15, 85.
13. STEWART II, W.E., deCLERCQ, E., BILLIAU, A., DESMYTER, J. &
    DeSOMER, P. (1972). Proc.Nat.Acad.Sci. USA, 69, 1851.

mRNA SPECIFIC INITIATION FACTORS IN THE CONTROL OF PROTEIN SYNTHESIS

M. Revel, Y. Groner, Y. Pollack, D. Cnaani, H. Zeller
and U. Nudel

Department of Biochemistry, Weizmann Institute of
Science, Rehovot, Israel

Before mRNA was discovered it was commonly accepted that ribosomes in cells are specialized for the synthesis of specific proteins. Following the demonstration that the information for the amino acid sequence is, in fact, in the mRNA, ribosomes began to be viewed as non-specific organelles, capable of translating indiscriminately all information brought to them by mRNA. If this concept is true, all the controls of gene expression which must come into action when a cell adapts to new environmental conditions should be exclusively at the level of mRNA synthesis (transcription and maturation). To determine if translation control is at all a possible mechanism for the control of gene expression, it is therefore important to establish whether or not ribosomes are capable of discriminating between mRNAs and of translating preferentially one or another of the mRNAs present in the cytoplasm. This question is of course most relevant for mammalian cells, in which we know that (1) stable mRNAs function for prolonged periods of time (1) and (2) that more mRNA is synthesized in the nucleus than is actually translated on the cytoplasmic polyribosomes (see Scherrer, this volume). Since, however, the mechanism of protein synthesis is known in more detail in E.coli, we have concentrated much of our efforts in studying mRNA discrimination by E.coli ribosomes. Our experiments over the past three years have clearly demonstrated the existence of ribosome-associated protein factors which make the ribosome specialized for specific mRNAs. Recently, we have isolated similar factors from mammalian cells; these results will be presented in the second part of this paper.

RECOGNITION OF mRNAs BY E. coli RIBOSOMES

The steps involved in the formation of an initiation complex
between free ribosomal subunits and mRNA are summarized in Fig. 1.
The various reactions involved in binding mRNA and formyl methionyl
tRNA to the ribosomal 30S subunit and the participation of the
three initiation factors have been established by several laboratories (2), essentially by using synthetic templates (the simplest
being the initiation codon ApUpG), or natural mRNAs (such as MS2
or T4 phage RNAs).

Studies on competition between synthetic templates and
natural mRNAs for binding to ribosomes have established that what
is recognized by the ribosome is more than the codon AUG (Ref.3
and Thach 1972, private communication). This additional information, which could be a nucleotide sequence of 6-10 bases (3,4),
or a region with a particular secondary structure near the AUG
codon (5), is designated as S ("initiation signal") in Fig. 1.
Our studies have also established that both initiation factors IF2
(a protein of 100,000 daltons) and IF3 (21,000 daltons) participate in the binding of RNA to the 30S ribosome by forming an IF2-
IF3 complex (6) on the surface of the ribosome (an IF3-IF1 complex
was also described by Hershey et al. (7)). IF3 is essential for
the specific recognition of natural mRNA (3,8) and since it possesses the ribosome dissociation activity (9) it appears that this
protein is the first to bind to the 30S subunit. Ribosomes without
initiation factors do not bind to mRNA. The roles of the 50S subunits and fmet tRNA binding in mRNA recognition are still unclear.

HETEROGENEITY OF INITIATION SIGNAL AND FACTORS

Messenger RNAs are not all translated uniformly by ribosomes.
Much information has, for example, been obtained on the discrimination between the three cistrons of RNA phage f2 (or R17, or MS2).
Some of these effects are due to the ribosome origin itself
(E.coli versus B. stearo) (10), some to the RNA secondary structure
(11) and some result from the action of initiation factors. These
will be reviewed here in detail.

The nucleotide sequence of the ribosomal binding sites of each
of the three cistrons is represented in Fig. 2. What parts of
these sequences serve for the specific recognition event is, however, not known. Our aim has been to study how E.coli ribosomes
recognize these different sites in comparison to other mRNAs, as
T4 and T7 mRNAs, and in particular to search for the existence of
protein factors which could confer on the ribosomes a higher
affinity for one or another of these sites.

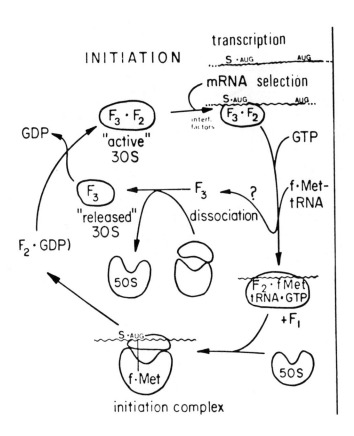

Fig. 1 A. Steps involved in the binding of mRNA to ribosomes
and initiation of translation.

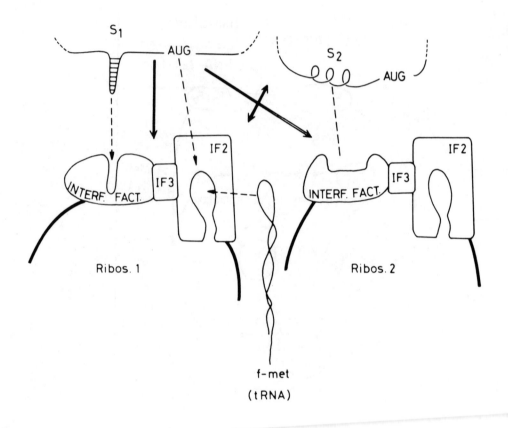

Fig. 1B.   Our present view of how interference factors select
mRNAs.

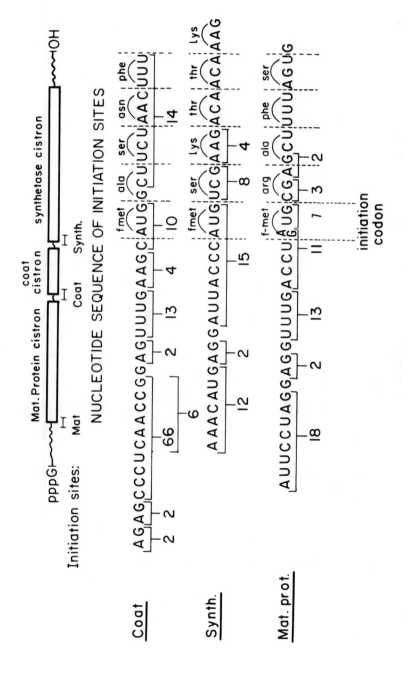

Fig. 2A. Nucleotide sequence of the three initiation sites of bacteriophages MS2 or R17 RNA. The numbers refer to the T1 oligonucleotides in 2B.

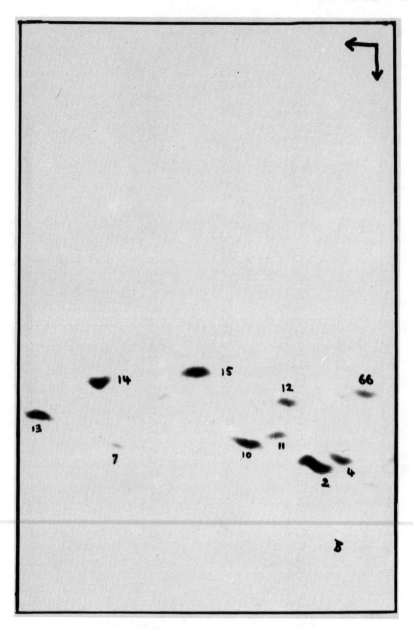

Fig. 2B. Autoradiograph of the T1 oligonucleotides from ribosome protected RNase A fragments of ^{32}P-MS2 RNA separated by electrophoresis at pH 3.5 on cellulose acetate in 6 M urea and by homochromatography in the second direction. Data from Steitz (5) and Revel *et al*. (4).

Our experimental system (12) consists of purified E.coli ribosomes, high speed supernatant after centrifugation at 150,000 x g (both free of initiation factors) and purified initiation factors. Initially we measured the incorporation of ^{14}C-valine into protein in response to MS2 and T4 mRNAs: this incorporation is completely dependent on the presence of IF3 and we could therefore compare the activity of the various IF3 fractions for the translation of these mRNAs.

To prepare IF3, ribosomes from 4-5 kg of E.coli MRE 600 were washed with a buffer solution containing 1 M NH$_4$Cl. On fractionation of the ribosome wash by successive chromatography on DEAE cellulose and DEAE Sephadex columns, the IF3 is separated into several subfractions which show very different relative activities for MS2 and T4 mRNA (Table 1) (13).

These subfractions were assayed also for their activity on the different cistrons of MS2 RNA, by analyzing ^{35}S-methionine incorporation into the characteristic tryptic/chymotryptic amino-terminal peptides from the coat, synthetase and maturation proteins, according to the method of Lodish (14). IF3-B2 was clearly most active on the coat protein cistron while IF3-B1 was very active on the synthetase cistron. This specificity of IF3-B2 for the coat cistron was confirmed by direct analysis of the sites on MS2 RNA to which ribosomes are attached in the presence and absence of IF3-B2. This is done by measuring the amount of each of the major oligonucleotides originating from the three initiation sequences (Fig. 2), found on the ribosomes after ribonuclease digestion of the non-bound regions. The data of Table 2 show that IF3-B2 stimulates exclusively ribosome binding to the coat protein cistron initiation site.

BASIS FOR THE HETEROGENEITY OF IF3 TOWARD DIFFERENT mRNAs

The separation of IF3 subfractions which differentiate between T4 and MS2 RNA and the different cistrons of this RNA, has been reported also by Lee-Huang and Ochoa (15) and by Yoshida and Rudland (16). This heterogeneity could be explained in two ways:

1) Several different IF3 exist in E.coli or

2) the various subfractions represent the same IF3 in combination with an mRNA specific co-factor.

Lee-Huang and Ochoa (15) have concluded that at least two IF3 species exist; one MS2 RNA-specific (IF3-α), active also on T4 early mRNA, and the other late T4 mRNA-specific (IF3-β). Of course these fraction could be active for many other mRNAs from

TABLE   1

FRACTIONATION OF IF3 ACTIVITY BY CHROMATOGRAPHY ON DEAE
SEPHADEX COLUMNS

Factors	NH_4Cl Molarity of elution (M)	Translation ratio $\dfrac{\text{T4 mRNA}}{\text{MS2 RNA}}$	Translation ratio $\dfrac{\text{MS2 coat}}{\text{MS2 synthetase}}$	Specific activity on T4 mRNA pmoles valine per µg protein
IF3-B1	0.05	1.9	0.6	32
IF3-B2	0.10	1.3	3.0	86
IF3-B3	0.15	3.8	1.0	70[*]
IF3-B4	0.20	31.0	-	21[**]

From Groner *et al*. (13), E.*coli* MRE 600 ribosomal wash is first
chromatographed on DEAE cellulose. Fractions containing IF3
activity are rechromatographed on DEAE Sephadex A50 with a NH_4Cl
gradient in 20 mM potassium phosphate buffer, pH 7.2, 0.2 mM
$MgCl_2$, 7 mM β-mercaptoethanol and 5 percent glycerol (Buffer P).

Overall amino acid incorporation: The assay mixture contains (in
0.065 ml): 50 mM Tris-HCl, pH 7.5, 50 mM NH_4Cl, 13 mM $MgCl_2$, 2 mM
ATP, 1 mM GTP, 5 mM phosphoenolpyruvate, 2 µg pyruvate kinase,
0.1 mM CTP and UTP, 0.15 mM 19 L-amino acids (minus valine), 6 mM
dithiothreitol, 0.5 µg formyltetrahydrofolate, 1.5 nmoles (^{14}C)-
valine (50 µc/µmole), 100 µg high salt-washed ribosomes, 5 µl
supernatant, 5 µg IF1, 15 µg IF2, 25 µg tRNA, 20 µg native MS2 RNA,
or 100 µg T4 mRNA (extracted from E.*coli* 20 min after T4 infection
at 30°C). After 30 minutes incubation at 37°C, the incorporation of
valine into hot trichloroacetic acid insoluble material is measured
by the filter paper disc method. The effect of adding various IF3
fractions is measured.

Study of the cistron specificity of IF3 activity by measure of N-
formyl-(^{35}S)-methionine incorporation into the specific aminoterminal peptides of each product. For these experiments, MS2 RNA
treated with 1 M formaldehyde at 37°C is used, to allow independent
initiation at the three cistrons. Protein synthesis is carried out
as above except that (^{35}S)-formyl methionyl tRNA (2×10^5 cpm, 25 µg,
free of unformylated species) is used as source of label. After
30 min incubation at 37°C, ribonuclease A (120 µg/ml) and 10 mM
EDTA are added and after 1 hour, proteins are acid-precipitated,
washed and digested with trypsin and chymotrypsin as described by
Lodish (14). Analysis of the peptides is carried out by electrophoresis at pH 1.9 or by a two dimensional system of electrophoresis at pH 3.5 and chromatography in isoamylalcohol-pyridine-
water (35:35:30). The effect of adding various IF3 fractions to
IF1 and IF2 on the synthesis of each peptide is measured.

[**]Further purified on hydroxylapatite.
[*]Further purified on phosphocellulose.

TABLE   2

EFFECTS OF IF3 AND INTERFERENCE FACTOR i ON RIBOSOME BINDING TO
THE INITIATION SITES OF THE THREE CISTRONS OF MS2 RNA

	Effect on ribosome binding, percent[*]		
Factor Assayed	Maturation cistron	Coat protein cistron	Synthetase cistron
IF3-B2	-10 percent	+130 percent	-10 percent
factor i	-25 "	- 50 "	+80 "

[*] Percent of control without the factor.

  Computed from published data on IF3-B2 (17) and factor i (12).
  The data express the variation in percent of oligonucleotides
from each binding site protected from nuclease digestion by
ribosomes in the presence of IF1 + IF2 + IF3 versus IF1 + IF2
and IF1 + IF2 + IF3 + factor i versus IF1 + IF2 + IF3. The
values represent an average of the variations of the following
oligonucleotides (Fig. 2): Maturation cistron: 18, 11, 7; Coat
cistron: 14, 10, 66, 6; Synthetase: 15, 12, 8; common maturation
and coat: 13.

E.$coli$ which have not been tested.

Although we were of the opinion (17) that IF3-B2 represents
a homogenous preparation of IF3 which is specific for MS2 coat
cistron, our more recent work (18) has shown that in many cases
the mRNA specificity of IF3 subfractions results from the presence
of other proteins which interfere with IF3 activity. An antiserum
against IF3-B2 cross-reacted with other IF3 subfractions of different template specificities. Moreover, from a T4 mRNA specific
subfraction, comparable to IF3-B4 of Table 1, we have been able
to recover a purified IF3 active for MS2 RNA, and an interference
factor. This has led us to favor the second alternative above and
to attribute the mRNA specificity of IF3 to its association with
"interference" factors.

INTERFERENCE FACTORS

The fractionation of a T4 mRNA specific IF3 subfraction,
devoid of MS2 translation activity (insert) on a phosphocellulose
column is shown in Fig. 3. This subfraction is separated into IF3
active for MS2 RNA and a factor J which inhibits preferentially
MS2 RNA translation when recombined with their IF3 (Table 3).
Factor J inhibits fmet-tRNA binding in response to MS2 RNA, but
not with poly AUG as template. It also inhibits the translation
of early T4 mRNA (synthesized in $vitro$ with E.$coli$ RNA polymerase
on T4 DNA) to a greater extent than that of late T4 mRNA (extracted
from E.$coli$-infected cells late after phage infection) (18). Since
it has a high tendency to stick to IF3 during purification, it may
be present in the late T4 mRNA specific IF3 fractions of Lee-Huang
and Ochoa (15). But this cannot be stated yet with certainty.

The interference factor may be responsible also for the
stimulation of R17 maturation cistron initiation observed by
Yoshida and Rudland (16) in a T4 RNA-specific IF3. This is shown
in Table 4, in which data on the synthesis of formyl methionyl
dipeptides directed by MS2 RNA unfolded with formaldehyde (11) are
presented. Addition of factor J markedly increases the synthesis
of fmet-arg (originating from the maturation cistron) over that of
fmet-ala originating from the coat cistron (Fig. 1).

Several other interference factors have been isolated. Factor
K (which on the column represented in Fig. 3 elutes before IF3)
inhibits T4 mRNA translation more than that of MS2 and in combination with IF3 can give an MS2 RNA specific subfraction. An
activity which inhibits histidine incorporation in response to
MS2 RNA (histidine is present only in the synthetase and maturation
proteins), but stimulates valine incorporation, has also been

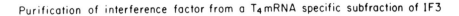

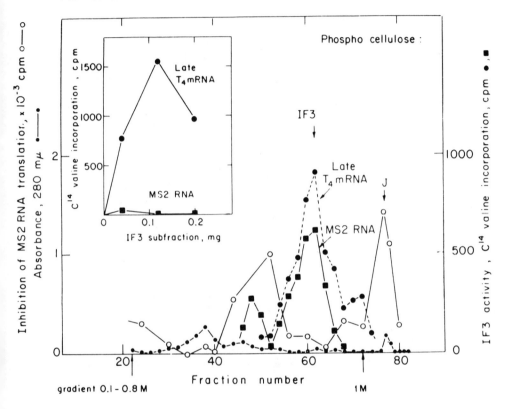

Fig. 3. Fractionation of T4 specific IF3 subfraction.
An IF3 subfraction from DEAE Sephadex (as IF3-B4) was chromatographed on a phosphocellulose column with NH$_4$Cl in buffer P (if
a phosphate gradient is used as in Table 1, no separation is
seen). Fractions were assayed for IF3 activity or for inhibition
of MS2 RNA translation in the presence of purified IF3. The
insert shows the activity of the subfraction before the phosphocellulose step.

TABLE 3

EFFECT OF INTERFERENCE FACTORS ON MS2 AND T4 mRNA TRANSLATION

Conditions	C^{14} - Valine Incorporation	
	Late T4 mRNA	MS2 RNA cpm
Expt. 1 Control with IF3	7,000 (100)	7,000 (100)
+ factor i, 5µg	7,100 (101)	2,600 (37)
" 7.5µg	7,450 (106)	1,150 (16)
Expt. 2 Control with IF3	7,865 (100)	4,550 (100)
+ factor J, 3µg	6,767 (86)	1,250 (27)
" 5µg	1,851 (24)	160 (4)

Protein synthesis measured as in Table 1.   Factor J is obtained
as in Fig. 3.   Factor i is purified as in Fig. 4.   A background
of 1,500 cpm in the absence of template was subtracted from all
values.   Figures in brackets represent percent of control.

TABLE 4

MS2 RNA DIRECTED DIPEPTIDE SYNTHESIS

Cistron	Dipeptide	f-[^{35}S]-methionine incorporation into dipeptides cpm	
		IF3	IF3 + J
Maturation	fmet-arg	1,150(24)	2,150(32)
Coat	fmet-ala	1,060(23)	1,260(19)
Synthetase	fmet-ser	2,425(52)	3,255(48)

IF3 purified on phosphocellulose with 6 M urea (free of any interference factor), 6 μg, was added to 300 μg high salt washed ribosomes, purified IF1 and IF2 and T factor in saturating amounts, f-[^{35}S]-met tRNA (10^5 cpm), tRNA charged with 19 cold amino acids (40 μg) and 33 μg formaldehyde-treated MS2 RNA. After 10 min at 30°C, the tRNA was hydrolyzed by 0.44M triethylamine and the dipeptides separated by electrophoresis at pH 3.5 for 90 min at 3.5 KV.

detected (unpublished results). The existence of this fraction
could explain the template specificity of IF3-B2, since it would
make IF3 specific for the coat cistron.

However, the best studied interference factor is factor i,
which was also the first that we described (12,13). Studies of
factor i best illustrate the cistron specific properties and the
mode of action of interference factors.

INTERFERENCE FACTOR i

The acidic protein, of molecular weight 74,000 daltons, has
been purified to homogeneity as shown in Fig. 4. When added to
IF3, it inhibits initiation on MS2 RNA but not on T4 mRNA. It
discriminates between the cistrons of MS2 RNA, inhibiting the
coat cistron while stimulating the synthetase cistron. This was
shown (12) by three different methods. 1. Inhibition of valine
incorporation but stimulation of histidine incorporation with unfolded (formaldehyde-treated) RNA. Unfolding is required to make
the synthetase cistron available under conditions where initiation
at the coat cistron is prevented (11). 2. Analysis of formyl-
(^{35}S)-methionine incorporation into the aminoterminal peptides and
3. direct analysis of the oligonucleotides bound to the ribosome
in the presence and absence of factor i. Results of these latter
experiments are given in Table 2. It is clear that factor i
blocks ribosome binding to the coat initiation site while stimulating that to the synthetase initiation site.

Factor i requires IF3 for its effect on protein synthesis.
However, it binds also directly to the ribosome. Factor i makes
a complex with IF3 both *in vitro*, on mixing the two purified proteins, and also *in vivo*, since a natural IF3-i complex can be
isolated from the ribosomal wash (13). The presence of this complex probably explains the activity of fraction IF3-B1 on the
synthetase (Table 1).

Factor i binds to MS2 RNA *in vitro*, as shown by the fact that
the purified protein traps RNA on a Millipore filter (18). There
is evidence that the protein also recognizes the RNA *in vivo*;
Factor i is integrated in the phage RNA replicase (12) after phage
infection and with Q$_\beta$ RNA replicase Kämen *et al*. (19) demonstrated
that factor i was needed to recognize the phage RNA (+) strand.

While factor i does not affect overall T4 mRNA translation,
analysis of the aminoterminal peptides shows that certain cistrons
are in fact stimulated while others are inhibited (18). A cistron
specific effect of factor i on T7 mRNA has also recently been
discovered.

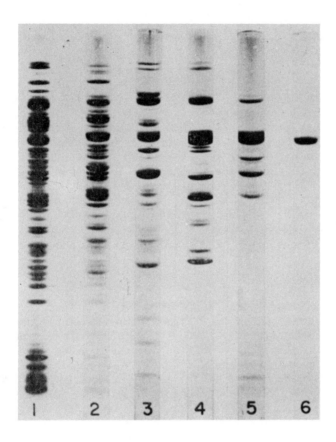

Fig. 4. Purification of interference factor i.
Factor i is purified by assaying its differential inhibitory
effect on native MS2 RNA but not T4 mRNA translation as in Table
3. Electrophoresis on 10-15 percent polyacrylamide gradient gels
in SDS shows (1) 1 M ribosomal wash; (2) fraction eluted from
DEAE cellulose at 0.22 M potassium phosphate; (3) phosphocellulose step; factor i is found in the non-adsorbed fraction; (4)
hydroxylapatite fraction eluted at 0.13-0.15 M phosphate; (5) DEAE
Sephadex fraction at 0.25 M NH_4Cl and (6) after equilibrium
sedimentation on a 5-20 percent glycerol gradient. Factor i,
MW = 7,400 sediments at 5.5 - 6S (18).

EFFECT OF FACTOR i ON INITIATION OF EARLY T7 mRNA TRANSLATION

Early T7 mRNA was transcribed with E.coli RNA polymerase from T7 DNA. This enzyme, in vitro, transcribes only a small region near the 5' end of the molecule. The mRNA produced codes for 4-5 proteins among which are the T7 RNA polymerase, the T7 ligase, some regulatory protein and possibly even the T7 lysozyme (20,21).

Figure 5 shows the dipeptides synthesized in response to this early T7 mRNA, and with late T7 mRNA (extracted from infected cells). With late T7 mRNA, Callahan and Leder (22) have shown that the main products are fmet-ala and fmet-ser. With early T7 mRNA, only little fmet-ala is formed and several other dipeptides appear. Addition of factor i inhibits the synthesis of three of these while stimulating the formation of three others. Formation of dipeptide II (Fig. 5) is almost factor i-dependent. The overall effect on early T7 mRNA translation is characterised by first stimulation (from 50-100 percent), followed by inhibition with larger amounts of i - probably reflecting the opposite effects observed on individual cistrons.

POSSIBLE FUNCTION IN TRANSLATION CONTROL

The discovery of interference factors shows that the ribosome possesses a mechanism (see Fig. 1) for translating more or less specific mRNA cistrons. As pointed out in the Introduction, this fulfills an essential condition for the existence of gene control at the level of translation.

Changes in the number of ribosomes having an IF3 molecule such as IF3-B2 (specific for MS2 coat cistron), or having the IF3-i complex (inactive for MS2 coat cistron), will drastically change the translation activity of the ribosomes. In stationary phase E.coli, we have observed a quantitative variation in the relative amounts of IF3 and an interference factor (23). We have also observed a chemical modification of factor i after T4 phage infection. This could lead to increased activity of the protein and explain the change in template specificity of T4-infected IF3 preparations (15,18).

DISCRIMINATION BETWEEN mRNAS BY MAMMALIAN INITIATION FACTOR

The activity of crude extracts of Krebs ascites cells for the translation of mammalian mRNA can be increased by the addition of ribosomal washes or supernatant fractions from various sources;

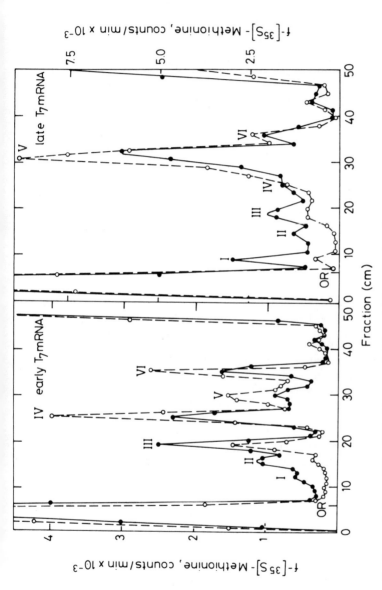

Fig. 5. Early and late T7 mRNA directed dipeptide synthesis.
Conditions were as described in Table 4 but with saturating amounts of early T7 mRNA (synthesized *in vitro* on T7 DNA with *E.coli* polymerase and phenol purified at 61.5°C) or late T7 mRNA (RNA extracted from T7 infected *E.coli* B, after 13 min at 30°C). When indicated, 60 μg factor i was added. Peptide V and VI are fmet-ala and fmet-ser respectively as established by comparison with known markers.

Table 5 shows that reticulocyte ribosomal wash stimulates hemoglobin mRNA translation, but not Mengo virus RNA translation,
while L cells ribosomal wash or supernatant fraction stimulates
Mengo RNA but not Hb mRNA translation. Such specific effects are
obtained only if the crude extracts are fully active. When partially inactivated extracts are used (as after freezing and
thawing several times) these are deficient in other soluble factors besides the mRNA specific ones, and in such cases reticulocyte ribosomal wash can stimulate also Mengo RNA activity. Such
non-specific stimulations are seen also if the assay is carried
out at high KCl concentrations.

     Purification of the Hb mRNA specific factor was achieved as
described in Fig. 6. After DEAE cellulose and phosphocellulose
chromatography, a highly purified preparation is obtained. The
activity is thermosensitive and the thermal transition is typical
of a protein. Upon sedimentation on a glycerol density gradient
the factor appears to have a molecular weight less than 100,000
daltons while on SDS gels after denaturation the protein has a
molecular weight of 60,000 daltons. This would indicate that
the factor differs from M3 (M.W. greater than 200,000 daltons)
described by Shafritz et al. (24) and considered to be the equivalent of bacterial IF3.

     The purified factor stimulates initiation of Hb mRNA transla-
tion. It also stimulates TMV RNA activity but even inhibits Mengo
RNA. The factor discriminates between the α and β chains of
globin mRNA. The amount of α and β globin synthesized is measured
by following the incorporation of ^{35}S-methionine into the unique
tryptic peptide present in each chain, as shown in Fig. 7. (Since
the initiator methionine is rapidly removed from the nascent
chain, only one internal methionine residue is found in each globin
chain.) Table 6 shows the effect of purified factor on the α/β
ratio. The Krebs extract synthesizes an excess of β chain. Addition of the factor stimulates almost exclusively α chain synthesis
and restores a normal α/β ratio.

     The Hb mRNA factor has not yet been found in other tissue,
Wigle and Smith (25) reported the isolation of an initiation
factor from Krebs ascites supernatant specific for EMC virus RNA
but which is inactive with Hb mRNA. This factor would require M3
for its activity (K. Marcker, personal communication). A similar
Mengo virus specific factor appears to be present also in L cells
(Table 5). A factor active for the translation of β globin mRNA
different from the EMC RNA factor was also detected in Krebs
supernatant (25).

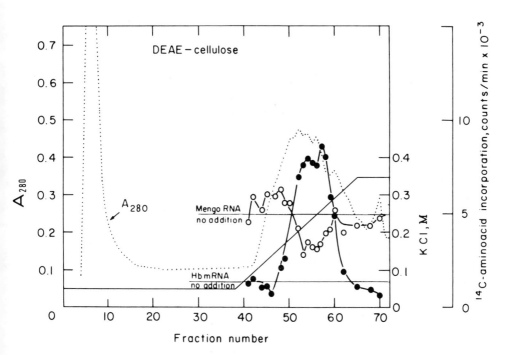

Fig. 6. Purification of Hemoglobin (Hb)mRNA stimulatory factor:
After DEAE cellulose chromatography of reticulocyte ribosomal wash
fraction (0.5 M KCl), fractions were tested for their effect on
mRNA translation in 0.3 A_{260} units Krebs S-30. Activity of factor
I_g was defined as the stimulation in the number of pmoles of
amino acid incorporated produced by 1 μg of protein when Hb mRNA
is used as template.

Step:	Specific activity:
I. Ribosomal wash	0.1
III. DEAE cellulose	1.8
IV. Phosphocellulose 0.3 M KCl fraction	14.0

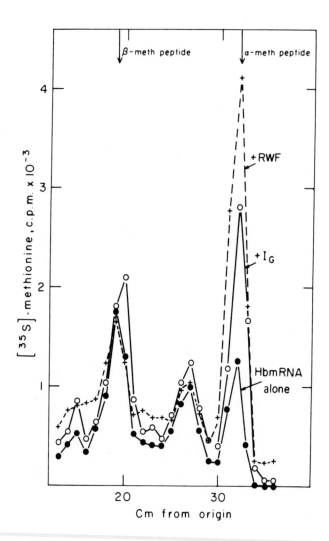

Fig. 7. Effect of ribosomal wash and purified I_g factor on α and β globin synthesis. Globin synthesis was performed in Krebs S-30 (1.5 A_{260} units) with (^{35}S)-methionine (33 mCi/µmole) with no addition (o), or with 600 µg reticulocyte ribosomal wash (+) or 6 µg purified I_g factor (o). After 60 min incubation at 30°C, the proteins were precipitated, digested with trypsin and analyzed by electrophoresis at pH 3.5. The position of marker peptides obtained from *in vivo* synthesized α and β chain (separated on CMC cellulose) is shown. Only one methionine-peptide is present in each rabbit globin chain.

T A B L E   5

EFFECT OF VARIOUS CRUDE FRACTIONS FROM RETICULOCYTE AND L CELLS ON KREBS ASCITES CELLS S-30 FRACTION

Expt.	Krebs S-30 fraction	Addition	Translation of	
			Mengo RNA	Hemoglobin mRNA
			^{14}C-Leucine incorporated, pmoles	
1	Fresh	None	7.2	5.8
		Retic.ribos. wash	3.9(0.55)	20.9(3.6)
	Frozen-thawed	None	2.4	2.8
		Retic.ribos. wash	3.3(1.34)	14.0(5.0)
2	Fresh	None	9.6	–
		L cell ribosomal wash	20.0(2.1)	–
		L cell supernatant	54.2(5.6)	–
3	Fresh	None	51.0	13.0
		L cell supernatant	74.0(1.5)	7.0(0.54)

A cell free system as described in Nudel et al. (26) was employed. All Krebs S-30 fractions were kept in liquid air. "Fresh" indicates an extract thawed once, "frozen-thawed" refers to extracts submitted to 3 cycles of freeze-thawing with liquid air. Amount of Krebs S-30 were 0.3 A_{260} units in expts. 1 and 2 and 0.6 A_{260} units in expt. 3. The reticulocyte or L cell ribosomal wash (100 μg) and L cell supernatant (150 μg) had no activity alone. Incorporation in the absence of mRNA was 0.5 pmoles without factor; 2.5 pmoles with reticulocyte ribosomal wash. The control values were subtracted appropriately. Figures in brackets represent ratios between values in the presence and absence of added factor.

TABLE   6

EFFECT OF RETICULOCYTES FACTORS ON α AND β GLOBIN SYNTHESIS
IN KREBS S-30

Conditions	(^{35}S)-methionine incorporated		α/β
	α globin peptide	β globin peptide	
1. Krebs S-30			
Total synthesis	4,600	8,600	0.5
2. Retic. ribosomal wash:			
Total synthesis	17,900	16,600	
Stimulation	13,300	8,000	1.6
3. Purified I_g factor			
Total synthesis	8,200	10,200	
Stimulation	3,600	1,600	2.2

Results computed from electrophoregram as in Fig. 7. Conditions
as in Legend to Fig. 7.

CONCLUSIONS

Our results already indicate that mammalian ribosomes use
mRNA specific initiation factors similar to those found in *E.coli*.
A study of the distribution, synthesis and variations in these
factors during differentiation, response to hormones and other
tissue-specific inducers should throw much light on the mechanisms
which regulate protein synthesis.

REFERENCES

1. M. REVEL & H.H. HIATT (1964). *Proc.Natl.Acad.Sci.USA*, *51*, 810.
2. M. REVEL, In: The mechanism of protein synthesis and its
   regulation, L. Bosh Ed., *North-Holland Publ.Co.*, *Amsterdam,
   London* (1972) pp.87-131.
3. M. REVEL, H. GREENSHPAN & M. HERZBERG (1970). *Eur.J.Biochem.*
   16, 117.
4. M. REVEL, Y. GRONER, Y. POLLACK, H. BERISSI & M. HERZBERG,
   In: Functional units in protein biosynthesis. (*FEBS
   SYMPOSIUM*) *Acad.Press,New York*, *23*, (1972a) 237.
5. J.A. STEITZ (1969). *Nature (London)*, *224*, 967.
6. Y. GRONER & M. REVEL (1971). *Eur.J.Biochem.* *22*, 144.
7. J.W.B. HERSHEY, E. REMOLD O'DONNELL, D. KOLAKOFSKY, K.F. DEWEY
   & R.E. THACH In: Methods in Enzymology, Moldave and
   Grossman Eds., *Acad.Press*, *New York*, *20*, (1971) 235.
8. S. OCHOA (1968). *Naturwissenschaften*, *11*, 505.
9. A.R. SUBRAMANIAN & B.D. DAVIS (1971). *Nature New Biol.*
   228, 1254.
10. H.F. LODISH (1970a). *Nature*, *226*, 705.
11. H.F. LODISH (1970b). *J.Mol.Biol.* *50*, 689.
12. Y. GRONER, Y. POLLACK, H. BERISSI & M. REVEL. (1972b).
    Nature New Biol. *239*, 16.
13. Y. GRONER, Y. POLLACK, H. BERISSI & M. REVEL (1972a).
    FEBS LETTERS, *21*, 223.
14. H.F. LODISH (1969). *Nature*, *224*, 867.
15. S. LEE-HUANG & S. OCHOA (1971). *Nature New Biol.* *234*, 236.
16. M. YOSHIDA & P.S. RUDLAND (1972). *J.Mol.Biol.* *68*, 465.
17. H. BERISSI, Y. GRONER & M. REVEL. (1971). *Nature New Biol.*
    234, 44.
18. M. REVEL, Y. POLLACK, Y. GRONER, R. SCHEPS, H. INOUYE, H.
    BERISSI & H. ZELLER In: Ribosomes, structures, function
    and biogenesis, *FEBS Symposium*, *Vol.* 27 (1972b) 261.
19. R. KAMEN, M. KONDO, W. ROMER & C. WEISSMANN (1972).
    Eur.J.Biochem. *31*, 44.

20. F.W. STUDIER (1972). *Science, 176,* 367.
21. P. HERRLICH, M. SCHWEIGER & W. SAUERBIER (1971). *Molec.Gen. Genetics, 112,* 152.
22. R.C. CALLAHAN & P. LEDER (1972). *Arch.Biochem.Biophys. 153,* 802.
23. R. SCHEPS & M. REVEL (1972). *Eur.J.Biochem. 29,* 319.
24. D.A. SHAFRITZ, P.M. PRICHARD & W.F. ANDERSON In: Methods in Molecular Biology, J.A. Last and A.I. Laskin, Eds., *Marcel Dekker Inc., New York, 2,* (1972) 265.
25. D.T. WIGGLE & A.E. SMITH (1973). *Eur.J.Biochem. in press.*
26. U. NUDEL, B. LEBLEU & M. REVEL (1973). *Proc.Natl.Acad.Sci. USA, in press.*

SOME CORRELATIONS BETWEEN RIBOSOMAL PROTEINS AND RIBOSOMAL

ACTIVITIES

A. Zamir, I. Ginzburg, N. Sonenberg, R. Miskin,
M. Wilchek and D. Elson

The Weizmann Institute of Science, Rehovot, Israel

INTRODUCTION

In order to understand the structural basis of ribosomal function in protein biosynthesis, it is necessary to amass a great deal
of information of many different kinds. In this communication we
describe two studies which pertain to one aspect of this problem,
the correlation of individual ribosomal proteins with ribosomal
activities.

AFFINITY LABELLING OF THE RIBOSOMAL CHLORAMPHENICOL BINDING SITE (1)

A number of approaches have been made to the problem of cor-
relating specific ribosomal proteins with specific ribosomal functions: e.g., the identification of an altered protein in a mutant
with an altered function (2); the observation of a change in some
function in reconstituted ribosomes which lack a particular protein
or carry it in an altered form (3); the correlation between the
loss of a certain activity and the chemical or enzymatic modification of a certain protein in the ribosome (4,5). Using such
approaches it can be shown that a protein affects a function, but
it is not established whether the protein is actually at the functional site in question, since it is always possible that the protein may exert its influence at a distance via an allosteric effect.

The technique of affinity labelling offers a way of eliminating this ambiguity (6). A close analogue of a known ligand of the ribosome is prepared which can form a covalent bond with proteins. It is necessary that the analogue bind to the same site as the ligand and that its physiological non-covalent binding be more rapid than the covalent attachment. If these conditions are met, there is reasonable assurance that the analogue will bind covalently to proteins at or adjacent to the functional site.

In the present study, this technique was employed to investigate the ribosomal binding site of chloramphenicol. This antibiotic interacts specifically with the 50S ribosomal subunit and inhibits peptidyl transferase activity, thus blocking protein synthesis. There is evidence which suggests that chloramphenicol binds at or near the peptidyl transferase site; however, this evidence is not conclusive (7,8). There is also evidence that chloramphenicol exhibits two modes of binding, one of high and the other of low affinity, possibly indicating two binding sites (9).

The affinity labelling analogue was prepared by replacing the dichloroacetyl group of chloramphenicol with a monobromoacetyl group. The resulting compound, bromamphenicol, attaches covalently to proteins in the ribosome and was shown, by amino acid analysis, to react exclusively with the sulfhydryl group of cysteine.

Before proceeding with the affinity labelling experiments, it was necessary to ascertain whether bromamphenicol is a true biological analogue of chloramphenicol. This was done by incubating both compounds with 50S subunits under conditions which exclude covalent binding, i.e., at pH 8.6 at 0° for times not exceeding 15 minutes. Under these conditions, the subunits catalyze the peptidyl transferase reaction and bind both compounds non-covalently, but the covalent binding of bromamphenicol is negligible. The double reciprocal plots of Fig. 1 show that bromamphenicol·inhibits peptidyl transferase activity, although less effectively than chloramphenicol. Figure 2 shows that the analogue competes with chloramphenicol for ribosomal binding sites. Thus, bromamphenicol is a valid analogue of chloramphenicol and can be used to investigate the antibiotic binding site.

For covalent affinity labelling, bromamphenicol was incubated with 50S subunits at the same pH, 8.6, but at 37°. At this temperature the covalent reaction, although much slower than non-covalent binding, proceeds at a significant rate. The rate and extent of the covalent reaction increased with rising analogue concentration, while peptidyl transferase activity diminished in parallel (Fig. 3).

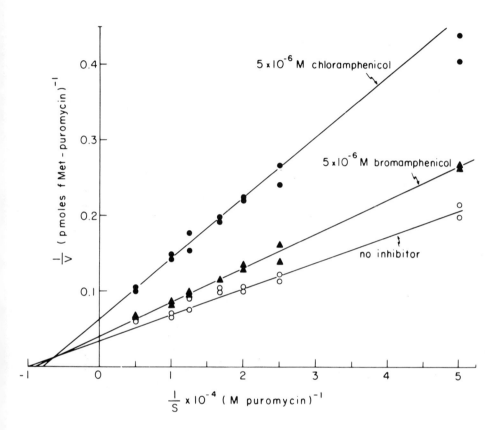

Fig. 1. Inhibition of peptidyl transferase activity by chloramphenicol and bromamphenicol. 50 S subunits were assayed under
conditions for non-covalent binding (1).

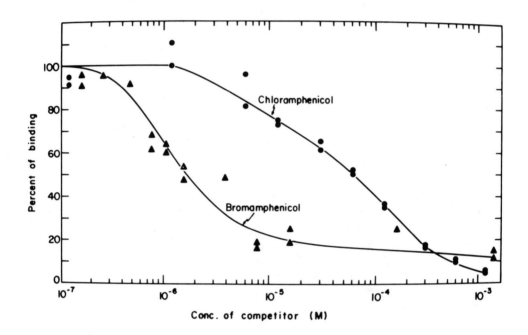

Fig. 2.   Competition between chloramphenicol and bromamphenicol in
binding to 50S subunits.   Binding of radioactive chloramphenicol
(●———●) or radioactive bromamphenicol (▲———▲) in the presence of
non-radioactive bromamphenicol or chloramphenicol, respectively.
The radioactive compound was at a fixed concentration of 10^{-5}M
and the concentration of the competitor was varied as shown. 100%
binding corresponded to 38.6 pmoles (^{14}C)-chloramphenicol or
15.3 pmoles (^{14}C)-bromamphenicol.   Assays were carried out under
conditions for non-covalent binding (1).

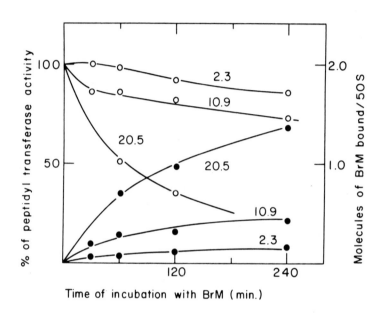

Fig. 3. Covalent binding of bromamphenicol to 50S subunits and inhibition of peptidyl transferase activity. 50S subunits were incubated with different concentrations of (^{14}C)-bromamphenicol (2.3, 10.9 or 20.5 molecules per ribosome) under conditions for covalent binding (1). Samples were dialyzed to remove excess reagent and assayed for uptake of bromamphenicol (●——●) and peptidyl transferase activity (o——o).

To identify the proteins which bind the analogue, 50S ribosomes were incubated with radioactive bromamphenicol at 37°. The
ribosomal proteins were extracted and separated by two-dimensional
gel electrophoresis (10). The individual proteins were located by
staining, cut out of the gel and combusted in a sample oxidizer.
Their radioactivity was determined (Table I); two proteins, L2 and
L27, were labelled about equally and to a much higher degree than
any others.

In order to test the specificity of the covalent binding reaction, similar reactions were carried out with two other radioactive compounds, N-bromoacetylphenylalanine methyl ester and N-
ethylmaleimide. Both of these reagents also form covalent bonds
with sulfhydryl groups and reacted with proteins in the intact 50S
ribosome. However, their labelling patterns (Table I) were significantly broader than that of bromamphenicol, both labelling a
number of proteins not labelled by the antibiotic. Although the
non-specific reagents bound to the ribosomes, they did not inhibit
the peptidyl transferase activity. Further, when subunits were
pretreated with non-radioactive N-ethylmaleimide and then exposed
to radioactive bromamphenicol, the uptake of radioactivity by L2
and L27 was greatly reduced and the peptidyl transferase activity
was not affected. This indicates that N-ethylmaleimide blocks the
attachment sites of bromamphenicol but that the blockage of the
sulfhydryl groups does not in itself cause inactivation. The inhibitory effect of covalently bound bromamphenicol must therefore
arise from a specific steric effect which would presumably occur
only at the effective antibiotic binding site. This strengthens
the evidence that bromamphenicol is covalently bound at this site
and that either L2 or L27 or both are at or adjacent to the site.

Several studies have reported the use of affinity labelling
with substituted Phe-tRNA to modify ribosomal components at the
peptidyl transferase center, but the labelled proteins have not
yet been clearly identified (11-13). It has more recently been
reported that an analogue of fMet-tRNA labels protein L2, showing
it to be at or near what is presumed to be the P site of the 50S
peptidyl transferase center (14). If this is so, then our finding
that bromamphenicol binds to L2 furnishes the first direct evidence
that chloramphenicol interacts with the ribosome at the peptidyl
transferase center.

DEMONSTRATION OF CONFORMATIONAL CHANGES IN THE 30S SUBUNIT, AND THEIR USE TO CORRELATE PROTEINS AND ACTIVITIES (15)

Ribosomes and their separated subunits may assume several different states of activity, depending not only on their current
environment but also on their past treatment. When the 30S subunit

TABLE   I

DISTRIBUTION OF LABEL IN PROTEINS OF 50S RIBOSOMAL SUBUNITS
TREATED WITH VARIOUS REAGENTS

Protein	T r e a t m e n t		
	Bromamphenicol	N-bromoacetyl-Phe methyl ester	N-ethylmaleimide
	R a d i o a c t i v i t y		(cpm)
L1	0	180	24
L2	480	170	965
L3	0	60	25
L4	0	40	17
L5	0	30	32
L6	40	95	81
L7+L12	0	20	10
L8+L9	10	10	41
L10	67	165	892
L11	50	145	286
L13	11	60	93
L14	71	85	43
L15	38	50	29
L16	11	35	26
L17	81	110	580
L18	6	55	43
L19	33	25	46
L21	2	10	0
L22	13	85	0
L23	0	75	0
L24	7	20	0
L25	0	25	0
L26	128	0	0
L27	446	50	750
L28	60	35	0
L29	0	10	0
L30	0	25	0
L32	0	10	0
L33	0	30	0

is depleted of K^+ and NH_4^+ ions or is exposed to a low concentration of Mg^{++} ions, it loses the ability to bind aminoacyl-tRNA in the presence of a suitable messenger, to bind streptomycin and dihydro-streptomycin, and to associate with the 50S subunit to form a 70S ribosome. These activities can be restored by supplying the depleted cations. However, the rate of reactivation is highly dependent on temperature and cation concentration. Thus, conditions can be found where the transition is very slow and active subunits remain active and inactive subunits remain inactive for extended periods of time. This shows that the difference in activity is not necessarily due to any difference in the ambient medium of temperature, which may be identical, but to a difference in the ribosomes themselves. No essential component is lost when ribosomes are inactivated in this way; therefore, the difference must be conformational. In agreement with this, 30S subunits have been found to differ in sedimentation constant and susceptibility to sulfhydryl oxidation (16-20).

The present study was undertaken in an attempt to provide additional and more definitive evidence for such a conformational difference. The results, described below, furnish such evidence, and also allow correlation of certain proteins with certain ribosomal activities.

In the technique employed, active and inactive 30S subunits were incubated under identical conditions (in which each type retained its original state of activity) with N-ethylmaleimide (NEM), a reagent that specifically reacts covalently with thiol groups in proteins and affects ribosomal activity (cf. 4,21). With radioactive NEM it was possible to measure quantitatively the uptake of the reagent. The ribosomal proteins that reacted with it were identified, using the two-dimensional gel electrophoretic technique mentioned above.

The total uptake of NEM by ribosomes increases as the concentration of NEM in the reaction mixture is raised (4). Figure 4 shows that active and inactive 30S subunits are indistinguishable by this criterion, both reacting with identical amounts of the reagent over a wide concentration range. However, extensive differences were seen when the labelled proteins were identified (Table II). When labelling was carried out at a concentration of 5 mM NEM, seven proteins were labelled in each activity state. Of these, only three reacted in both states. Four other proteins reacted only when the ribosomes were active, and a different set of four only when the ribosomes were inactive. These large differences in the labelling pattern clearly establish that the inactive and active 30S subunits differ in conformation.

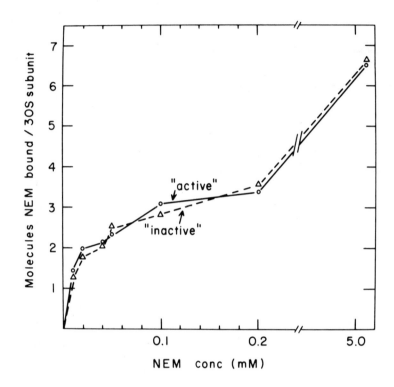

Fig. 4. Covalent binding of (^{14}C)-N-ethylmaleimide to active and inactive 30S subunits as a function of reagent concentration in the incubation mixture. See reference 15 for details.

TABLE   II

PROTEIN LABELLED IN ACTIVE AND INACTIVE 30S SUBUNITS TREATED
WITH (^{14}C)-NEM

NEM Concentration Activity State	0.02 mM		5 mM	
	Inactive	Active	Inactive	Active
Protein	R a d i o a c t i v i t y (cpm)			
S9	-	-	812	911
S13	1118	697	1969	1033
S19	-	1656	1795	2726
S2	-	-	-	2130
S4	-	-	-	612
S12	-	-	-	1228
S17	-	-	-	2381
S1	-	-	1446	-
S14	-	-	3417	-
S18	1566	-	1184	-
S21	639	-	1937	-

In another series of experiments, performed to test the effect of NEM uptake on four 30S activities, active and inactive subunits were incubated with different concentrations of the reagent and assayed. (The inactive ribosomes were subjected to a reactivating treatment before the assay.) Figure 5 shows the effect on three activities: the non-enzymatic binding of Phe-tRNA directed by poly U; the enzymatic binding of fMet-tRNA directed by poly AUG (formation of the initiation complex); and the binding of dihydrostreptomycin. In no case did active subunits lose activity when reacted with NEM at any of the concentrations tested. Inactive subunits, however, lost the ability to regain activity, with each of the three activities exhibiting a different inactivation pattern. The ability to bind fMet-tRNA was abolished at a low NEM concentration, while the ability to bind dihydrostreptomycin was affected only at high NEM concentrations. The ability to bind Phe-tRNA was lost in two distinctly separate stages. A fourth activity, the ability to associate with 50S subunits to form 70S ribosomes, was lost at a low NEM concentration when inactive subunits were reacted (Fig. 6), as in the case of fMet-tRNA binding. When labelled in the active state, the subunits retained the ability to form 70S ribosomes, as judged by their ability to polymerize phenylalanine in the presence of 50S subunits (data not shown).

These results show that blockage by NEM of sulfhydryl groups in proteins S2, S4, S9, S12, S13, S17 and S19 does not inhibit any of the four activities tested. (These were the proteins labelled when the subunits were in the active conformation, and their labelling caused no loss of activity.) Therefore, loss of activity is due to the reaction with NEM of one or more of the four proteins labelled only in the inactive conformation: S1, S14, S18 and S21.

No information on the nature of this inhibitory effect is provided by the data given so far. The protein or proteins involved might either (a) participate directly in the activity in question, or (b) be necessary for the restoration of the active ribosomal conformation, whether directly participating in the activity or not. It was possible to distinguish between these two possibilities by using the labelling pattern itself as a criterion of ribosomal conformation. Inactive subunits were labelled with radioactive NEM, and a portion was then subjected to a treatment which would convert unlabelled inactive subunits to the active conformation. These "reactivated" subunits were then again labelled with NEM to see if they now showed the labelling pattern of the active conformation. The reverse experiment was also done: active subunits were labelled, inactivated and again labelled.

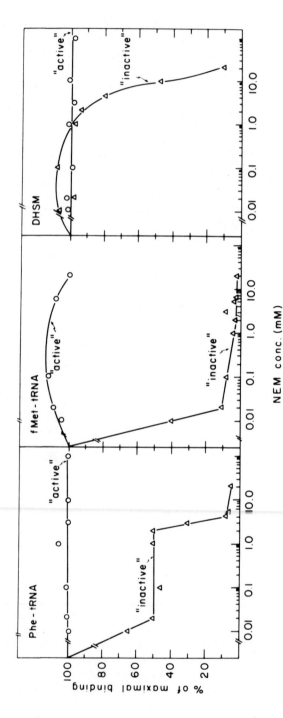

Fig. 5. The effect of N-ethylmaleimide on various activities of the 30S subunit.
Active and inactive subunits were incubated with different concentrations of NEM
and assayed for the binding of Phe-tRNA (non-enzymatic), fMet-tRNA (enzymatic),
and dihydrostreptomycin (DHSM). Initially inactive subunits were reactivated before
assay.

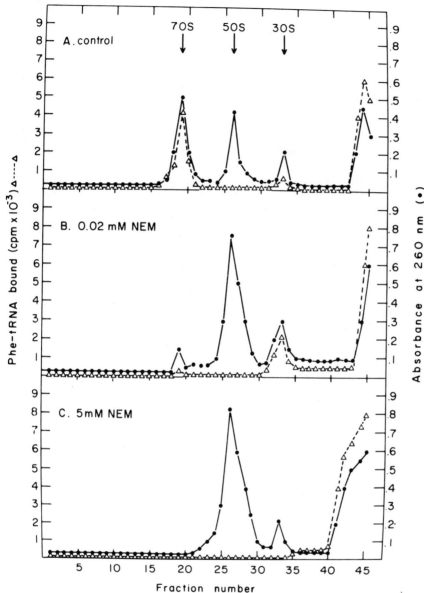

Fig. 6. Effect of N-ethylmaleimide on subunit association. Inactive 30S subunits were treated with 0.02 mM or 5 mM NEM, subjected to an activating treatment, and incubated with (^{14}C)-
Phe-tRNA in the presence of poly U. One equivalent of active 50S
subunits was added and the mixture was analyzed by sucrose gradient
centrifugation for absorbance at 260 nm (● ——— ●) and binding of
Phe-tRNA (Δ ——— Δ). The 50S peak is large relative to the 30S
peak because of the tendency of inactive 30S subunits to form 50S
dimers (20). See reference 15 for details.

The results (Table III) show that 30S subunits labelled with NEM
in either conformation are still able to assume the other conformation; such twice labelled ribosomes have the combined patterns
of both conformations. Thus, the reaction of NEM with those proteins whose labelling affects ribosomal activity does not block
the conversion to the active conformation, and therefore one or
more of the proteins must be directly involved in the activity
itself.

Some inferences can be drawn as to which proteins affect which
activities. Two activities, association with the 50S subunit and
the binding of fMet-tRNA, were fully abolished at a low NEM concentration (0.02 mM). Of the four proteins in question, only S18
and S21 were labelled at this reagent concentration and only they
can be responsible for the loss of these activities. Almost the
entire population of reactivated 30S subunits is competent to
combine with 50S subunits (20). Since S21 is only partly labelled
in 0.02 mM NEM, it is unlikely to be the target protein for abol-
ishing this activity, leaving S18, which is fully labelled, as
the only strong candidate. The same argument can be invoked to
implicate S18 in the binding of fMet-tRNA. However, S21 cannot be
ruled out in this case since only a fraction of the ribosomes was
capable of this activity and it is conceivable that S21 may be
preferentially labelled in this fraction.

Figure 5 indicates that the inactivation of phenylalanine
binding activity occurs in two discrete steps, and the same was
observed with the poly A directed binding of lysine (data not
shown). It is therefore possible that two different sites are involved, one inactivated at low and the other at high NEM concentration. The site inactivated at low NEM concentration might then
be the same site that binds fMet-tRNA, presumably the P site
(22,23), with S18 as the most likely target protein for its inactivation and S21 as a less probable candidate. With this in
mind, the Phe-tRNA binding activity remaining after treatment with
0.02 mM NEM was examined and found to exhibit properties associated
with the A site in 70S ribosomes; compared with the total binding
activity it showed a higher Mg^{++} requirement (24) and a lower
affinity for deacylated tRNA (25) (data not shown). S18 was clearly not involved in the inactivation of this site; therefore, one
or more of the protein S1, S14 and S21 was involved. The same
applied to the dihydrostreptomycin binding activity, which was also
inactivated only at high NEM concentrations.

The above results are in accord with earlier reports which
implicated S18 as the target protein in the NEM inhibition of phenylalanine polymerization (4) and suggested that S14 might be involved in the binding of streptomycin (5).

TABLE III

LABELLING PATTERNS OF 30S SUBUNITS TREATED WITH (^{14}C)-NEM BEFORE
AND AFTER "ACTIVATION" OR "INACTIVATION"

NEM Concentration Activity State	0.02 mM				5 mM			
	I	A	I→A	A→I	I	A	I→A	A→I
Protein	R a d i o a c t i v i t y (cpm)							
S9	-	-	-	-	935	1011	878	1226
S13	1130	956	1050	805	1216	1126	1096	967
S19	-	1765	1625	1937	1926	3016	2626	3228
S2	-	-	-	-	-	2327	2169	2196
S4	-	-	-	-	-	819	617	915
S12	-	-	-	-	-	1372	1467	1427
S17	-	-	-	-	-	2116	2548	1960
S1	-	-	-	-	1627	-	1785	1436
S14	-	-	-	-	3326	-	2929	3628
S18	1576	-	1982	1678	1326	-	2167	2976
S21	980	-	820	1135	1726	-	1528	1676

Labelling treatments: I, labelled only in inactive state; A,
labelled only in active state; I→A, labelled in inactive state;
"reactivated", labelled again; A→I, labelled in active state,
inactivated, labelled again.

What emerges from these experiments is that protein S18 is involved in subunit association and probably in the binding of aminoacyl-tRNA and the formation of the initiation complex, where its influence may be restricted to the P site. One or more of the proteins S1, S14 and S21 affect the binding of dihydrostreptomycin and of aminoacyl-tRNA, perhaps at the A site.

ACKNOWLEDGEMENTS

We are grateful to Mr. S. Avital for instruction and help in gel electrophoresis techniques, and to Mr. D. Haik for ribosome preparations.

REFERENCES

1. SONENBERG, N., WILCHEK, M. & ZAMIR, A. (1973). Proc.Nat.Acad. Sci. USA. 70, 1423.
2. DAVIES, J. & NOMURA, M. (1972). Ann.Rev.Genetics, 6, 203.
3. NOMURA, M. (1973). Science, 179, 864.
4. MOORE, P.B. (1971). J.Mol.Biol. 60, 169.
5. CHANG, F.N. & FLAKS, J.G. (1970). Proc.Nat.Acad.Sci.USA, 67, 1321.
6. SINGER, S.J. (1967). Adv.Prot.Chem. 22, 1.
7. PESTKA, S. (1971). Ann.Rev.Microbiol. 25, 487.
8. MONRO, R.E. & VAZQUEZ, D. (1967). J.Mol.Biol. 28, 161.
9. PESTKA, S. (1972). J.Biol.Chem. 247, 4669.
10. KALTSCHMIDT, E. & WITTMANN, H.G. (1970). Proc.Nat.Acad.Sci. USA, 67, 1276.
11. BOCHKAREVA, E.S., BUDKER, V.G., GIRSHOVICH, A.S., KNORRE, D.G. & TEPLOVA, N.M. (1971). FEBS Letters, 19, 121.
12. PELLEGRINI, M., OEN, H. & CANTOR, C. (1972). Proc.Nat.Acad. Sci. USA, 69, 837.
13. CZERNILOFSKY, A.P. & KUECHLER, E. (1972). Biochim.Biophys. Acta, 272, 667.
14. LENGYEL, P., lecture at this symposium; C. Cantor, cited in ref.4.
15. GINZBURG, I., MISKIN, R. & ZAMIR, A. (1973). J.Mol.Biol. in press.
16. ZAMIR, A., MISKIN, R. & ELSON, D. (1971). J.Mol.Biol. 60, 347.
17. VOGEL, Z., VOGEL, T., ZAMIR, A. & ELSON, D. (1970). J.Mol.Biol. 54, 369.
18. SPITNIK-ELSON, P., ZAMIR, A., MISKIN, R., KAUFMANN, Y., EHRLICH, Y.H., GINZBURG, I. & ELSON, D. (1972). FEBS Symp. 27, 251.

19. MISKIN, R. & ZAMIR, A.   (1972). Nature New Biol. 238, 78.
20. ZAMIR, A., MISKIN, R., VOGEL, Z. & ELSON, D. (1973). Methods
        in Enzymology, Vol.30, in press.
21. TRAUT, R.R. & HAENNI, A.L. (1967). Eur.J.Biochem. 2, 64.
22. THACH, S.S. & THACH, R.E. (1971). Proc.Nat.Acad.Sci.USA,
        68, 1791.
23. KUECHLER, E. (1971). Nature New Biol. 234, 216.
24. IGARASHI, K. & KAJI, A. (1970). Eur.J.Biochem. 14, 41.
25. DeGROOT, N., PANET, A. & LAPIDOT, Y. (1971). Eur.J.Biochem.
        23, 523.

DNA COMPLEMENTARY TO GLOBIN AND IMMUNOGLOBULIN mRNA:

A PROBE TO STUDY GENE EXPRESSION

H. Aviv, S. Packman, J. Ross, D. Swan, J. Gielen and
P. Leder

National Institutes of Health
Bethesda, Maryland, USA

During the development of an embryo, various processes occur
which induce the formation of differentiated tissues. Some of
these processes can be observed at a molecular level, for example,
myosin is synthesized in muscle cells, crystaline in lens tissue,
keratin in skin, immunoglobulin in lymphocytes and hemoglobin in
reticulocytes (1,2).

The molecular mechanisms of these differentiation processes
are not clear - theoretically, the cell may control its expression
in the following different ways:

(a) Gene amplification or gene deletion. The genes for a
tissue-specific protein may be amplified during the process of
differentiation. Alternatively, genes which are not expressed in
the differentiated tissue may be deleted during differentiation.
The loss of the gene would be an irreversible process.

(b) Gene activation or inactivation. The transcription of
messenger RNA which codes for a tissue-specific protein may be
initiated in the differentiating process, or, alternatively, non-
relevant genes may not be transcribed. The inactivation process
may be reversible, and transcription may initiate in another
developmental stage, or it may be irreversible, in which case a
particular gene may never be transcribed again.

(c) Post-transcriptional control. The expression of a specific messenger RNA can be controlled by its stability to degradation
processes or by its selective transportation from the nucleus.
Alternatively, messenger-specific initiation factors may affect its
translation.

The isolation of a messenger for a specific protein and its transcription into complementary DNA provides a general approach to study the control of gene expression.

ISOLATION OF MESSENGER RNA

In order to isolate mRNA for a specific protein, one needs a cell-free system which will translate messenger RNA faithfully into the specific protein. It is convenient if the system is also efficient and multipotential, namely, messenger from any type or species can be translated. Krebs ascites cells (3) provide such a source although they may not be unique; other cells may have similar properties (4). Preincubated extracts from Krebs ascites have a very low endogenous messenger activity - 0.1 - 0.5 μg of pure mRNA can be detected. Messengers of many types and species have been translated: mRNA for globin from duck, rabbit, mouse and humans (5-8); immunoglobulin light chain (9,10), lens crystaline (11), histones (12); and RNA from EMC, Mengo (3,13), Qβ and R17 viruses (14,15).

If messenger is present in a very low concentration and is contaminated by polynucleotides which inhibit its translations, it is also important to purify the messenger. This was done utilizing the existence of polyadenylic sequences present in many messenger RNA species from eukaryotic cells. We have synthesized oligo-thymidylate-cellulose (7,16) which can be used for chromatographic column separation. Only poly-(A) containing mRNA will anneal to oligo-(dt)cellulose under conditions favorable for hydrogen bond formation (i.e., high salt concentration), while other polynucleo-tides such as ribosomal RNA, tRNA, double-stranded RNA and histone mRNA will not bind. Washing the column with a buffer of low salt concentration will elute the poly(A) containing mRNA (Fig. 1). Using this method we have purified mRNA for globin from duck, rabbit, mouse and human reticulocytes (7), and messenger for immu-noglobulin light chain from myeloma MOPC 41 (a).

SYNTHESIS OF DNA COMPLEMENTARY TO mRNA

Pure mRNA can be used also as a template for reverse trans-criptase (17-20). Fortunately, the existence of poly(A) on the 3' end of many eukaryotic mRNAs is useful in phasing reverse trans-cription. Oligo (dT) will form a hybrid with the poly(A), and thus serve as a primer for the enzyme (Fig. 2). The reaction yields a DNA product complementary to messenger, labelled to a high specific activity and therefore useful for quantitation of both gene and messenger molecules. DNA complementary to globin mRNA is about 5-600 nucleotides long as measured in alkaline sucrose gradients

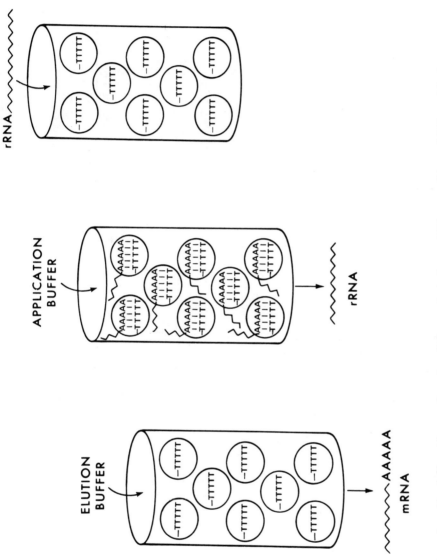

Fig. 1   Purification of poly-(A) containing mRNA on oligo (dT)-cellulose.

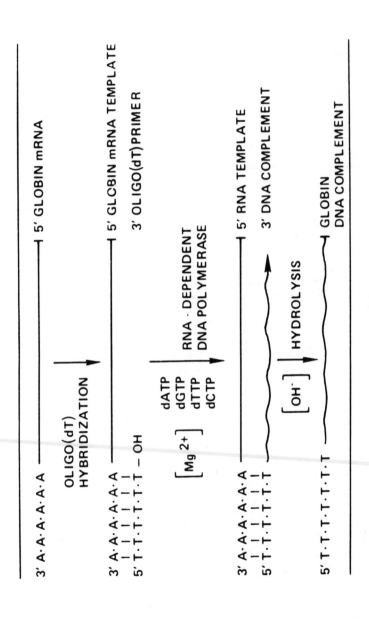

Fig. 2   Synthesis of DNA complementary to rabbit globin mRNA.

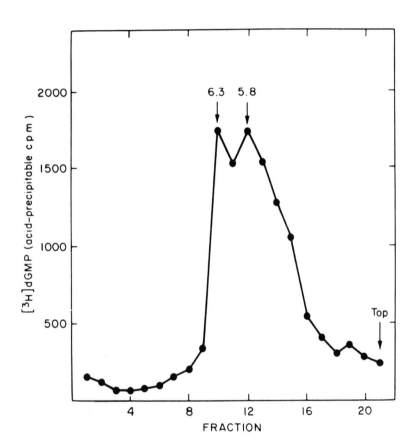

Fig. 3.   Alkaline sucrose gradient analysis of DNA product
by sucrose gradient.

$S_{20,w}$ values of DNA standards are indicated by the
arrows.

(Fig. 3), which is enough to contain the information for globin. Its hybridization properties are species-specific; RNA complementary to rabbit globin does not hybridize to RNA from duck reticulocytes and only slightly to RNA from human reticulocytes (Fig. 4A). On the other hand, DNA complementary to duck globin mRNA does not hybridize to RNA from rabbit or human reticulocytes (Fig. 4B).

DNA complementary to mRNA derived from myeloma MOPC 41 is approximately 325 nucleotides long which is only 40 percent the size of its template. Assuming oligo(A) is on the 3' - OH end of the messenger, we would expect the DNA synthesized to be complementary to the constant region of immunoglobulin light chains. Comparing the hybridization properties of the DNA with RNA from two different myelomas, MOPC 41 and MOPC 315 (Fig. 5), we can see that at low concentrations of RNA, MOPC 41 RNA is more efficient than RNA from MOPC 315. The percentage of hybridization found suggests that 50 percent of the synthesized DNA contains sequences complementary to immunoglobulin light chain mRNA, but in addition the DNA also contains sequences complementary to a variety of many other myeloma RNAs.

THE USE OF DNA COMPLEMENTARY TO mRNA

Highly radioactive DNA complementary to specific mRNA provides a probe for the determination of (a) the relative frequencies of one specific gene in differentiated as compared to non-differentiated cells, (b) the concentration of specific mRNA molecules during the process of differentiation.

The number of globin genes in duck reticulocytes was found to be in the range of 2-3 (21,22); moreover, there is no difference between the number of globin genes in duck reticulocytes and duck liver (Fig. 6). Thus in a differentiated cell such as liver, which in avians is not an erythropoietic organ, the genes for globin were not deleted, they are present but not expressed, excluding a gene deletion mechanism. The question remains whether this is a general phenomenon in differentiated cells.

Concluding that the globin genes are not amplified during erythroid cell differentiation, this leads to the question whether there is an induction of globin gene transcription or is the control post-transcriptional? Erythroblastic cells isolated by C. Friend provide an interesting model for these studies. When treated with 2% dimethyl sulfoxide DMSO these cells start to produce mouse α and β globin (23). The question arises whether globin mRNA is present in these cells before DMSO treatment or does globin mRNA accumulate only after the DMSO treatment? Using

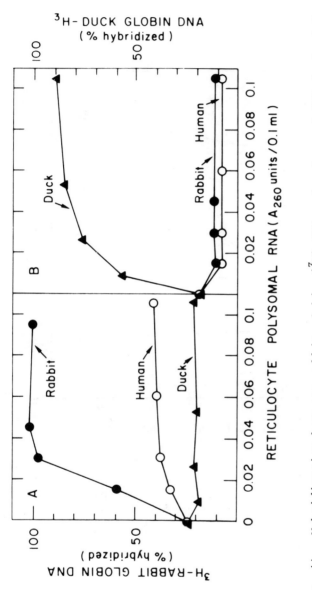

Fig. 4A. Hybridization between rabbit globin (^{3}H) DNA and polysomal RNA derived from: (●——●) rabbit, (O——O) human and (▲——▲) duck reticulocytes.

Fig. 4B. Hybridization between duck globin (^{3}H) DNA and polysomal RNA derived from: (▲——▲) duck, (O——O) human and (●——●) rabbit reticulocytes.

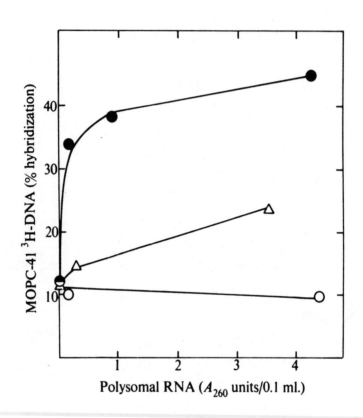

Fig. 5   Hybridization between MOPC 41 DNA and polysomal RNA
          derived from: MOPC 41 (●———●),
          MOPC 315 (△———△) and duck reticulocytes (0———0) (20).

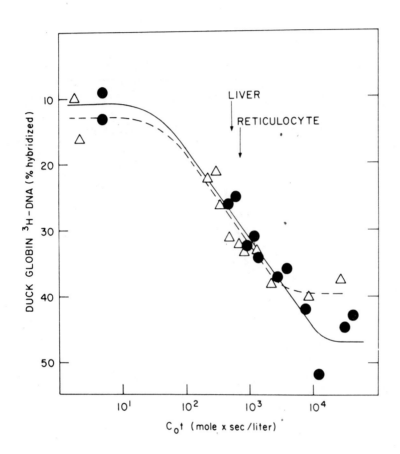

<u>Fig. 6</u>   Reassociation kinetics of single-stranded ^{3}H
        duck globin DNA in the presence of duck reticu-
        locyte or liver DNA   (21).

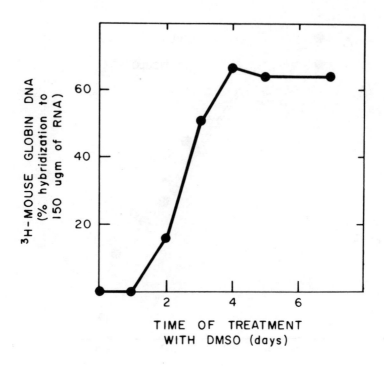

Fig. 7   Time course of induction of globin mRNA after
treatment with Me$_2$SO   (24).

purified DNA complementary to mouse globin mRNA, an increase in the amount of globin mRNA copies was detected (Fig. 7) (24). Since globin mRNA seems to be stable we think that these experiments indicate that the control of globin gene expression is transcriptional; however, the effect of DMSO on globin mRNA stabilization cannot be ruled out.

Assuming that the control of globin genes during differentiation is transcriptional, we have started to study cell free transcription of chromatin. Hopefully, such studies will help to identify the elements controlling transcription of a specific gene.

ACKNOWLEDGEMENTS

We appreciate the assistance of Dr. Carol Prives and Aviva Bokish for their help in preparing this manuscript.

The present address of H. Aviv is the Biochemistry Department, Weizmann Institute of Science, Rehovot, Israel.

REFERENCES

1. GROBSTEIN, C.; (1964) *Science 143*, 643.
2. EBERT, J. D.; (1965) Interacting systems in development (Holt, Rinhart and Winston.
3. MATHEWS, M. B. & KORNER, A.; (1970) *Eur. J. Biochem. 17*, 328.
4. ROBERTS, B. & PATTERSON, B.; *Proc. Nat. Acad. Sci.* (In press)
5. PACKMAN, S., AVIV, H. & LEDER, P. (Unpublished).
6. HOUSMAN, D., PEMBERTON, R. & TABER, R.; (1971) *Proc. Nat. Acad. Sci. USA 68*, 2716.
7. AVIV, H. & LEDER, P.; (1972) *Proc. Nat. Acad. Sci. USA 69*, 1408.
8. MATHEWS, M. B., OSBORN, M. & LINGREL, J. B.; (1971) *Nature New Biol. 233*, 206.
9. SWAN, D., AVIV, H. & LEDER, P.; (1972) *Proc. Nat. Acad. Sci. USA 69*, 1967.
10. MACH, B., FAUST, C. & VASSALLI, P.; (1973) *Proc. Nat. Acad. Sci. USA 70*, 451.
11. PIYATAGORSKIJ ET AL., (In preparation).
12. GROSS, K., RUDERMAN, J., JACOBS-LORENA, M., BAGLIONI, C., & GROSS, P.R.; (1973) *Nature New Biol. 241*, 272.
13. AVIV, H., BOIME, J. & LEDER, P.; (1971) *Proc. Nat. Acad. Sci. USA 68*, 2303.
14. AVIV, H., BOIME, J., LOYD, B. & LEDER, P.; (1972) *Science 178*, 1293.

15. MORRISON, T. G., LODISH, H. F.; (1973) *Proc. Nat. Acad. Sci.*
     USA 70, 315.

16. GILHAM, P.; (1964) *J. Amer. Chem. Soc. 86*, 4982.

17. ROSS, J., AVIV, H., SCOLNICK, E., & LEDER, P.; (1972) *Proc.*
     Nat. Acad. Sci. USA 69, 264.

18. VERMA, J. M., TEMPLE, G. F., FAN, H. & BALTIMORE, D.; (1972)
     Nature New Biol. 235, 163.

19. KACIAN, D. L., SPIEGELMAN, S., BANK, A., TERADA, M., METAFORA,
     S., DOW, L. & MARKS, P. A.; (1972) *Nature New Biol. 235*,
     167.

20. AVIV, H., PACKMAN, S., SWAN, D., ROSS, J. & LEDER, P.; (1973)
     Nature New Biol. 241, 173.

21. PACKMAN, S., AVIV, H., ROSS, J. & LEDER, P.; (1972) *Biochem.*
     Biophys. Res. Commun. 49, 813.

22. BISHOP, J. O., ROSBACK, M.; (1973) *Nature New Biol. 241*, 204.

23. FRIEND, C., SCHER, W., HOLLAND, J. G. & SATO, T.; (1971)
     Proc. Nat. Acad. Sci. USA 68, 378.

24. ROSS, J., IKAWA, Y., & LEDER, P.; (1972) *Proc. Nat. Acad.*
     Sci 69, 3620.

DEFECTIVE TRANSLATIONAL CONTROL IN THE β-THALASSEMIA OF FERRARA

Francesco Conconi and Laura del Senno

Centro di Studi Biochimici sul Morbo di Cooley
Cassa di Risparmio di Ferrara c/o Instituto di Chimica
Biologica dell'Università degli Studi di Ferrara
Ferrara, Italy

β-Thalassemia is a genetically determined anemia of man, characterized by a decreased synthesis of β-globin (and consequently of hemoglobin A) and a relative excess of α-globin synthesis.

The form of the disease described in the region of Ferrara (1,2) differs from most thalassemias in that β-globin synthesis is completely abolished.

Fig. 1 shows a typical globin synthetic pattern obtained after incubation of the intact reticulocytes of a homozygous subject from Ferrara with labelled amino acid. The patient had never received any transfusions. It is very evident that β-globin, which migrates on CM cellulose column chromatography (3) after the peak of γ-globin (see Fig. 3), is absent both as the pre-existing and as the newly synthesized radioactive molecule.

In this paper we will not consider the excess of α-globin synthesis (4,5) which although typical of the disease is secondary to the defect of β-globin synthesis (6). We will instead present our more recent experiments, through which we have been able to elucidate in part the alteration causing the absence of β-globin synthesis.

Proposed Theoretical Mechanisms for the Absence of β-globin
Synthesis in Ferrara β-Thalassemia

The failure to synthesize β-globin which is typical of our thalassemic population, may originate from:

153

(a)   lack of transcription of the gene for β-globin;
(b)   lack of translation of β-globin mRNA;
(c)   incomplete translation of β-globin mRNA.

It has been recently shown (7) that the transcription process of the globin genes in rabbit reticulocytes does not lead directly to mRNA synthesis, but to the synthesis of a high molecular weight RNA, called HRNA. In view of this finding, one may well speculate that the absence of β-globin synthesis may arise from an inability to transform HRNA into mRNA for β-globin.

The analysis of the transcriptional process in thalassemia would require the use of large amounts of bone marrow samples and is, therefore, technically difficult. For this reason we have examined experimentally possibilities (b) and (c), i.e., the two translational alterations which are hypothetical causes of the absence of β-globin synthesis.

Lack of Translation of β-globin mRNA

The lack of β-globin synthesis could result from an incomplete translation of the β-messenger due to a "nonsense" mutation of the messenger itself, with insertion of signals for chain termination or chain initiation (Fig. 2) instead of one of the 146 amino acids constituting β-globin.

In fact, the insertion of a terminating triplet (TER) would result in the release from the ribosomes of an amino-terminal β-globin fragment, while the carboxy-terminal part of the genetic message would not be translated. In the case of the insertion of an initiating signal (INI), on the contrary only a carboxy-terminal fragment would be translated and regularly released in the cytoplasm. Very recently (8), we have demonstrated that the reticulocytes of β-thalassemic subjects from Ferrara do not incorporate labelled amino acids in the β-T_1 peptide (which is the amino-terminal) nor in the β-T_{14} peptide (which is immediately adjacent to the carboxy-terminal). This result excludes the insertion of a terminating triplet after the codon for the 8th amino acid, or the insertion of an initiating triplet before the codon for the 133rd amino acid. It can be therefore concluded that the absence of β-globin synthesis in Ferrara thalassemia is due either to the non-synthesis or to the non-translation of β-globin mRNA.

Non-Translation of Normal β-globin mRNA in Ferrara β-Thalassemia

We have recently investigated the problem of the absence of β-globin synthesis in our thalassemic population in cell-free conditions (9). The results obtained in a typical experiment are presented in Fig. 3. The upper curve shows the chromatographic

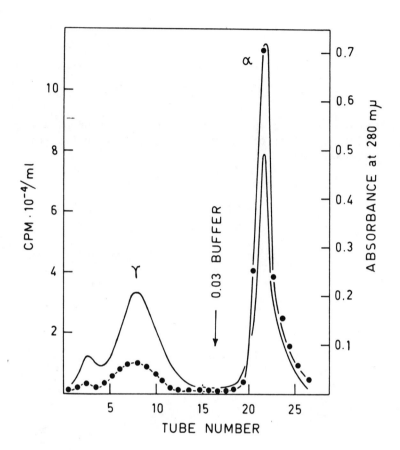

Chromatographic pattern on CM cellulose column of the labelled globin chains present in the reticulocytes of a homozygous β-thalassemic subject, after incubation with ^{3}H leucine (1).

Fig. 1   Chromatographic separation was performed according to the procedure of Clegg and coworkers (3). ——, O.D. pattern; ● —— ●, radioactivity.
From Bargellesi and coworkers (1), reprinted with permission.

Fig. 2   Scheme showing the effect of the insertion of a termina-
         ting signal or of an initiating signal on β-globin mRNA
         translation.

         (A)   normal β-globin mRNA translation;

         (B)   insertion of a terminating signal (TER);

         (C)   insertion of an initiating signal (INI).

         From J. Dreyfus and coworkers (8), reprinted with
         permission.

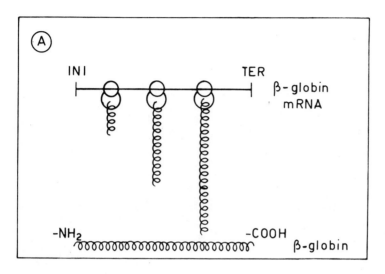

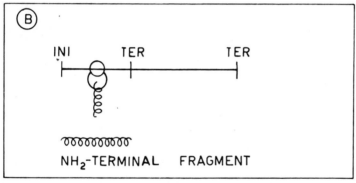

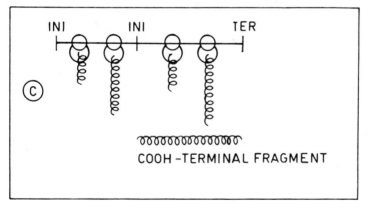

Fig. 3   Chromatographic patterns on CM cellulose columns of
            the newly synthesized globins obtained from a poly-
            transfused homozygous β-thalassemic subject from
            Ferrara, under different experimental conditions.

            Upper curve: intact cell incubation;

            Middle curve: cell-free incubation of homozygous
                           β-thalassemic ribosomes with
                           thalassemic supernatants;

            Lower curve: cell-free incubation of thalassemic
                           ribosomes with non-thalassemic
                           supernatants.

            From Conconi and coworkers (9), reprinted with
            permission.

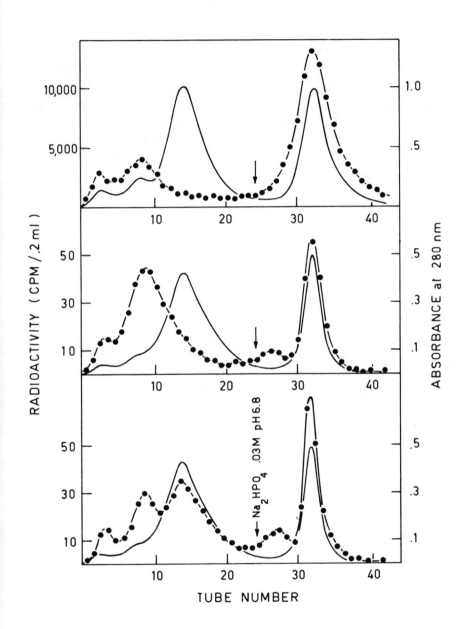

TUBE NUMBER

separation of the radioactive globins present in the reticulocytes
of a homozygous polytransfused β-thalassemic subject, after incubation with labelled amino acids; the two other curves represent
the results obtained in cell-free conditions with the ribosomes of
the same thalassemic subject incubated in the presence of supernatant from the same cells (middle curve) or in the presence of
the supernatant from the cells of a normal subject (lower curve).
It is evident that the peak of β-globin is not radioactive in the
two upper figures, but becomes radioactive in the "crossed" cell-
free incubation (thalassemic ribosomes + normal supernatant). The
appearance of radioactive proteins in the β-globin region has been
constantly observed in all cases in which the total radioactivity
was adequate for analysis. In the crossed cell-free incubation,
reported in Table 1, for example, the amount of induced β-globin
synthesis varied from 19 to 70 percent.

TABLE 1

^{3}H-LEUCINE INCORPORATION INTO α- β- AND γ-GLOBIN
BY β-THALASSEMIC RIBOSOMES AND NORMAL SUPERNATANT

Subject	Total Radioactivity (c.p.m.)			
	α-globin	β-globin	γ-globin	% of β-globin synthesis
1	4,931	2,666	11,190	19.2
2	2,075	2,500	2,150	35.5
3	4,250	5,500	12,250	30.9
4	775	640	1,180	35.1
5	10,882	9,186	3,882	70.2
6	2,180	1,047	1,418	42.5

The radioactivity migrating in the β-globin region is not derived from contaminating γ-chains. HbA was purified from thalassemic and "crossed" cell-free mixtures and then chromatographed on CM cellulose columns to separate α- and β-globin. As shown in Fig. 4, the purified β-globin peak was not radioactive in the thalassemic mixtures, and radioactive in the "crossed" cell-free mixtures. The radioactive proteins migrating in the β-globin region after "crossed" cell-free incubation have been analyzed and shown to be newly synthesized β-globin molecules. The β-globin tryptic peptides isolated from the incubation mixture, some of which typical of β-globin as opposed to α-, γ- and σ-globin, were radioactive. In addition, the specific activities of the various peptides were very close to those theoretically expected (9).

Incorporation of radioactivity into β-globin was also obtained after incubation of thalassemic ribosomes with red blood cell supernatants from HbS homozygous subjects, thus showing that β-globin synthesis is not induced by the β- mRNA present in the normal supernatants added to thalassemic ribosomes, in "crossed" cell-free incubations. The fingerprinting analysis of the radioactive proteins synthesized by thalassemic ribosomes, in the presence of HbS supernatant, also showed the presence of radioactive β-globin peptides; peptide β-S-T_1, isolated from the same incubation mixture, was not radioactive (9).

Our results therefore show that (a) normal red blood cell supernatants induce Ferrara homozygous β-thalassemic ribosomes to synthesize β-globin; and (b) that β-globin mRNA is not responsible for the inducing effect, since supernatants from HbS homozygous subjects are just as effective as supernatants from normal individuals in promoting β-globin synthesis. Ribosomes from thalassemic homozygotes from Ferrara, therefore, contain functional β-globin mRNA, whose translation requires a factor present in normal red blood cells and lacking or not functioning in thalassemic erythrocytes.

Nature of the Factor Inducing β-globin Synthesis

The β-globin inducing factor could be a tRNA or an aminoacyl tRNA synthetase; an argument against these two hypotheses is the lack of evidence in thalassemia of altered protein synthesis in other tissues. We have preliminary evidence that normal supernatants maintain their inducing capacity after RNAse treatment, but lose it after trypsin digestion (10).

It is possible, therefore, that the defect in Ferrara β-thalassemia may involve a previously unrecognized protein factor, specific for β-globin synthesis. Analogous specific translational

Fig. 4   Chromatographic patterns on CM cellulose columns of
          α- and β-globin of HbA, purified from a thalassemic
          cell-free system.

          Upper curve: thalassemic ribosomes and thalassemic
                          supernatant;

          Lower curve: thalassemic ribosomes and non-thalassemic
                          supernatant.

          ● ——— ●, radioactivity;

          —————————, absorbance at 280 mμ;

          From Conconi and coworkers (9), reprinted with
          permission.

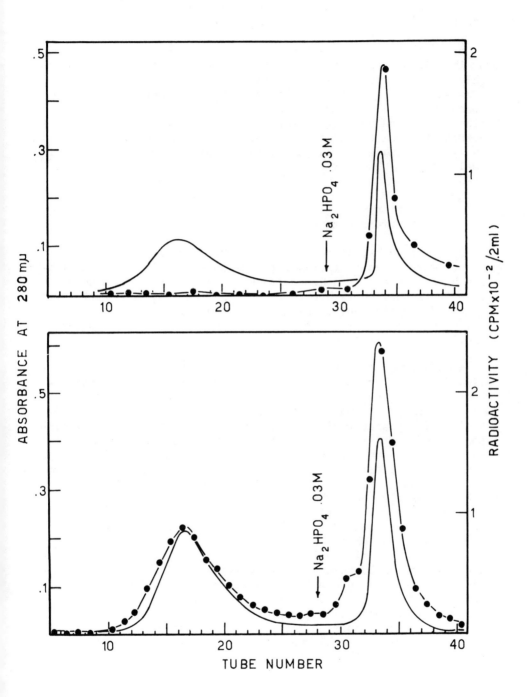

control have been reported by a number of authors in several
systems (11-14).

Very recently, we have further confirmed the existence of the
protein molecule specific for human β-globin synthesis (10).
Highly purified ribosomes from normal individuals do synthesize
α-, β- and γ-globin, when incubated in the presence of their own
supernatant; but β-globin synthesis does not occur when the incubation is carried out with normal ribosomes in the presence of
supernatants from erythroid cells of never-transfused homozygous
β-thalassemic subjects, while α- and γ-globin were synthesized at
normal rates.

Induction of β-globin Synthesis by Transfusion in Ferrara Homozygote β-thalassemia Subjects

In recent years, blood transfusions to Ferrara thalassemic
patients were given as infrequently as possible; lately, pediatri-
cians have switched to a hyper-transfusion regimen. As a consequence it is now impossible to examine patients 90 days after their
last blood transfusion, as we did in the past. In this new situation, we have made the observation that now most of our thalassemic
subjects do synthesize β-globin (15).

As is evident from Fig. 5, in which β-globin synthesis is
followed in a homozygous β-thalassemic subject, a progressive increase in β-globin specific activity occurs after blood transfusion, reaching its maximum approximately at the 15th day. This
kinetics of appearance of β-globin synthesis is not in accord with
a postulated synthesis of β-globin by the transfused normal reticulocytes. In such a case, one would expect the maximum of β-
synthesis immediately after transfusion and a progressive decrease
in the following one or two days. The same kinetics of β-globin
synthesis has also been observed in a plot obtained from the
analysis of several cases; it has also been noted that β-synthesis
disappears between the 30th and 60th day after blood transfusion.
The percent of β-globin synthesis relative to total counterpart
(β+γ) globin synthesis varies from case to case, but can reach
values as high as 50 percent. In addition, in the same subject,
different amounts of β-globin synthesis can be attained after different transfusions. In a few cases, we have separated thalassemic red blood cells of A group from normal transfused erythrocytes of O group by means of lectine precipitation (17). We were
able to demonstrate in this way that β-globin synthesis occurred,
as expected, within the non-agglutinated thalassemic red blood
cells.

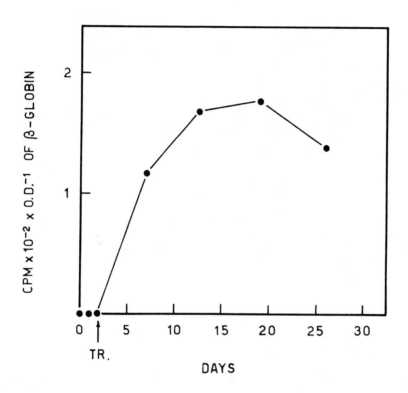

<u>Fig. 5</u>   Incorporation of radioactivity into purified β-globin in
a homozygous β-thalassemic subject from Ferrara before and after
transfusion.   After incubation with ³H-leucine, cells were lysed
and stroma removed by centrifugation (1); lysates were chromatographed on Amberlite CG-50 (16); purified HbA was then submitted
to CMC column chromatography (3) and the specific activity of
purified β-globin calculated from the O.D. and radioactivity
chromatographic patterns.   TR.:   blood transfusion.

The newly synthesized radioactive molecules present in
thalassemic reticulocytes after lectine agglutation, and migrating
with the peak of cold β-globin on CM cellulose chromatography,
have been characterized by the fingerprinting technique and shown
to be newly synthesized β-globin molecules. These data suggest
that the inducing molecule may be able to turn on β-globin synthesis not only *in vitro*, but also *in vivo*, after crossing the
red cell walls of thalassemic erythroid cells.

A Model for Ferrara β-Thalassemia

In conclusion, on the basis of these findings, we propose
that Ferrara β-thalassemia is due to a mutation affecting a gene
for a previously unrecognized protein factor, specifically involved
in β-globin mRNA translation. From available data (18-21) it is
possible to hypothesize that the action of this specific protein
is in the formation of the β-globin initiating complex. This
hypothesis is in contrast with several findings that the translation of purified mRNA, including rabbit globin mRNA, is not
specific, and can be obtained in heterologous systems (22-31).
In this regard, it may be emphasized that our system does not
require the isolation of β-globin mRNA, and β-globin synthesis
is induced on untreated ribosomal material. On the contrary, for
the exogenous translation, mRNA is purified as 9S RNA, through
procedures that could cause conformational alterations and possibly
loss of specificity of the genetic message.

Wherever the site of action of the molecule lacking in
Ferrara β-thalassemia may be, its demonstration is of importance
in that it proposes the existence in mammals of factors specifically controlling the translation of certain mRNAs. The same type
of alteration shown in the Ferrara β-thalassemia may conceivably
be the basis of other human hereditary diseases.

REFERENCES

1. BARGELLESI, A., PONTREMOLI, S. AND CONCONI, F; 1967, *Europ. J.
       Biochem. 1*, 73.
2. CONCONI, F., BARGELLESI, A., PONTREMOLI, S., VIGI, V., VOLPATO,
       S. & GABURRO, D; 1968, *Nature 217*, 259.
3. CLEGG, J.B., NAUGHTON, M.A. & WEATHERALL, D.J; 1965, *Nature
       207*, 945.
4. BARGELLESI, A., PONTREMOLI, S., MENINI, C. & CONCONI, F.: 1968,
       Europ. J. Biochem. 3, 364.
5. VIGI, V., VOLPATO, S., GABURRO, D., CONCONI, F., BARGELLESI, A.
       & PONTREMOLI, S.: 1969, *British J. Haematol. 16*, 25.

6. BANK, A., BRAVERMAN, A., O'DONNEL, J. V. & MARKS, P. A.; 1968, *Blood 31*, 226.
7. WILLIAMNSON, R., DREWIENKIEWICZ, C., & PAUL, J.; 1973, *Nature New Biol. 241*, 66.
8. DREYFUS, J. C., LABIE, D., VIBERT, M. & CONCONI, F.; 1972, *Europ. J. Biochem. 27*, 291.
9. CONCONI, F., ROWLEY, P. T. del SENNO, L., PONTREMOLI, S. & VOLPATO, S.; 1972, *Nature New Biol. 238*, 83.
10. Del SENNO, L., BUZZONI, D. & CONCONI, F. To be published.
11. REVEL, M., AVIV, H. (Greenshpan), GRONER, Y., POLLACK, Y.; 1970, *FEBS Letters 9*, 213.
12. POLLACK, Y., GRONER, Y., AVIV, H. (Greenshpan), & REVEL, M.: 1970, *FEBS Letters 9*, 218.
13. HEYWOOD, S. M.; 1970, *Proc. U. S. Nat. Acad. Sci. 67*, 1782.
14. LEE-HUANG, S., & OCHOA, S.: 1971, *Nature New Biol. 234*, 236.
15. CONCONI, F., del SENNO, L., MENINI, C. & VULLO, C. To be published.
16. ALLEN, D. D., SCHROEDER, W. A. & BALOG, G.: 1958, *J. Amer. Chem. Soc. 80*, 1628.
17. RACE, R. R. & SANGER, R. in "Blood Groups in Man". Blackwell Scientific Publications, Oxford, England, 1962.
18. HUNT, T., HUNTER, R. & MUNRO, A.: 1968, *J. Mol. Biol. 36*, 31.
19. LUPPIS, B., BARGELLESI, A. & CONCONI, F.; 1970, *Biochemistry 9*, 4175.
20. LEBLEU, B., NUDEL, U., FALCOFF, E., PRIVES, C. & REVEL, M.; 1972, *FEBS Letters 25*, 97.
21. NUDEL, U., LEBLEU, B., TOVA, Z. W. & REVEL, M.; 1973, *Europ. J. Biochem. 33*, 314.
22. STRAVNEZER, J. & HUANG, R.C.C.; 1971, *Nature New Biol. 230*, 172.
23. MATTHEWS, M. B., OSBORN, M. & LINGREL, J. B.; 1971, *Nature New Biol. 223*, 206.
24. HOUSMAN, D., PEMBERTON, R. & TABER, R.; 1971, *Proc. Nat. Acad. Sci., U.S.A. 68*, 2716.
25. RHOADS, R. E., McKNIGHT, G. S. & SCHIMKE, R. T.; 1971, *J. Biol. Chem. 246*, 7407.
26. MATTHEWS, M. B., OSBORN, M. BERNS, A.J.M. & BLOE-MENDAL, H.; 1972, *Nature New Biol. 236*, 5.
27. BERNS, A.J.M., STROUS & BLOE-MENDAL, H.; 1972, *Nature New Biol. 236*, 7.
28. LOCKARD, R. E. & LINGREL, J. B.; 1972, *J. Biol. Chem. 247*, 4174.
29. LANE, C. D., MARBAIX, G. & GURDON, J.B.; 1971, *J. Mol. Biol. 61*, 73.
30. PICCIANO, J. D., PRICHARD, P. M., MERRICK, W. C., SHAFRITZ, D. A., GRAF, H., CRYSTAL, R. G. & ANDERSON, W. F.; 1973, *J. Biol. Chem. 248*, 204.
31. SHREIER, M. H. & STAEHELIN, T.; 1973, *Proc. Nat. Acad. Sci. U.S.A. 70*, 462.

CONTROL OF GENE EXPRESSION IN ANIMAL CELLS: THE CASCADE REGULATION
HYPOTHESIS REVISITED

K. Scherrer

Molecular Biology Department
Swiss Institute for Experimental Cancer Research
Lausanne, Switzerland

ABBREVIATIONS

IIT : Intra-cellular information transfer; mRNA : messenger RNA; pre-mRNA : precursor to mRNA (used synonymously
with the formerly used terms, messenger-like RNA (mlRNA),
DNA-like RNA (D-RNA) and heterogeneous nuclear RNA
(HnRNA); RNP : ribonucleoprotein complex; mRNP : RNP
containing mRNA.

I.   INTRODUCTION

More than 10 years have passed since the publication of
the first comprehensive theory of gene regulation in bacteria (1).
Since that time, we have witnessed spectacular progress in studies
of the genetics and biochemistry of regulation in prokaryotes.
However the fact is often overlooked that in neither the Lac operon
nor the Lamda phage - not to speak of E.coli as a whole - has the
mechanics of regulation been revealed in sufficient detail to
enable us to really comprehend the "wiring" diagrams and all the
mechanisms of the regulatory circuits.

The interest of many molecular biologists has started
to focus on the animal cell and, in particular, on problems of
regulation and differentiation. However, knowledge and comprehension in this field are much less developed than in prokaryotes.
Some reasons for this state of affairs are evident: e.g. the considerably greater size of the eukaryotic genome and the greatly
reduced practicality of the genetic approach which was so immensely
useful in understanding bacterial regulation. In fact, the

analytical approach to regulation in animal cells was for many
years almost completely biochemically oriented.

However some other - possibly not so evident - facts made
progress difficult in the investigation of eukaryotic regulation.
Two of these reasons may be mentioned here and considered as "psychological" factors.

One was the fixation of ideas on the bacterial model. It
took a long time for the idea to develop that an axiom like
"what is valid for E.coli is also valid for the elephant", is of
limited validity and should be replaced by its corollary "the
elephant is qualitatively (and not only quantitatively) different -
although some fundamental mechanisms discovered in E.coli may still
be valid".

The second major "psychological block" could be found in a
feeling of desperation - even hybris - when facing the formidable
task of trying to investigate the flow of information and its regulation in eukaryotes. One of the fathers of molecular biology
declared ten years ago that anybody studying molecular biology in
animal cells was "either a hero - or a fool"; and it was not all
evident if he felt there was any difference between the two!

Nevertheless, at present a major effort has been invested in
the analysis of regulation in higher cells. With the idea in mind
that "to do little is better than doing nothing at all" the author
attempted several years ago with the Cascade Regulation hypothesis
(2,3) to put into a scheme at least some of the very basic facts
concerning intra-cellular information transfer (IIT) in animal
cells. It was hoped that this effort - in spite of the risk of
being basically wrong due to lack of sufficient experimental data -
would help at the same time to break the bonds of the bacterial
model and the fear of entering the field.

The moment may now have come to re-evaluate this earlier
attempt to comprehend the regulation of gene expression in animal
cells and - in case of a positive judgement - to develop the model
further in the light of present theoretical and experimental knowledge.

Starting this reevaluation by theoretical considerations,
the author will break a principle rule in scientific statement
which calls for an exposition of the experimental evidence first
and only then allows one to proceed to theoretical deductions. The
reasons for applying this inverse approach are essentially the
following.

This paper can be considered as a theoretical analysis within the framework of the general theme of this symposium "Strategies of Gene Regulation in Eukaryotes"; we will try to test if certain theoretical predictions concerning mRNA formation and its regulation are reflected in the experimentally confirmed reality. I have recently written two reviews (4,5) that report more extensively the experimental evidence serving as the basis for my reflections.

However, the main reason for the somewhat different scheme of this paper is the desire to show that many of the rather surprising findings about the biochemical mechanisms involved in the system of gene expression in eukaryotes can actually be predicted on purely formal, theoretical grounds.

2. THE CASCADE REGULATION HYPOTHESIS

Based on the pattern of RNA formation in animal cells, cytogenetic data, and theoretical considerations, the Cascade Regulation hypothesis of control of gene expression in animal cells was formulated in 1967-68 (2,3). This theory proposed a multistep model for the regulation of Intra-cellular information transfer from the gene encoded in DNA to its phenotypic expression by protein synthesis.

The process of IIT includes two clearly distinct phases (cf. Table 1): the first is messenger-linked, starts with transcription and ends with the termination of the polypeptide; the second comprises the assembly of the polypeptide into a biologically active protein and thereafter the phenotypic expression secured by this protein. To distinguish the fundamental differences with respect to regulation in these two phases of IIT we proposed to distinguish between primary (or messenger-linked) and secondary regulation (3). Although the scheme of Cascade Regulation encompasses logically both of these phases, we will restrict here our considerations essentially to primary regulation which concerns directly the formation and expression of mRNA.

TABLE 1

Regulation and Intra-Cellular Information Transfer (IIT) in Animal Cells

Flow of information from the gene to phenotypic expression →

	transcription	processing of pre-mRNA and transport	translation	phenotypic expression
Type of regulation	Primary regulation		Secondary regulation	
Level of regulation	transcriptional regulation	post-transcriptional regulation		
		intermediary	translational	post-translational
Phase of IIT	transcription	processing of pre-mRNA and transport	translation	phenotypic expression
Information carrier	nascent pre-mRNA	intermediary pre-mRNA	functional mRNA	polypeptide, protein
Biochem.form of inform. carrier	nascent pre-mRNP	transfer RNP's (Informofer-RNA and Informosome)	mRNP (Polyribosome)	protein and protein associations
Cellular compartment	Chromatin and nucleoplasm	Nucleoplasm and cytoplasm	Cytoplasm	total cell

The basic characteristics of the original scheme of Cascade Regulation included two kinds of propositions: one concerned the organisational structure of the regulation system and the other the structural organisation, the physical structure and the metabolism of the immediate transcription products. These two aspects of IIT were linked by the idea that the physical structure of the immediate transcription product and of its metabolic forms must be understood as the direct consequence of the organisational structure of the regulation system.

The principal proposition relating to regulation was, that the specificity of gene expression in animal cells is secured by a multiplicity of consecutive regulation steps ("cascade" of regulation) rather than by a single step mechanism selecting directly a specific message in the genome. Implicit in this proposition was that transcriptional regulation is only a first step of selection which can be considered to be of relatively low specificity compared to the finally selected and expressed information. Thus, transcription yields not the expressed mRNA exclusively but an RNA which contains, in addition, untranslated message as well as other types of information directing RNA processing, and finally no-sense (spacer) RNA. The regulation of the expression of the message is a post-transcriptional multistep process (Fig.1b). This model represented a close analogy to the scheme of formation of ribosomal RNA in animal cells (6,7,8).

This proposition conflicted with the then current views on regulation which were reflections of the bacterial model. In fact, prokaryotes regulate the expression of genetic information by a single step selection at the transcriptional level; the transcribed information is necessarily expressed by translation. Fig.1 reproduces the original schematic comparison of the bacterial single-step selection model with the - then purely hypothetical - eukaryotic model (3). In the former, the transcribed information potential is fully expressed by the compulsory translation of the transcribed mRNA. According to the latter, the transcribed information potential is gradually reduced to the expressed information, and final specificity is obtained only at the end of the cascade of selection.

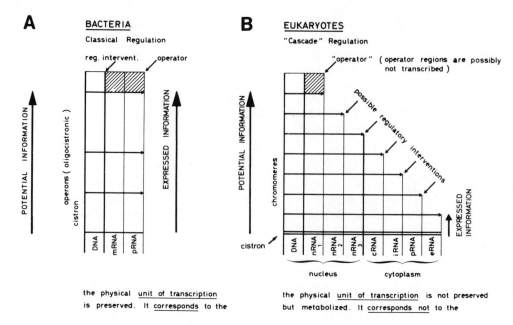

FIGURE 1 The Original Schematic Representation of the Cascade
         Regulation hypothesis: Theoretical Models of Gene
         Regulation and Expression.

Bacteria: The information of one operon is transcribed from the
DNA into one oligocistronic mRNA molecule which is in its totality
translated into the corresponding proteins. The total information of the operon is thus phenotypically expressed. The information content of the regulatory unit of the DNA within the operon
corresponds to that of the transcription product (mRNA) and to
that of the RNA being translated in the polyribosome (pRNA).
Operator regions (shadowed area) are or are not transcribed.

Eukaryotes: The information content of the units of gene transcription (corresponding to the totality or to fractions of the
DNA in the regulatory unit of transcription) is transcribed into
a polycistronic mRNA molecule which may contain one or several
cistrons (probably unrelated to each other in respect to biological function). On its way from the chromosome to the site of
translation in the polyribosome, the nascent RNA may be broken
down into oligocistronic or cistronic functional segments. Con-

comitantly or subsequently, a fraction of the originally transcribed information may be eliminated or neutralized by regulatory interventions which could interfere with the flow of information at various stages of RNA metabolism.

Such a process of "Cascade Regulation" may reduce in many
steps the information potential already transcribed to that actually expressed. The physical units of transcription and of
translation (and thus of regulation) would be different in information content and in size.

A further proposition of the Cascade Regulation hypothesis
attempted to give a rational explanation for this apparently im-
precise and wasteful multistep selection process which implied
that, at any moment of cellular life, much more RNA is synthesized
than is acted on by the translation apparatus. We pointed out that
in information processing, a multistep mechanism may be more economical than a single step process (3). In other words, the effort
required to select one specific unit out of a large number of units
of information is less if a multistep process pertains, since the
energy required for selection can be reduced by the organisation
of the system. We will discuss this in detail later.

In complicated biological systems, another equally important basic advantage of a multistep selection process is that it
allows for multiple interventions at all levels of mRNA formation
and transport. Thus, it confers on the cell more flexibility and
more subtle possibilities of control than an all-transcriptional
control system and the compulsory expression of the transcribed
mRNA.

Quite in general, we have to consider that the degree of
selectivity necessary to regulate a system such as the animal cell
(estimated selectivity 10^{-5}) is in practice not realisable by
physical means in a single step manner. The classical solution
to such problems is to put in series multiple, relatively simple
mechanisms which may be of low selectivity. In addition, these
mechanisms have to be linked by feed-back loops which allow for
adaptation of the consecutive selection steps. These considerations lead us to conceive a system of linked regulatory <u>circuits</u>

(as an example we may point to systems of high selectivity in radio technology).

A further proposition concerns the coordination of function in higher cells and organisms in eukaryotic systems, cistrons which are closely related functionally are in general not genetically linked.

Moreover, such loci as those of the two mammalian globin chains are distributed among different chromosomes. Hence, the coordination of function in animal systems cannot operate as in bacteria by the polycistronic linkage of functionally related mRNA (1). Within the frame of a multistep selection system, this fact leads to the deduction that the coordination of function must operate to a large extent by the post-transcriptional regulation of the expression of individual mRNA's.

If post-transcriptional control and coordination are accepted as a model of regulation, then we must expect that the biochemical system involved in securing such controls is linked to the message during its passage through the cascade of regulation. This recalls the view already expressed in the beginning of this section, that the structure of the transcription products, including mRNA, must be expected to be structured as a function of the regulation system.

This consideration leads us to the second set of propositions presented in the Cascade Regulation hypothesis, relating to the structure and metabolism of the initial forms of mRNA. As we have seen, the biochemical structure of the transcription products and of their metabolic forms must reflect the necessities of the multistep selection system. Thus, giant precursor molecules are produced rather than functional RNA; the organisation of the regulating mechanism which leads to this apparent waste in RNA size and excessive turnover is compensated for by the economical structure and function as well as the increased potentialities of the controlling system.

The following features of the nascent transcription products of genes, and of the functional mRNA were proposed: a) in animal cells, the majority of genes are transcribed into giant $(1-30 \times 10^6$ MW) pre-mRNA molecules, which eventually give rise to functional mRNA after passing through a complex processing scheme; b) pre-mRNA and mRNA molecules contain, in addition to coding sequences, "signal sequences", these are either the transcripts of signals in the DNA related to the control of transcription (operator sequences), or govern and regulate(and/or are directly involved in) the biochemical mechanisms of post-

transcriptional processing and transport of pre-mRNA. In addition,
there are signals involved in translation of mRNA; c) as a consequence of the organization of the chromosome in polycistronic
transcription units, which may include physically linked but
functionally unrelated mRNA sequences, "idle" messenger sequences
may be transcribed which would have no function at a given time
in a given cell. Linked in the pre-mRNA to expressed mRNA
sequences, this "idle" mRNA may be separated by processing from
the expressed mRNA and be broken down or stored for later use;
d) "signal" sequences having no further function in processing
may be destroyed; e) as a consequence of the "architectural" organization of the transcriptional unit, true no-sense sequences
with spacer or linker function exist; their break-down during
processing may also account for part of the observed turnover of
nascent pre-mRNA. All these elements are contained in the model depicted in Fig.2 which is taken from our original publication (3).

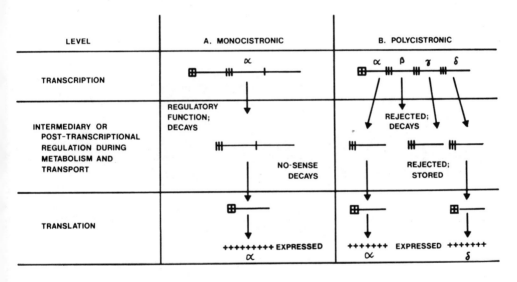

·FIGURE 2 The Original Interpretation of pre-mRNA Structure
(original, slightly abbreviated legend from ref.3). mlRNA (= pre-
mRNA) contains information for protein synthesis in cytoplasmic
polyribosomes and reaches functional state through a metabolic
process. If mlRNA (1-10 x 10⁶ MW) contains information for structural genes that correspond to polypeptides (α,β,γ,δ), two basically different arrangements can be considered.

A. Monocistronic Transcriptional Unit. The RNA molecule contains
only one cistron (α) which will be translated. The excess RNA
contains no information but may have a structural or regulatory
function prior to decay.

B. Polycistronic Transcriptional Unit. Several cistrons ($\alpha,\beta,\gamma,\delta$)
linked together in the genome, are transcribed into a single RNA
molecule. It may correspond to an operon or to several independent cistrons which become separated during metabolism. Some of
these individual cistrons reach the polyribosomes and are translated independently; some are immediately rejected and destroyed,
while others are rejected but stored at the intermediary level.
The decay of the immediately rejected cistrons accounts for part
of the observed nuclear turnover of mlRNA. The polycistronic
molecule may contain, in addition, sequences without structural
information, such as those proposed for the monocistronic unit.
(|||| signals relating to processing).

        The Cascade Regulation hypothesis was based on one key
assumption: the prediction that nascent nuclear RNA molecules
of 1- 30 x 10^6 MW contain in their covalent nucleotide chain true
messenger sequences. For many years, only indirect evidence
could be found in support of this proposition. However, recently
we could show conclusively that giant nuclear RNA from duck erythroblasts contain the globin messenger sequence (9).
Other laboratories working with different methods and systems have
come to similar conclusions (10,11).

        This demonstration and other recent results from our labo-
ratory made it possible to draw for the first time an outline of
the "life-history" from transcription to translation of a specific
eukaryotic mRNA, the duck globin mRNA. This outline is presented
in a recent paper (4). It is concerned with the pattern of mRNA
formation and the presently known biochemical steps of processing
of pre-mRNA, transport and translation.

        Here we will consider primarily problems relating to the
regulation of these processes. Reviewing general and specific
features of the regulation of gene expression in animal cells, we
will attempt to analyse critically - and bring up to date - the
Cascade Regulation hypothesis.

        Several other models of gene regulation were proposed with-
in the last few years. Within the framework of this analysis we
would like to evaluate them in relation to the Cascade model.

One such model which has been formulated by G.Georgiev (12,13) shares several essential elements with the Cascade hypothesis (giant pre-mRNA , "signal" sequences, etc.). One particular feature is a row of signal sequences (acceptor sites) relating to transcriptional regulation placed at the beginning of a transcriptional unit which has one (or several) mRNA sequences at its 3'- end. The experimentally observed rapid breakdown of part of the transcription product is accounted for exclusively by the immediate decay of the transcript of these signal sequences which are placed at the five-prime end of pre-mRNA; this metabolism would leave behind the stabilized functional mRNA(s) in its final form to be exported to the cytoplasm. Essentially the same proposition as that of Georgiev is contained in the chromosome model of F.Crick (14) who, placing one messenger sequence at the three-prime end of pre-mRNA, explains the rest of the giant pre-mRNA molecules by the organization and transcription of the operator sequence(s) in the chromosome. Recently J.Paul (15) proposed that the giant size and break-down of pre-mRNA were due to degenerate but physically conserved mRNA sequences. R. Britten and E. Davidson (16) describe their model in terms of an integrating multi-key system (cf p.185)of transcriptional regulation as applied specifically to the animal cell systems.

All these models share one feature, namely, that the control of gene expression and, therefore, the regulation of messenger formation, operates at the transcriptional level exclusively: in this they are closely related to the Jacob-Monod model (1) of pro-karyotic gene regulation. In contrast, one of the essential propositions of the Cascade Regulation hypothesis was that, although transcriptional regulation is essential as a first step of control, a large part of the regulation of IIT in animal cells (including the process of differentiation) is regulated at post-transcriptional levels. In this respect the model of a post-transcriptional regulation loop as proposed by G.Tomkins shares the same view (17).

From a biochemical viewpoint, it should be kept in mind that a living cell cannot be compared to a machine in the sense that a machine is a stringent and absolute integration of unique mechanisms. All biochemical processes observed represent the integration of statistical probabilities around possible outcomes for a given reaction mechanism. Hence, no rigid machine-like structure of the mechanisms of regulation should be considered. In a rigid system, the potential barriers encountered by evolu-tive pressure would be too high to allow smooth adaptation. However, many cases are known in nature where organisms adapt rapidly even to moderate selective pressure. (Even molecules may adapt in vitro as shown recently by Spiegelman's group (18).

We must expect the expression of this fundamental condition
in the structure of biological molecules and in biochemical
mechanisms.

2. THEORETICAL REQUIREMENTS OF A SYSTEM OF GENE REGULATION IN ANIMAL CELLS

The Necessity for Peripheral Memories

The qualitative difference between the organisational
structure (in the structuralistic sense) of the regulation systems
in prokaryotes and eukaryotes may be best summarized by the statement that we deal in the former with a "point" system of control
whereas in the latter we are confronted with a "multi-dimensional"
system (Fig.3)

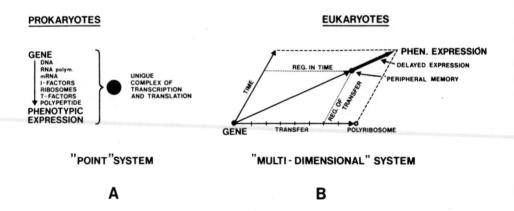

PROKARYOTES   EUKARYOTES

"POINT"SYSTEM   "MULTI - DIMENSIONAL" SYSTEM

A   B

FIGURE 3 The Organisational Structure of Intra-cellular Information Transfer in Bacterial and Animal Cells

A. Bacteria. The transcription-translation complex includes all
elements necessary for the information transfer from the DNA to
the finished polypeptides. The stringent coupling of the physical and biochemical entities involved in IIT leads to the

compulsory synthesis of a polypeptide once the synthesis of its
mRNA is induced. To a first approximation, we may say that no vectors exist, neither in space nor in time, that would delay or
disrupt the flow of information. Hence this system is "unidi-
mensional"; in other terms, it represents a "point" system.

B. Eukaryotic cells. The sites of transcription and translation
are separated in space. Hence, a vector in space results, along
which the information is transported from the DNA in the nucleus
to the polyribosome in the cytoplasm (and finally to the phenotypic expression of the genetic information). This vector crea-
tes instantly a second vector in time. Hence, the point system
is disrupted and the expression of the genetic information is the
resultant of the two vectors in space and time. Both these vectors can be cut short by one of the multiple mechanisms that control the formation, transport and translation of mRNA as well as
its temporal expression. This regulation of physical transfer
and temporal expression leads to the formation of peripheral memories from which the information can be drawn, and be expressed
rapidly upon a signal controlling the post-transcriptional steps
of regulation.

If we draw a schematic representation of a bacterial operon in
function, we can localize within one complex structure of linked
elements all features regulating transcription and translation.
In fact, the transcription-translation complex in bacteria comprises the DNA-genome, inactivated repressor, RNA polymerase,
messenger RNA, ribosomes with initiation and translation factors,
activated tRNA, and the growing and finally the complete polypeptide chain.

All biochemical mechanisms involved in the phenotypic expression
of a gene by the synthesis of specific proteins are encompassed
in this transcription-translation complex; organisationally, it
has no dimension and, hence, represents a "point" system. As a
consequence, gene activation and expression are rigidly coupled;
the activation of an operon leads necessarily to the phenotypic
expression of its information. Hence, from the point of view of
regulation also, it represents a "point" system. As a consequence
of these two statements, we may conclude that it represents a
"point" system also in time. Although there is necessarily a
delay between the induction of the operon and the termination of
the polypeptide chain, this time-lag is short and, to a first
approximation, constant. The transcription-translation complex
also allows for the possibility of direct feed-back effects;
events interfering with translation may influence the further
transcription of the DNA.

Thus, in such a system, the unit of genetic regulation (operon) equals the unit of transcription (DNA in operon) and the unit of translation (polycistronic mRNA). The structuralistic characterization of such a regulation system derives from the physical structure of the transcription-translation complex (Fig.3a).

In eukaryotic cells, such a system is impossible. As shown diagramatically in Fig.3b, the transport of the information carrier from the central memory, the DNA-genome, to the translation complex in the cytoplasm, introduces necessarily a time delay in the expression of the genomic information. Breaking up the point system in space, the regulative- and the time-coupling are immediately destroyed. Thus a time-dimension enters the structure of the regulational system.

The transport of mRNA through the cell necessitates the participation of a multitude of biochemical mechanisms involved in stabilization of RNA, of pre-mRNA processing, transfer to the nuclear membrane, association (or not) with the endoplasmic reticulum and finally the formation of the translation complex. Since all these processes must be regulated, the possibility arises of interrupting the information transfer at many instances throughout this process, leading necessarily to a corresponding time delay in the phenotypic expression of the gene. Thus, regulation of transport implies regulation in time.

The pools of pre-mRNA or mRNA held back during their transport would constitute what I have designated-in analogy to a term in computer terminology - a peripheral memory (Fig.3b)

As an example of such a situation, we may recall the mRNA stored in the mature egg awaiting during days, or months the moment of fertilization. This stored mRNA represents such a peripheral memory. Quite generally, the temporal regulation of gene expression necessary for all differentiating organisms may operate post-transcriptionally as well as at the level of transcription and, thus, involve such peripheral memories.

Having shown the theoretical possibility of peripheral memories and having given an example of their real existence in the animal cell, it may be interesting to discuss two basically different formal reasons for their existence.

The first relates to the requirements of efficiency and versatility of regulation in a multi-cell (or multi-organ) system which must adapt locally and rapidly to changes in physio-

logical or functional state. We may recall, as a contrast, the
well-known phenomenon of diauxic growth of E.coli (19); here, the
bacterial regulation system has to retrieve new information from
the central genetic memory in order to adapt to new growth requirements. It takes a bacterial population about 20 minutes to adapt
its enzyme systems to a new substrate. Such a time-lag would be
ruinous to a higher organism. For instance, had the human organism to retrieve new information from its genome in order to
switch from carbohydrate to protein digestion, a considerable
time-lag would result (which would take all the fun out of eating
and living!) The structures of the regulational systems of the
organism adapted to this by storing the genetic information for
the corresponding proteases at the very periphery (i.e. in the form
of trypsinogen or chymotrypsinogen), allowing the expression of
the genetic information upon a signal from the environment.
Similarly, it will be more efficient to activate an mRNA already
present in the cytoplasm than to produce a new message through
transcription and the whole assembly line of processing. Thus, in
the formal consideration of optimal function, there is an advantage to storing genetic information in peripheral memories rather
than having to call always upon the central memory.

The second theoretical requirement for the existence of
peripheral memories relates to the possibility that the export to
and the storage of genetic information in peripheral memories
represents an essential mechanism of the processes of development and differentiation. In fact, the passage of the genomic information from one cell generation to the other, and - more important - from one generation to the next, in sexually reproducing
systems, - necessitates the peripheral storage of information.
This requirement stems from the formal impossibility for a transcriptional unit in the genome to activate itself. DNA by itself
is silent; that part of the genetic information which contains the
program to retrieve information from the DNA in the daughter cell,
or in the next generation, must be stored peripherally in the
environment into which the newly made DNA will be placed. (One
can imagine the possibility that between generations most of the
information in the genome may be stored peripherally as well as
in the DNA). Thus, two systems of information transfer between
generations can be postulated as depicted in the schematic representation of Fig.4. Furthermore, we are led to the interesting
theoretical deduction that the programming of the expression of
the genetic information in the next generation, at least during
the initial phases of embryonic development, is reserved to the
maternal genome, the sperm adding essentially "silent" DNA. In
fact, the phenomenon of parthenogenesis shows that the male DNA
may not even be necessary at all for normal development.

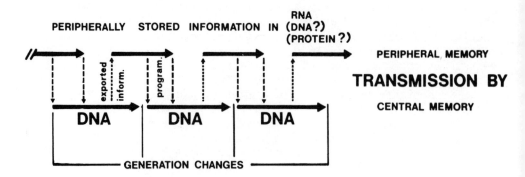

FIGURE 4   Transfer of Genetic Information between Generations
            of Cells and Organisms.

        The genetic information is transferred from one genera-
tion to the other by the replication of DNA. However the DNA by
itself is silent; thus, a program is necessary to call upon the
genetic information by activation of specific DNA segments which
are stored in peripheral memories. These may be localized in
the nucleoplasm or cytoplasm of the daughter cell, or of the
mature oocyte in sexually reproducing systems into which the DNA
of the central genetic memory will be placed in the next generation or during development. Thus, in addition to DNA, a second
system of information transfer between generations exists in the
form of peripheral memories which bridge the "generation gap".

        Extrapolating from present day experimental knowledge, one
may assume that this second system of inheritance is carried by
RNA (20,21). Peripheral memories in the form of stored mRNA may
be situated at every step of the biochemical processing of pre-
mRNA into mRNA. However, it is by no means excluded that part of
this peripherally stored programming or structural information
may exist also in the form of DNA or protein.

        Concluding this section, we may postulate that peripheral
memories are theoretically necessary for the regulation mechanisms
of the eukaryotic cell. They add to the efficiency and versatility of the control system and permit the regulation and temporal
expression of genes. The existence of such peripheral memories
has been experimentally demonstrated in several cases.

Programming Sequences in Pre-mRNA and mRNA, a Consequence of an
Integrating Multi-key System of Control

    In the original definition of the Cascade Regulation hypo-
thesis, we pointed out the importance of a multi-step control
system for the regulation of gene expression in highly developed
organisms. The Cascade model of multi-step regulation combines
two fundamental requirements of control: 1) the necessity of a
multi-key * system of control capable of handling economically
the high number of units of information in the animal genome;
2) an integrator function necessary to coordinate the simultaneous
expression of functionally related but physically non-continuous
genes.

    Both requirements may lead to the same biochemical pheno-
menon: the excessive synthesis of coding and non-coding RNA as a
result of a) the transcription of operator sequences in the DNA
relating to transcriptional regulation, b) the synthesis of
programming sequences containing signals for the post-transcriptional formation of mRNA from pre-mRNA and the regulation of this
processing as well as of translation, and c) the idle transcription of untranslated coding[xx] (messenger) sequences combined in
transcriptional units with translated but functionally unrelated
mRNA.

* A Multi-key System may be exemplified by a system of locks
which can be opened only by a combination of k keys out of a
total of n. Thus a given key - but in different combinations -
would be used to open many doors. As a further possibility,
the system may call for a given sequence in the turning of the
individual keys of a given combination, allowing different per-
mutations to open different locks. To such systems the laws of
variation apply, hence n^k locks can be handled by n keys in sets
of k.

** Since eukaryotic mRNA has been found to contain non-coding
sequences as poly(A) of repetitive sequences, we have to distinguish between the mRNA as a whole and its actually translated
fraction. Throughout this paper we will call the latter the
coding sequence of mRNA.

The production of all this excessive RNA would be related
to the organization and, hence, to the economy of the regulational
system per se. It is an expression of the low specificity of the
initial selection steps, leading to the transcription not only of
temporarily unused RNA, but also of RNA securing the programming
of processing and final selection. The energy loss involved in the
synthesis of this RNA with only transient or no actual function
at all is compensated for by the economy realized through an efficient organization of the regulational system.

The essential feature of a multi-key system of control is
its potential to govern in an economical way a multiplicity of
units of information. Applied to the regulation of gene expression, such a system theoretically allows the control of a very
high number of signals in the DNA or RNA, each one recognized by
a specific repressor or activator.

A multi-step selection process, as proposed in the Cascade Regulation hypothesis, can be considered analogous to a
multi-key control system in which the keys would be turned conse-
cutively. As shown in fig.5, the energy required to select one
unit of information out of 10^5 units, can be dramatically reduced if the direct, single step selection of one in 10^5 is replaced by five successive selection steps of one in ten. The turning of a single key of a given set amounts to one step of selection in the multistep system. Necessarily, a single key or selection step confers little specificity initially. Selectivity
can only be obtained by the operation of all keys of a given set,
or by passing through the entire cascade of selection.

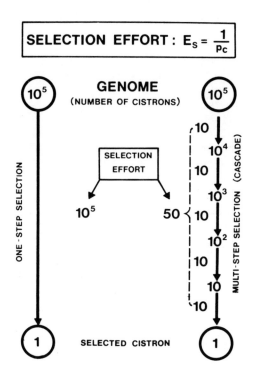

FIGURE 5 <u>The Energy Required for the Selection of Information.</u>

According to an earlier proposition (3), the energy required to select one unit of information, i.e. the selection
effort $\underline{E}$, is by definition inversely proportional to the probability of finding a given unit of information by chance (P_c). Hence,
to find one unit of information among 10^5 ($P_c = 10^{-5}$) an effort
of 10^5 is necessary. If the system is organised in a manner
allowing the selection of this information by a stepwise process,
involving consecutive choices of 1 in 10 ($E = 10$), the total selection effort is reduced to 50. This is an expression of the
fact that part of the selection energy is fixed potentially by
the organisation of the system and may be drawn upon at any
instant. Hence, the additional energy necessary for an individual
operation of selection is considerably reduced (cf ref.3).

Simple multi-key selection systems are intrinsic to the models proposed by Georgiev (12) Britten & Davidson (16) and by Crick (14). Considering biochemical mechanisms, it is evident that in such systems the activation of a specific messenger sequence results also - assuming negative control - in excessive RNA production by the transcription of the operator sequences containing the signals of the multi-key system.

These models suggest all-transcriptional systems of regulation. However, we discussed in the preceding section the possible existence of peripheral memories which would give the opportunity for post-transcriptional regulation. Therefore, we have to postulate that the multi-key system operates according to a multi-step version in which the keys of a given set are turned in a specific sequence. Hence, the mechanism of the multi-key system has to be linked to the messenger sequence in what we may characterize as a programming sequence, and be transported with it to the peripheral memories and to the translation system. The selection of a specific message could then be realized at a relatively late stage of transport, after processing and intermediate storage of the message. As a consequence, we should observe at the level of transcription a rather non-specific activation of genes, resulting possibly in the production of pre-mRNA with messenger sequences that will not necessarily be expressed at a given time in a given cell ("idle" mRNA). Parts of each pre-mRNA molecule would contain signal recognition sites relating to the mechanism of consecutive selection and constituting the programming sequences. With each successive selection step part of these sequences are rendered useless and may be disposed of by degradation to mononucleotides.

The integrator function of the regulational system in eukaryotes is necessary to coordinate the function of many polypeptides which compound a given biochemical mechanism or pathway. It is clear that coordination is required over the whole range of cellular protein synthesis, from the relatively simple case of hemoglobin as a multi-peptide protein, to complicated metabolic chains involving more than ten enzymes (e.g. the citric acid cycle). The most simple biochemical realization of such an integration of function is the polycistronic messenger occuring in bacterial operons (1). However, in animal cells, the operon, corresponding to a single unit of transcription and translation as a regulative unit (polycistronic mRNA) is unknown. In fact, such closely related polypeptides as alpha and beta chains of human hemoglobin are widely separated in the genome (22,23).

The physical separation of genetically related cistrons in the eukaryotic chromosome may be attributed simply to random evolutionary divergence. However, considering cellular economy, the separations of individual cistrons became of selective advantage from the moment that a given polypeptide chain was shared by more than one functional protein (e.g. hemoglobin of types $\alpha_2\beta_2$, $\alpha_2\gamma_2$, α_2, δ_2). Thus a selective pressure must have developed to separate physically functionally related genes and, hence, destroy the "classical" operon. As a consequence, other means of biochemical control must have evolved to achieve the coordination of gene function.

In their extensive analysis, Britten and Davidson (16) discuss the formal requirements of a multi-key integrating system restricted, however, to transcriptional control. Although many elements of this model may still have to pass experimental screening, their formal considerations are valid for any system of control. The cascade regulation principle may introduce additional potentialities to such a relatively simple multi-key integrating system. The basic problem, however, is the same, i.e. the integration of signals into programs which govern in a sequential pattern a given number of coordinate functions.

It may be premature to speculate about the biochemical nature of the active signals. However, in view of the consideration already discussed, it is evident that the passive receptors of these signals must be part of the DNA, of pre-mRNA and mRNA. The organization of signals and their receptors according to the requirements of a multi-key system raises the question of the existence of a distinct programming code.

In fact, the very concept of a multi-key system implies the existence of a number of distinct "keys" or signals. For example, in the genetic code, 4 signals exist which provide organized in sets of 3, 64 possible programs (under the restrictions imposed by base pairing). By analogy, as little as 7 distinct signals organized in sets of 6 (this is a possible figure for the number of selection steps in IIT) could provide specific selection for the $\sim 10^7$ cistrons that can be expected to exist in an animal genome. Although the signals in the programming of IIT are necessarily more elaborate than those of the genetic code (having to recognize nucleotide sequences or a resulting secondary or tertiary structure of the nucleic acid) a certain probability exists that through evolution and selection, at least some of these signals became genetically fixed and common to many branches of the tree of evolution. Thus a program could be composed by a set of more or less universal signal-sequences which would be present many times in the genome but in various combinations.

Summarizing, we may postulate that the messenger sequence has to be physically linked to a programming sequence which contains recognition sites for signals relating to the stepwise selection of a given piece of information. The organization of these signal sites obeys the requirements of a multi-key, multi-step selection system and of an integrative function relating to the coordination of the synthesis of functionally related polypeptides. These programs may be written in a more or less universal, more or less degenerate, specific programming code.

Necessity for a communication system between the information carriers and their environment

As already pointed out, a nucleic acid per se is silent. Only by receiving signals from, and interacting with, the intracellular environment, can it deliver its information and prime in turn the definition of this environment. To do this according to a program, this interaction must be highly specific and subject to regulative modulation. This latter requirement is of particular importance since it is known that the living cell responds very rapidly to environmental changes and to a wide spectrum of chemical substances. Thus, a rather elaborate communication system, relating signals of many kinds, must exist between the nucleic acid and its cellular environment.

The Cascade principle implies that this communication system must accompany the messenger-linked program through all stages of IIT, from the genome to the peripheral memories and the translation machinery.

In view of the bacterial repressor-DNA interaction, it is a simple extrapolation to expect proteins to act as signal-carriers within such a system. Also quite general biochemical considerations lead to the conclusion that, even if nucleic acids satisfy the requirements of selective specificity (and of stability), they are rather poorly suited to act as communication signals from the milieu. Our knowledge concerning the possible biochemical nature of such signals, which can be of macromolecular, ionic, steric or chemical nature, leave as the most likely candidates the proteins, which combine all the required properties with their variable but characteristic intrinsic biochemical stability.

Thus, the theoretical requirement for the existence of a system of communication between the information carriers and their environment leads to the conclusion that at least some of the signals for the programming of gene expression must be transmitted by the proteins. Thus, under the conditions of Cascade Regulation, the mRNA should be expected to be associated during

its whole life time with specific proteins. As we will see, this
is indeed the case.

The necessity for retroactive c ontrol loops

A further requirement of any system regulating gene expression is the necessity that somehow the central memory has to be
informed of the situation at the periphery, in order to be able to
react and to adapt to changing metabolic or physiological conditions.

Feed-back mechanisms of control are well known in prokaryotic cells, where, in view of the close coupling of transcription
and translation in the DNA-mRNA-ribosome complex, any interference
with peptide synthesis can have a direct biochemical effect on the
movement of the RNA polymerase. However, the biochemical formulation of such feed-back mechanisms is much more difficult in the
case of the eukaryotic cell. Again this difficulty resides in
the physical separation in space (and, hence, in time) of the sites
of translation from the chromosome, the central genetic memory.
Under the conditions of cascade regulation, at any time of its
transfer through the animal cell the mRNA must be able to receive
signals which relate to the expression of its message and direct
its further progress. Somehow, a retroactive regulative loop has
to include not only phenotypic expression and genetic information
(direct retroaction of product or substrate levels on the activity
of the chromatin) but also must be able to control the peripheral
memories, the mRNA during its transfer (Fig.6).

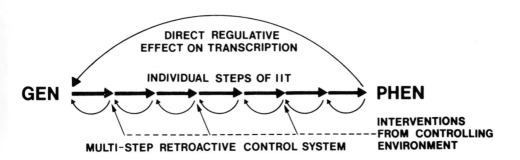

FIGURE 6 Possible Schemes of Retroactive Control.   Assuming a
multistep regulation of IIT, there are two basically different
possible schemes for influencing the flow of information by feed-
back control: 1) the direct arrest of transcription by signals

from the periphery (product or substrate levels, hormones,etc);
2) a multistep feed back mechanism bearing on the individual phases of IIT, i.e. the biochemical equilibria governing the individual reactions of processing, transport and translation, and
the respective pool sizes of intermediates and products. In this
manner a feed back effect from the very periphery could "climb
back up" the cascade of individual regulative steps. Furthermore, regulative effects from the intra-cellular environment may
induce at intermediate level such a chain of feed back reactions
which ultimately reach the level of transcription. (As an example
of such an individual peripheral feed back effect, we may mention
the direct regulative effect of the intra-cellular concentration
of a given polypeptide on its messenger's translation.

        Such a system of multiple linked regulation circuits is
in accordance with the theoretical requirements of a highly selective control system.

        In addition, there must exist a dynamic equilibrium bet-
ween the consecutive pools of pre-mRNA and mRNA. That is,a retroaction of control through all the steps of the Cascade must be
envisaged, which ultimately may also influence regulation at the
transcriptional level. The easiest biochemical formulation of a
retroactive controlling mechanism involves the individual reaction equilibria regulating each step of processing, transport or
activation/inactivation. Thus, a feed-back signal could "climb
back up" the Cascade.

        At the very end of the Cascade, a direct product-mRNA
interaction could take place; such a case has been reported recently, in which it has been shown that immunoglobulins can form a
complex with their mRNA (24). However, also more elaborate models
of retroactive control circuits have to be considered. As an
example, we may recall the system proposed by G.Tomkins (17) for
the regulation of the hepatic enzyme, tyrosin aminotransferase.

3. THE PATTERN OF MESSENGER RNA FORMATION IN ANIMAL CELLS IN
    RELATION TO THE CASCADE REGULATION HYPOTHESIS

        We will now discuss the experimentally derived pattern of

transcription, processing of pre-mRNA, transport and translation
of messenger RNA, keeping in mind our theoretically formulated
requirements for a control system regulating gene expression in
animal cells. No attempts are made here to give a complete picture
of messenger RNA formation; we have treated this topic more fully
in two other current reviews (4,5). Only those elements which
seem necessary for the critical evaluation of some aspects of the
Cascade Regulation hypothesis are dealt with here.

Transcriptional Units and their Products; Transcriptional Control

Two of the predictions of the Cascade Regulation hypothesis
concerning transcription are of particular importance: one concerns the subdivision of the genome into transcriptional units
(containing one or several cistrons) and the second relates to
the seeming randomness of the transcription products, i.e. the
low specificity of transcriptional control as compared to the specific functional requirements of a given cell.

Three principal definitions of a transcriptional unit in
animal cells exist. The first concerns the morphological units
of activity in giant dipteran chromosomes. The chromosomal bands
(chromomeres) develop into "puffs" upon a "signal" (e.g. the
hormone Ecdyson) and produce RNA in an orderly sequence (as originally shown by uridine incorporation and autoradiography).
Hence, these morphological units correspond to units of transcriptional regulation. The second, a genetic definition of this observed chromosomal transcription unit, relates to the fact that
specific phenotypic characters can be attributed to the individual
chromosome bands. An extensive genetic analysis showed that these
bands correspond to units of genetic complementation (25,26).
Thus we can consider that the unit of transcription, the unit of
regulation and the unit of genetic complementation are identical.

The third definition of the transcriptional unit is given
by the properties - in particular, the size - of its product, the
nascent pre-mRNA (9). The observation that the non-ribosomal
transcription products consist of RNA molecules of $1-20 \times 10^6$ MW
(18, 27, 28, 29) - as confirmed by electron microscopy (30) -
led us to estimate the amount of DNA in the transcriptional unit
as being of the order of 50,000 base pairs. This amount of DNA
is of the same order of magnitude as that present in a band of
the giant dipteran chromosomes (dividing the haploid DNA contents
of the organism by the number of bands). Hence, we concluded that
the giant nascent RNA represented the full transcript of the DNA
in a puff, and that the apparent heterogeneity of pre-mRNA in
animal cells can be attributed to the joining of the nascent products of many units of transcription. This idea was confirmed

recently by Daneholt's group (31) who extracted the nascent RNA
from a single chromosome puff of Chironomus by micro-manipulation.
They found, as the exclusive transcription product, a homogeneous
giant RNA with (in the case of Balbiani Ring 2 RNA) a sedimentation constant of 75S and, hence, a MW of about 7x 10^7.

That messenger RNA must be contained in such a gene-speci-
fic transcript was originally inferred from the fact that the
transcriptional units in giant chromosomes could be genetically
mapped and, thus, necessarily contained phenotypically expressed
genetic information. However, the direct demonstration of a messenger RNA sequence in giant nascent pre-mRNA was only recently .
made by Imaizumi et al. (9) in the case of the pre-mRNA for duck
globin mRNA.

This result confirmed what had seemed originally a rather
unlikely suggestion: that messenger RNA was transcribed as an integral part of a precursor molecule of almost 100 times its size.
In view of the theoretical considerations developed above, this
may not be so paradoxical any more. However, one essential question remains unanswered at the present time: it is not known if
several messenger sequences-identical or unrelated - exist within
such a transcription unit. In other words, the fraction of coding
(messenger) sequence in this giant RNA is totally unknown.

The linkage of identical messenger sequences to a giant
precursor within the globin transcriptional unit is ruled out
a priori, since the genome seems to contain only one gene per globin chain. This conclusion can be drawn from the existence of
point mutations in animal globins (22) as well as from the recent
findings of Bishop and Rosbash (32), who determined the number of
globin genes in duck and other animal DNA and found, as a rule,
one sequence per globin chain.

At present it is impossible to prove or disprove the linkage of several unrelated messenger sequences in one transcriptional unit. The only argument that can be made in this respect
relates to the relatively small total number of bands, and, hence,
of genes which can be observed in dipteran chromosomes (2,000-
5,000 bands). Since I would consider unlikely the notion that an
entire organism could be compounded from only 2-5,000 polypeptides,
I tend to stress the polycistronic nature of the transcriptional
unit, and of pre-mRNA. However the definitive resolution of this
problem needs further biochemical and genetical experimentation.

The genetic approach may supply quite rapidly new answers
concerning this question; as already mentioned, the genetic analysis of Drosophila led to the conclusion that chromosome bands
correspond to the genetic complementation groups. However, some

recent observations can be interpreted as pointing to intra-band complementation and, hence, the existence of several individual cistrons within the transcriptional unit (Judd, pers.comm.1973). The linkage of human β and δ hemoglobin chains may also be interpreted in this manner. (33).

The low specificity of transcriptional control is a further prediction of the Cascade Regulation hypothesis. Several experimental approaches have led to the conclusion that, in all animal cells examined so far, between 5-10% of the DNA is transcribed; this corresponds to 10-20% of the genome (McCarthy, this volume). This relatively high figure was particularly striking in such cells as the avian erythroblasts (3) which devote 80-90% of their protein synthesis to the production of hemoglobin, and where the polyribosomal messenger population consists of 40-50% 9S globin mRNA (28,29,34).

Although part of the excess RNA transcribed may correspond to no-sense and programming sequences, or to the transcript of the operator sequences in the DNA relating to transcriptional control, the large fraction of activated DNA in highly specialized cells leads to the quite stringent conclusion that untranslated ("idle") mRNA must be transcribed.

High C_ot hybridization experiments showed that the nuclear pre-mRNA from HeLa cells is complementary to ten times more DNA than the cytoplasmic mRNA population (35). Low C_ot competition/hybridization experiments gave similar results (3, 36, 37, 38).

It is difficult to compensate in such experiments for the participation of repetitive and unique (messenger) sequences and, hence, to know if the reduction of the spectrum of RNA in the cytoplasm, relative to the nucleus, concerns messenger sequences as well as repetitive RNA. However, considering the vast excess of unique sequences in animal cell DNA and the interspersion of repetitive and unique sequences (37), we are led to conclude that repetitive sequences in pre-mRNA must be linked to structural genes and that the above related experiments involved mRNA as well as repetitive sequences. Thus, the suggestion seems justified that the relatively large fraction of transcribed DNA in highly specialized cells includes messenger sequences which are actually not translated.

Recent experiments appear to confirm this concept. In duck erythroblasts, 10% of the genome (8 x 10^{11} MW DNA) is transcribed, representing 8 x 10^{10} MW of double stranded DNA or 4 x 10^{10} MW RNA equivalent. Hence, the 6 x 10^5 MW of the 3 adult

globin mRNA sequences would represent a fraction of 1.5×10^{-5} of
the transcribed DNA. The fraction of globin messenger sequences in
nascent pre-mRNA ($1-3 \times 10^{-4}$) is only about ten times higher (9).
Hence, taking into account the rapid turnover rate of nascent pre-
mRNA, we find the expected amount of globin mRNA among the total
transcribed RNA. We are led to conclude that the same proportion
of messenger sequences must be represented in the non-globin pre-
mRNA. Thus, about $10^3 - 10^4$ messenger types are transcribed in
this highly specialized cell, which translates at best several
hundred of them.

An even better demonstration that genes can be transcribed
in the absence of subsequent translation is found given in erythroid
cells that do not synthesize hemoglobin at all. Avian erythroblas-
tosis virus "transformed" erythroblast-like cells originating in
the peripheral blood of infected animals can be grown in tissue
culture. These cells, incapable of either normal or inducible
(in contrast to the Friend system; c.f. ref. 40) globin synthesis,
contain in their nuclear RNA the same proportion of globin messenger
sequences as the nascent pre-mRNA in the normal erythroblast
(Therwath, A. & Scherrer, K., unpubl). This system represents,
thus, the clear cut case of a cell in which a specific gene is
transcribed but its expression is suppressed at an early post-
transcriptional level.

A recent paper concerning the newt oocyte (41) provides a
perfect example combining three of the principles we are discussing:
the subdivision of the genome in transcriptional units, the low
specificity of transcriptional control, and the storage of information in peripheral memories. During the lampbrush state of oocyte maturation a large fraction - if not all - of the genome is
transcribed on thousands of lampbrush chromosome loops which, by
regulative and genetic criteria, represent transcriptional units.
The products of transcription constitute giant pre-mRNA molecules
of more than 5×10^6 MW which accumulate predominantly in the
nucleoplasm but also directly on the lampbrush loops (rendering
them visible in the light microscope). Since it is unlikely that
in this cell all this transcribed information is also translated,
and since an actual storage in the nucleus of pre-mRNA in the form
of RNP-particles can be observed, this situation represents the
example of an early peripheral memory still containing a major
fraction of the genetic information. Thus, the transcriptional
unit produces in this case, with little regulative selection at
the transcriptional level, a pre-mRNA which remains stored for
some time. This situation represents a perfect illustration of
the first steps of control within the framework of the Cascade
Regulation scheme (Fig.1b).

Concluding this section, we may consider several of the predictions of the Cascade Regulation hypothesis as being confirmed. The genome is subdivided into transcriptional units producing giant pre-mRNA. Regulation at the transcriptional level is of low specificity; genes that are not expressed in a given cell at a given time can be transcribed, but the transcription product, the pre-mRNA, may be stored or destroyed at the post-transcriptional level.

The Processing of pre-mRNA

Two outstanding properties of pre-mRNA are fundamental in considering the role of this RNA class; one relates to its size-spectrum, the other to the rapidity of its overall decay. Exponential polyacrylamide gel electrophoresis (42) allows us to estimate quite precisely the maximal MW of pre-mRNA as being approximately 5×10^7 (43). Labeled into apparent steady-state (80 min.), 30% of the pre-mRNA decays rapidly with a half-life of about 30 min; the rest is considerably more stable (44). The rapidity of this initial decay is even more striking considering the relatively long time needed to synthesize such giant molecules: it takes about 20 min to form a molecule of 5×10^7 MW (Edström,pers.comm.; c.f. also Ref.(45). Since labeling and decay times of the unstable fraction are of the same magnitude, it follows that the pool of nascent molecules must be very small.

The size pattern and the kinetics of labeling and decay evaluated by exponential polyacrylamide gel electrophoresis permit the definition of three distinct classes among the nuclear pre-mRNA (35, 43). 1) The nascent pre-mRNA, of $5-30 \times 10^6$ MW, represents the immediate transcription product. In HeLa cells and avian erythroblasts, this RNA class is rapidly labeled into steady-state (in about 80 min) and decays with a half-life of about 30 min. 2) The intermediate-size pre-mRNA consists of molecules of $1 - 5 \times 10^6$ MW. In HeLa cells it takes about 3 hours to label this class into steady-state; correspondingly, the turnover time is quite slow (half-life: 3-7 hours). 3) The small or messenger-size pre-mRNA migrates electrophoretically in the same zone as polyribosomal mRNA ($1 - 10 \times 10^5$ MW). This RNA is only slowly labeled; its decay is very slow also and, hence, difficult to measure. Its half-life must be estimated as more than 15 hours. The relative amounts of the three nuclear pre-mRNA classes in order of decreasing MW are estimated by steady-state labeling as 4: 5: 1 respectively.

Some interesting deductions are possible on considering these quantitative relations between the three pre-mRNA fractions in the light of their respective turnover. The intermediate-size pre-mRNA must accumulate, since its half-life is relatively long; its absolute amount in the nucleus (as estimated by steady-state labeling) is similar, however, to that of the nascent class. It follows that the nascent pre-mRNA must represent a wider spectrum of RNA types than the intermediate size molecules. However, the labeling and decay kinetics of this latter class show that it contains also a small fraction of rapidly decaying molecules. Furthermore, hybridization shows the same saturation level as the nascent pre-mRNA (35), although the initial rate is slower.

From all these considerations, we can construct a processing model where the nascent pre-mRNA molecules are cleaved rapidly to smaller size. A fraction of these cleavage products are solubilized rapidly, leaving behind a pool of selected and stabilized intermediate-size pre-mRNA molecules. This pool represents the major concentration of messenger-containing molecules in the cell. Its spectrum is much larger qualitatively and quantitatively than that of the small nuclear pre-mRNA and of the cytoplasmic mRNA cf.previous section).

In terms of the Cascade Regulation hypothesis, we may interpret the three pre-mRNA fractions as representing three distinct steps of IIT and, hence, of regulation. This purely formal classification is independent of the detailed mechanism of processing. However, the actual biochemical mechanisms of information processing may play a role. The straightforward scheme of pre-mRNA processing given above has to be taken with a grain of salt; the cell may still hide major surprises in regard to mRNA formation. Therefore we have to present a word of caution.

Although there is no doubt - at least in the case of duck globin mRNA - that the three classes of pre-mRNA represent informational precursors of functional mRNA there is at present no stringent evidence that they are also the direct physical precursors. The straightforward processing model involving a simple reduction in size of the nascent pre-mRNA, and selective stabilization, excision and final regulative selection of the functional message is far from proven. This is due to the unfortunate fact that the quantitative relations between the three pre-mRNA classes - and between them and the cytoplasmic mRNA - are such that no net transfer of RNA from one compartment to the other can be stringently established, at any time of labeling and chase. The same holds true for the poly(A) sequence attached to pre-mRNA although here a stronger case has been made (46) for the relationship between the nuclear and the cytoplasmic fraction. Thus, no firm conclusions can be drawn with respect tr the direct physical precursorship of pre-mRNA; alternative schemes of processing, such as RNA/RNA replication of pre-mRNA, or reverse transcription and

re-transcription (RNA/DNA/RNA) of the initial nascent pre-mRNA
cannot be excluded at present.

In duck erythroblasts, all three classes of nuclear pre-
mRNA contain globin messenger sequences (9,43,44). However, no
accumulation of final 9S globin mRNA can be observed in the nucleus;
the electrophoretic migration properties of small size pre-mRNA is
different from that of the polyribosomal 9S mRNA (4, 43).

The pre-mRNA of intermediate size, i.e. the bulk of accumulating nuclear pre-mRNA, consists of about 1% globin messenger
sequences (9). This represents a higher percentage than that in
the nascent pre-mRNA (about 0.03%). Thus, the first processing
step, which is accompanied by the decay of about 40% of the synthesized RNA, results in a selection for one of the expressed messenger sequences. This decay can be interpreted as a destruction
(or rather non-stabilization) of programming sequences related
to transcriptional control and might be accompanied (as discussed
in the previous section) by the decay of some not-translated,
"idly" transcribed messenger sequences.

Since the nucleus contains as little as 2% of the total
cellular globin messenger sequences (Imaizumi, T., Spohr, G. and
Scherrer,K.; unpubl.results) it is difficult to estimate the true
content of small nuclear pre-mRNA since the slighest contamina-
tion of nuclei by cytoplasmic messenger RNA would completely con-
fuse such an estimation. Thus it is not now possible to decide
if, between intermediate- and small-size pre-mRNA, a further selection of the expressed mRNA sequences takes place.

We may conclude that the observed pattern of pre-mRNA
formation and decay in the nucleus is compatible with our stated
theoretical requirements for the transcription, in addition to the
translated mRNA, of (repetitive) programming sequences and untranslated messenger sequences which both decay gradually.in the
initial phases of regulative selection.

The structure of pre-mRNA

Nuclear pre-mRNA has certain structural characteristics
which should be considered in a discussion of possible regulation
mechanisms. Most important among these are oligo(A) and poly(A)
sequences. Short homopolymer sequences of adenosine can be identified in the nascent transcription product and in nuclear DNA
(28, 47, 48). Of particular interest is the post-transcriptional
addition of a long poly(A) sequence, 100-200 nucleotides long,
in nuclear pre-mRNA (cf.review by Weinberg, Ref.49). In the
experiments leading to these observations, no distinction was

made between nascent and intermediate-size pre-mRNA (50). Sedimentation properties and the kinetics of synthesis of pre-mRNA
relative to those of the poly(A)-carrying molecules lead us to
suspect that the probable targets of polyadenylation are the intermediate-size molecules rather than the nascent pre-mRNA.

In addition to oligo(A) and poly(A), the pre-mRNA contains
short oligo(U) sequences which occur about once in every intermediate-size pre-mRNA molecule (51). Furthermore, double-stranded
RNA segments about 1,000 nucleotides long are present in pre-
mRNA, which may be subdivided into series of smaller regions forming double-stranded hairpin loops.

It is evident that neither oligo(A), poly(A), nor oligo(U),
or double-stranded sequences per se, could be considered as signals
related to the specific post-transcriptional control of individual
messenger sequences. However, they may participate in such functions as the stabilization of pre-mRNA, release from the chromatin,
and transport to the nuclear membrane.

Perhaps more closely related to programming sequences in
pre-mRNA and mRNA than these quasi-universal structural features
are the rapidly hybridizing sequences observed in several laboratories. In fact, hybridization experiments with steady-state la=
beled nuclear pre-mRNA show that two distinct classes of RNA exist:
one hybridizes rapidly at low $C_o t$ and, hence, corresponds to repetitive sequences; the second represents intermediate frequency
or unique sequence RNA (35,38,52; Davidson, E.H. pers.comm).
The mRNA, however, contains little repetitive, rapidly hybridizing
RNA (35; Davidson, E.H. pers.comm). There is no a priori necessity that the hypothetical programming sequences should be transcribed from repetitive DNA. Signals that can be recognized by
control factors (proteins or nucleic acids) could as well be
superimposed on a (unique) messenger sequence or be contained in
unique programming sequences linked to mRNA. However, the very
principle of a multi-key system calls for the repetitiveness of
the individual signal. A system of unique controlling elements -
if applied on a general scale - would destroy the merits of the
multi-key system and, hence, infringe on the economy principle
(unless the product of an mRNA regulated its own synthesis by
direct interaction with its pre-mRNA or mRNA. Therefore, it
seems reasonable to consider the repetitive segments in pre-mRNA
as possible elements of a system of control.

Recent observations in Darnell's laboratory show that
the ratio of repetitive to unique sequences in pre-mRNA increases
with increasing polynucleotide length, from the three-prime end
up to a certain length of the RNA molecule; thereafter, this ratio
remains constant (Jelinek, W.; pers.comm). Interestingly enough,

this threshold length corresponds to the size of the intermediate-size pre-mRNA (1-5 x 10^6 MW). Hence, this class of pre-mRNA seems to include several unit features: one unit length of unique and repetitive sequence, one poly(U) segment, one oligo(A) and one poly(A) sequence and one large double-stranded region. Thus, the intermediate-size pre-mRNA, including a messenger and programming sequence as well as the general signals related above, may represent a subunit of the unit of transcription according to the model of Fig.7.

UNIT OF TRANSCRIPTION AND pre-mRNA

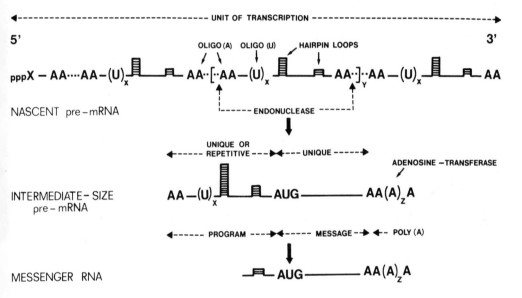

FIGURE 7   Tentative scheme of pre-mRNA Structure and Processing

According to this model, the nascent pre-mRNA contains one or several segments of intermediate-size pre-mRNA which are excised by the processing enzymes. Each intermediate-size pre-mRNA molecule may contain one (or several) mRNA sequences which are excised (or further processed by re-transcription) and transported to the cytoplasm, or are stored in the nucleus as small pre-mRNA.

The pre-mRNA is composed of messenger sequences, true no-sense segments and programming sequences. The latter contain regulative signals directing, through association with proteins,

the stabilization of pre-mRNA, and its processing and transport
to the cytoplasm, as well as its translation. Thus, the extra
nucleotide sequence observed in many mRNA's, in addition to the
coding sequence, may represent the remaining part of the programming sequences(s).

The regulative signals in pre-mRNA and mRNA may reside in
particular RNA sequences as oligo(U), oligo(A), and poly(A) or in
regions of particular secondary structure leading eventually to
the formation of hairpin loops. These regions are recognized by
specific proteins which constitute the communicating system with
the intra-cellular environment.

No-sense and programming sequences of no further use would
be solubilized and could account in part for the decay of pre-
mRNA. In addition, entire units composed of programming and
messenger sequence may be destroyed in such cases where an mRNA,
transcribed as part of a unit of transcription, is not needed in
a given cell at a given time ("idle" mRNA).

The last structural feature of pre-mRNA to be discussed
here relates to its ribonucleoprotein nature. As first observed by
Samarina et al. (53) and confirmed in many other systems, including avian erythroblasts (54), nuclear pre-mRNA is associated with
a specific type of protein termed "Informofer" (cf Ref.55). The
Informofer protein seemed at first to be unique and universal within the animal kingdom, representing a specific class of protein,
homogeneous in charge and size. However, more recently several
groups of investigators found the Informofer proteins to be heterogeneous; more than 10 bands could be identified by SDS-polyacrylamide gel electrophoresis (Morel, C. & Scherrer,K. unpublished
results; Pogo, A., pers.comm.;Sekeris, C., pers. comm.). Although
according to published data the proteins associated with pre-mRNA
are different from those associated with mRNA (54, 56), we have
to bear in mind that present techniques would not allow the detection of a messenger-specific protein represented only once per
pre-mRNA-protein complex. This consideration, as well as the
recently discovered heterogeneity of Informofer proteins, leaves
open the question if the pre-mRNA associated proteins serve a
strictly structural or metabolic function, or if they have a regulative function . If mRNA specific proteins could be detected
among the major pre-mRNA-proteins, then we could speculate that
they may act as factors selectively stabilizing specific messenger
sequences in pre-mRNA, and accompany them to the cytoplasm. Thus,
these factors could represent part of the communication system

between information carrier and the controlling environment proposed above on purely theoretical grounds.

A particular case of pre-mRNA-protein complexes is represented by the RNP particles accumulating in the nucleoplasm of
lampbrush stage oocytes,e.g. in the newt (44). These structures
are of particular interest since they are likely to constitute, as
already mentioned, a pool of stored nuclear pre-mRNP representing
an early peripheral memory. These particles contain much more
protein (95%) than the average nuclear pre-mRNP in growing or
differentiating cells (75% protein).

In summary, we may recall that the structure of pre-mRNA
molecules is compatible with the notion of a linkage of messenger
sequences to programming and no-sense ("architectural") sequences.
The programming sequences contain some common "signals" as oligo(U),
oligo(A) and poly(A). In addition, there are intermediate repetitive sequences which may serve as more selective controlling elements. The pre-mRNA is always associated with proteins; these may
play a role as biochemical mediators of processing of pre-mRNA and
of the control of the initial steps of Cascade Regulation.

The Cytoplasmic Phase of Intra-Cellular Information Transfer

The cytoplasm of animal cells contains little or no pre-mRNA
of sizes larger than functional mRNA. An apparent exception is
represented by the 75S Balbiani Ring 2 RNA of Chironomus which is
transported to the cytoplasm as a giant molecule. However, in this
case, the giant RNA represents a true mRNA for a giant protein
(a protein of 570,000 MW has been isolated from the salivary
gland (57)). Although we still could argue that a very rapid
processing of the immediate precursors to translated mRNA may obscure a cytoplasmic phase of pre-mRNA, present evidence indicates
that the bulk of mRNA has reached its final form upon entering
the cytoplasm.

For example, duck erythroblast cytoplasm contains no globin
specific pre-mRNA larger than polyribosomal mRNA. However, two
distinct populations of functional globin mRNA exist, one free
from ribosomes in the cytoplasm and the other ribosome-associated
in the polyribosome. Messenger RNA isolated from both compartments can be translated in vitro. Hence, we conclude that the
globin mRNA has found its final and functional form once liberated
from the nucleus.

However, processing does not end with the integration of
mRNA into the polyribosome. Purified and translatable duck globin
mRNA has a heterogeneous pattern on polyacrylamide gels,spreading

from about 1.6 to 2.2 x 10^5 MW. Upon pulse labeling, only the 2.2 x
10^5 MW trailing edge of this pattern incorporates radioactivity (4).
Thus, we must conclude that the mRNA enters the polyribosome as
a molecule of 2.2 x 10^5 MW and is reduced in size during transla-
tion.A shortening of the poly(A) sequence was observed in duck
globin mRNA (58).

The occurrence of free mRNA outside the polyribosome complex can be considered as a general feature of animal cells(cf.
Refs. 34, 59). In HeLa cells, up to 40% of the total cytoplasmic
mRNA can be in free form as ribonucleoprotein (RNP) complexes (59);
in duck erythroblasts 25% of the translatable globin mRNA is in
the free pool (60, Spohr,G., Imaizumi, T., and Scherrer, K.
unpublished).

Comparing the electrophoretic migration pattern of total
free and polyribosomal mRNA, it is evident that the free cytoplasmic mRNA represents a larger spectrum of mRNA types, qualitatively and quantitatively different from that of polyribosomal
mRNA (34). Hence, a control mechanism seems to select among the
total free cytoplasmic mRNA for the types and amounts of mRNA to
be translated.

Free and polyribosome bound messenger RNA are both associated with specific proteins in a messenger-ribonucleoprotein com-
plex(cf.Ref.61). It is of particular interest that the globin
mRNA in the two compartments is associated with distinctly different proteins (62). Hence, these proteins may correspond to mediators of signals relating to a late step in pre-translational
control.

A consideration of both the differing content of messenger
RNA molecules in the two cytoplasmic compartments and the different types of proteins associated with a specific message present
in the two compartments lead to the idea that a regulative mechanism must operate to discriminate between stored and actually
translated mRNA, and to control quantitatively the translation of
a specific mRNA.

Of particular interest in this respect is the recent report
of Stevens and Williamson (24) who observed in myeloma cells a
direct feed back effect of the intra-cellular pool of immunoglobulin on the translation of its mRNA. Moreover, the immunoglobulin seems to bind directly to its mRNA, constituting an RNP-
complex. (Interestingly enough, we find in the free, untranslated
globin mRNA-protein complex several proteins which, by size, could
be globins (62). However, proof of identity cannot yet be given).
It is evident that such a direct feed back effect of product concentration on mRNA translation would represent the most economical

mechanism to control quantitatively, in a late phase of Cascade
Regulation, the flow of information from a peripheral pool to its
expression. How would one expect mRNA to interact specifically
with proteins? Messenger RNA molecules are known to contain
(with the exception of histone mRNA) a large poly(A) sequence at
their three-prime end (63, 64, 65, 66). This poly(A) sequence
may be associated with a specific protein (67). Furthermore, Ilan
and Ilan (68) reported recently that in five-prime of insect polyribosomal mRNA, a short (15 nucleotide long) sequence exists, common to all insect mRNA and containing up to 50% of a A.

The size of duck globin mRNA exceeds the sequence needed to
code (coding sequence) for a duck globin by about 70,000 MW. Thus
there is space within this molecule to accommodate, in addition
to poly(A) and the Ilan-type of common sequence, other signal receptor sites. Electron micrographs of globin mRNP (Fig.8) show
that the proteins in the mRNP are distributed over the full length
of the duck globin mRNA (69). Hence, it is possible that signal
receptor sites are not only present in specific sequences at the
five- and three-prime ends of the coding sequence. Superimposed
on the coding sequence itself, there may exist sequence specific
recognition sites for the interaction with proteins.

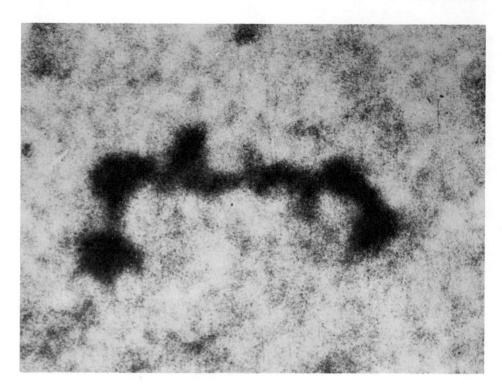

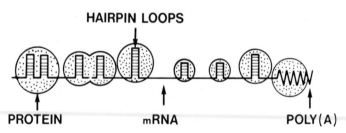

FIGURE 8 <u>Electron Micrographs and Schematic Drawing of a Polyribosomal Globin Messenger Ribonucleoprotein Particle.</u>

      mRNP particles from duck erythroblasts were isolated by
EDTA dissociation of polyribosomes according to Morel et al.
(54, 61), prepared for electron microscopy and visualized as
described by Dubochet et al.(1973).

      The schematic drawing is based on the electron micrographs
and the structural analysis of Favre et al (46) who demonstrated
extensive regions of double-strandedness in the RNA contained in
the particle. These proteins associate preferentially with
regions of high secondary structure.

Such mRNA-bound proteins may play the role of initiation factors for protein synthesis which have been reported in many systems. However, indirect evidence leads to the conclusion that there is no absolute factor specificity for a given globin mRNA (70,71). Rather, we have to consider that a given type of factor has a differential capacity to act on different types of mRNA. Thus the notion of an only relative specificity in the signal-mRNA interaction arises. This would be compatible with the formal requirements of a multi-key, multi-step integrating selection system, such as that theoretical system presented in this review. The partial redundancy of the signals in a programming sequence would allow the expectation that a protein binding with optimal efficiency to its true recognition site would interact also - but with less efficiency - with programming sequences containing the same signals but in different combinations.

The facts about cytoplasmic mRNA most pertinent to the Cascade Regulation hypothesis may be summarized as follows: the spectrum of cytoplasmic mRNA is much smaller than that of nuclear pre-mRNA; this spectrum is further reduced in the poly-ribosomal mRNA population. Hence, a pre-translational control of mRNA takes place, selecting qualitatively and quantitatively the mRNA to be translated. The mediators of this selection may be the specific proteins attached to mRNA which are different in the two compartments, the free and the translated mRNA. These mRNA-associated proteins may represent the communication system between mRNA and the controlling cellular environment envisaged in the first section of this review, on theoretical grounds.

The processing of mRNA continues throughout the translation process, resulting in a progressive reduction in size. If the newly synthesized mRNA has about 200 nucleotides in addition to the coding sequence, the smallest translatable globin mRNA may be reduced to the coding sequences and about 50 extra nucleotides. Thus, the decay of signals (poly(A)) and of the programming sequence may continue during translation, representing a last mRNA-linked control mechanism within the frame of Cascade Regulation.

4. THE CASCADE REGULATION HYPOTHESIS REVISITED

In the schematic representation of Fig.9 we attempt to summarize our present knowledge of mRNA formation in animal cells. Although many of the details of this scheme must at present remain hypothetical (e.g. the direct physical precursorship of pre-mRNA to mRNA), all depicted fractions and compartments containing pre-mRNA or mRNA are experimentally characterized. It follows that IIT in animal cells is a complicated multi-step process, involving a multiplicity of transformations of the information carriers and, hence, many biochemical reactions which necessitate multiple regulative controls (indicated in Fig.9 by vertical bars).

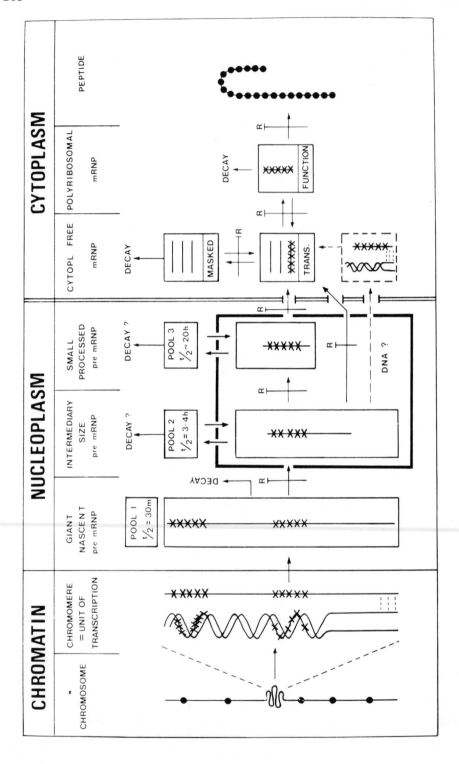

FIGURE 9   <u>Flow Schema of Messenger RNA Formation and Intra-Cel-</u>
           <u>lular Information Transfer in Eukaryotic Cells from</u>
           <u>the DNA to the Polypeptide.</u>

The transcriptional unit in the DNA corresponding to the
chromomere is transcribed into giant pre-mRNA molecules, including
one or several messenger sequences. This nascent pre-mRNA is
rapidly (ca.30 min·half-life) cleaved into intermediate size
pre-mRNA (cf. Fig.7) which has a half-life of 3-7 hours. During
this process, about 50% of the nascent pre-mRNA decays to acid
soluble products. The further processing until the appearance
of the functional mRNA in the cytoplasm is hypothetical and therefore place in a "black box". However it is certain that in addition to the pool of intermediate size pre-mRNA, a pool of quite
stable (half-life > 15 hours) small pre-mRNA exists (cf.Ref.4).
The mRNA appears in the cytoplasm first in a transient pool from
which the mRNA is either transferred into polyribosomes and translated, or stored in the "Informosome" (21) pool.

In order to draw attention to the fact that the "black box"
may conceal alternative ways of information processing, we depict
as an example the possibility of the transfer of DNA to the cytoplasm following the proposition of Bell (1970). (Vertical bars
headed by the letter R indicate possible thresholds of regulation).

←———

Comparing this flow scheme of IIT with the graphical representation of Cascade Regulation (Fig.1B) it becomes evident
that both schemes, in structuralistic terms, are perfectly super-
imposable. In fact, the thresholds of regulation (Fig.1B) of
mRNA formation proposed in 1967/68 (2,3) may be easily correlated
with the presently known steps of metabolic conversion of the
information carriers during IIT (Fig.9).

According to the Cascade Regulation Scheme (Fig.1B), the
total information potential of the animal genome is reduced
stepwise to that expressed in a given cell, at a given time. The
individual selection thresholds reflect the biochemical conversion
of the information carrier along the pathway of IIT: transcription
of DNA into nascent pre-mRNA ($nRNA_1$ in Fig.1B) and the conversion
of this primary transcript into various metabolic forms ($nRNA_{2+3}$);
the exportation of the information to the cytoplasm (cRNA)
and the passage of inactive mRNA (IRNA) to the mRNA of the polyribosome (pRNA); and, finally, its expression (eRNA). Thus, the
formal, theoretical considerations presented early in this review,
and the experimental observations reported in later sections, show

that this scheme may at present still be adequate to describe
the basic pattern of regulation in the eukaryotic cell.

We have seen that a stepwise selection process is compatible
with the theoretical necessity of a multi-key control system, as
well as with the theoretically necessary and experimentally observed existence of peripheral memories in the form of pre-mRNA and
masked mRNA, or of programming information in the form of RNA, DNA
or protein. The programming sequences in DNA, pre-mRNA and mRNA
containing the recognition sites for the regulational signals permit the permanent control of equilibrium and specificity in the
flow of information from the genome to phenotypic expression.

Screening other models of regulation in the light of the
pattern of mRNA synthesis, we may present the following reflections:

Although negative evidence is never compelling, we must
point out that among the known classes of nuclear RNA, no easy
candidate is in view to serve the Integrator-RNA function proposed
by Britten and Davidson (16). Such a class of RNA may simply have
escaped analysis by present day techniques. Alternatively, the
principal class of nuclear RNA, the pre-mRNA itself, may exert such
a function. However, the recent in vitro transcription of specific
messenger sequences from chromatin leads to the conclusion that
proteins rather than RNA play the determinant role in transcriptional regulation (72, Gilmour, S., pers.comm).

Considering Georgiev's (12,13) model of pre-mRNA structure,
processing and regulation we find many common features with the
Cascade Regulation hypothesis. The explanation of the decay of
part of the pre-mRNA by the solubilisation of the transcript of
operator sequences in the DNA (2,3), as well as its placement in
five-prime of the messenger sequence, is logical. There is,
however, one major discrepancy. In Georgiev's model (12,13) the
decay of pre-mRNA is due exclusively to the decay of such operator
sequences leaving behind the stabilized mRNA. This view conflicts
with the fact that the intermediate-size pre-mRNA is quite
stable and thus represents a storage form of mRNA in the form of
a precursor, and not of finished, translatable molecules. Hence,
it must include programming sequences for post-transcriptional
control. A further discrepancy relates to the fact that this
model excludes the possible "idle" transcription of mRNA sequences
and their post-transcriptional elimination or storage; we consider
this possibility in the Cascade hypothesis. At present, there is
no direct experimental evidence to confirm the validity of either
model in this respect.

However, the most serious discrepancy between the Cascade Regulation hypothesis and G. Tomkin's scheme of regulation (17) on the one side, and most other models on the other, is the total neglect of post-transcriptional regulation in the latter. If many aspects of the Cascade Regulation scheme remain hypothetical, I feel that the concept of post-transcriptional regulation in eukaryotic cells has left the status of a hypothesis and has become a firm fact.

While well aware of the tentative value of all our schemes of regulation at the present state of experimental knowledge, nevertheless I think them valid as a basis of further reflection and experimentation. It may well be that the living cell is still hiding theoretical and biochemical principles beyond even the start of our comprehension.

One essential problem unsolved in our model of regulation relates to its integrative function to, i.e. to the mechanisms which coordinate the synthesis of peptides that secure a given biological function. We have seen that the classical operon does not exist in eukaryotes, and that it may have proven a selective advantage to disperse functionally related cistrons throughout the genome. Thus a coordination by translation of polycistronic mRNA cannot be envisaged (with the exception of many RNA viruses). However, there are two distinct ways in which the Cascade Regulation Scheme may allow this coordination of function.

As a first possibility, we may imagine that there are special transcription units which integrate the information controlling a particular program of genetic expression (Fig.10A). Should such groups of programming signals exist, the selective pressure would not act to disperse the individual signals but, on the contrary, would tend to keep them physically linked. Such sequences reflect operationally the integrator RNA proposed by Britten and Davidson (16). However, since such an RNA has not been identified thus far, we have to consider the possibility of some DNA or - most likely - protein acting as control factors; in fact, DNA, pre-mRNA and mRNA are always found in close association with a variety of proteins. In this case, the sequences in the integrating transcriptional unit would represent true messenger RNA for regulative proteins. Tomkin's (17) observation of superinduction of enzyme synthesis by actinomycin D may be interpreted - assuming negative control - by the arrest of synthesis of mRNA for such regulative proteins, in this case a repressor.

A

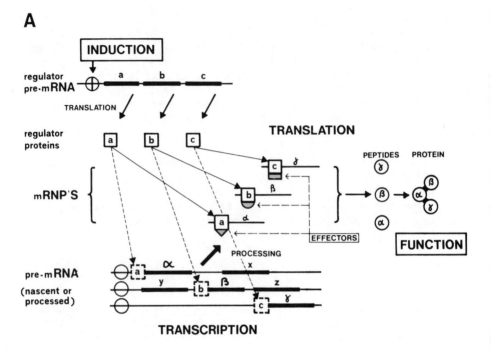

B

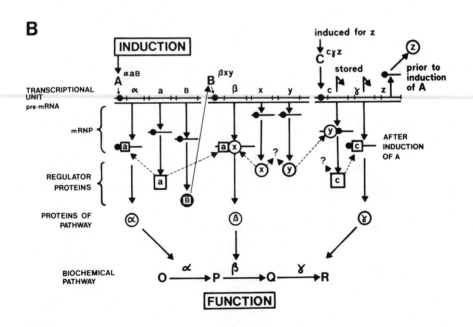

FIGURE 10 Hypothetical Schemes of Coordinative Control Systems

In order to form multi-peptide proteins (e.g. hemoglobin), or ascertain the synthesis of the enzymes of an enzymatic pathway (e.g. citric acid cycle) in a coordinate manner, the regulation system has to provide an integrative function. This may be possible by the coordinate or sequential synthesis of the factors of control (which are likely - but not necessarily or exclusively - to be proteins). Two basically different mechanisms may be considered:

FIGURE 10a Integrating Transcriptional Units.

The factors regulating the expression of a biological function are encoded in one (or a few) transcriptional units. After induction, the corresponding pre-mRNA is synthesized and the RNA sequences corresponding to the regulative factors are translated into proteins (or act, possibly, directly as RNA). The factors - once functional - induce the synthesis of pre-mRNA and regulate its processing into the mRNA's which must be translated in a coordinate manner to ascertain the expression of the biological function. Alternatively, such pre-mRNA or mRNAs may already exist in peripheral memories at the time of induction, and simply be activated by regulative factors.

FIGURE 10b Coupling of Controlling Factors to Structural Messenger Sequences in pre-mRNA.

The induction of a specific biological function (e.g. the enzymatic pathway ($0 \rightarrow R$) starts with the induction of a pre-mRNA which contains one of the necessary cistrons (α) as well as information for controlling factors (a,B) which permit the regulation of the expression of α (a), or induce the synthesis of another pre-mRNA (B). This second pre-mRNA may include the mRNA for another of the pathways proteins (ρ) as well as more regulative factors (x,y). Factors may have unique (B) or multiple functions (a,c,x,y) and they may act alone (B) or in cooperation with other regulative proteins ($\bullet$) on an mRNA.

In this example, the third cistron of the pathway is thought to be preinduced as a consequence its physical linkage in the DNA to a different function (Z). In such a case, the third message for the pathway is stored until the sequential induction of A and B permit, through a regulative factor (y), the expression of γ.

These schemes are thought to show some possibilities of regulative circuits and should not be considered as formal propositions. Although schema A is more clear and has the potentiality of coordinate control it lacks a major advantage of scheme B, which allows not only a global but also the temporal coordination of the synthesis of individual proteins.

There exists however a second theoretical possibility of coordinative control. Messenger sequences for regulative proteins might be linked in the transcriptional unit - and thus in pre-mRNA - to mRNA carrying information for cellular functions. Thus, the transcription of a specific message could automatically entail the synthesis of elements regulating its own expression as well as the programming of subsequent or correlated functions (Fig.10B)

Both models of the coordinate synthesis of regulative proteins (or of regulative RNA - the formalism being almost the same) would result in either a direct expression of regulative or programming signals or simply confer upon the nucleic acid-protein complex the potentiality of being regulated. This could occur presumably by the modulation of the activity of the nucleic acids through chemical, allosteric or ionic modification of the mRNA associated regulative proteins.

It may be premature to carry speculation thus far. All I can hope to achieve is to show that there are ways to comprehend the theoretical problems of regulation in higher organisms compatible with present day experimental knowledge. Entirely different models of regulation may arise and replace the present attempt at generalization. All we can attempt to do is push our thinking and our comprehension of current experimental knowledge to that limit where new ideas and new experiments may be stimulated.

ACKNOWLEDGMENTS

I wish to thank R. Eisenman for critically reading the manuscript and T. Imaizumi, J. Villa and P. Dubied for their help during its preparation.

REFERENCES

1. Jacob, F. and Monod, J. (1961) J.Mol.Biol. 3, 318

2. Scherrer, K. (1967) in: Int. Symp.Reinhardsbrunn on Biochemistry of ribosomes and mRNA. Abhandl.Deutsch. Akad. Wiss. Berlin (Medizin) 1968, 259.

3. Scherrer, K. and Marcaud, L. (1968) J. Cell Physiol. 72, 181.

4. Scherrer, K. (1973) in E. Diczfalusy Ed. "Protein synthesis in Reproductive Tissue". Sixth Karolinska Symposium on Research Methods in Reproductive Endocrinology, Bogtrykkeriet Forum, Copenhagen.

5. Scherrer, K. (1973) in: Regulators of gene expression in cultured cells. Fogarty conference.

6. Scherrer, K. and Darnell, J.E. (1962) Biochem. Biophys.Res. Comm. 7, 486

7. Scherrer, K., Latham, H. and Darnell, J.E. (1963) Proc.Natl. Acad. Sci. USA 49, 240.

8. Weinberg, R., Loening, U.,Willems, M. and Penman, S. (1967) Proc. Natl. Acad.Sci. USA 58, 1088.

9. Imaizumi, T., Diggelmann, H. and Scherrer, K. (1973) Proc. Natl. Acad.Sci. USA 70, 1122

10. Beato, M. (1973) Proc. Natl. Acad.Sci.USA, in press

11. Firtel, R.A. and Lodish, H.F. (1973) J. Mol. Biol. 79, 295

12. Georgiev, G.P. (1969) J. Theoret.Biol. 25, 473.

13. Georgiev, G.P. (1972) In: Moscona, A.A. and Monroy, A., Eds. Current Topics in Developmental Biology, Academic Press,Inc., New York, pg. 1-60.

14. Crick, F. (1972) Nature 234, 25

15. Paul, J. (1972) Nature, 238, 444.

16. Britten, R.J. and Davidson, E.H. (1969) Science, 165, 349.

17. TOMKINS, G.M., GELEHRTER, T.D., GRANNER, D.M., SAMUELS,H.H. AND THOMPSON, E.B. (1969) Science 166, 1474.

18. MILLS, D.R., PETERSON, R.L. and SPIEGELMAN, S.(1967) Proc. Nat.Acad.Sci. USA 58, 217-224.

19. MONOD, J. and COHN, M. (1952) Advances in Enzymology, 13, 67.

20. GROSS, P.R., GROSS, K.W., SKOULTCHI, A.I. and RUDERMAN, J.V. (1973) in: E. Diczfalusy Ed. "Protein Synthesis in Reproductive Tissue" . Sixth Karolinska Symposium on Research Methods in Reproductive Endocrinology. Bogtrykkeriet Forum, Copenhagen.

21. SPIRIN, A.S. (1969) Europ. J. Biochem. 10, 20.

22. INGRAM, V.M. (1963) in "The Hemoglobins in Genetics and Evolution". Columbia University Press, New York.

23. EPSTEIN, A.G. and MODULSKI, C.G. (1965) Prog.Med.Genet.4, 97

24. STEVENS, R.H. and WILLIAMSON, A.R. (1973). J. Mol.Biol. 78, 517

25. KAUFMANN, T.C., SHEN, M.W. and JUDD, B.H. (1969), Genetics 61, Suppl., 30.

26. SHANNON, M.P., KAUFMANN, T.C. and JUDD, B.H. (1970) Genetics 64, Suppl., 58

27. SCHERRER, K., MARCAUD, L., ZAJDELA, F., LONDON, I. and GROS, F. (1966a) Proc. Natl. Acad. Sci. USA 56, 1571

28. SCHERRER, K., MARCAUD, L., ZAJDELA, F., BRECKENRIDGE, B. and GROS, F. (1966b) Bull. Soc. Chim. Biol. 48, 1037.

29. SCHERRER, K., and MARCAUD, L. (1965) Bull. Soc. Chim. Biol. 47 1697.

30. GRANBOULAN, N. and SCHERRER, K. (1969). Europ. J.Biochem.9, 1.

31. DANEHOLT, B. and HOSICK, H. (1973) Proc. Natl.Acad.Sci.USA. 70, 442

32. BISHOP, J.O. and ROSBASH, M. (1973) Nature New Biology 241, 204.

33. BAGLIONI, C. (1963) in J.H.TAYLOR Ed. "Molecular Genetics"
    Part I. 405-469. Academic Press. London - New York

34. SPOHR, G., KAYIBANDA, B. and SCHERRER, K. (1972) Eur.J. Bio-
    chem. 31, 194.

35. SCHERRER, K., SPOHR, G., GRANBOULAN, N., MOREL, C., GROSCLAUDE,
    J. and CHEZZI, C.(1970) Cold Spring Harbor Symp. Quant. Biol.
    35, 539.

36. SHEARER, R.W. and McCARTHY, B.J. (1970) J. Cell. Physiol. 75,
    97.

37. SOEIRO, R. and DARNELL, J.E. (1970) J. Cell. Biol. 44, 467.

38. GREENBERG, J.R. and PERRY, R.P. (1971) J. Cell. Biol. 50,774

39. DAVIDSON, E.H., HOUGH, B.R., AMENSON, C.S. and BRITTEN, R.J.
    (1973) J. Mol. Biol. 77, 1.

40. SCHER, W., PREISLER, H.D. and FRIEND, C. (1973) J. Cell.Physiol.
    81, 61.

41. SOMMERVILLE, J. (1973) J. Mol. Biol. 78, 487.

42. MIRAULT, M.E. and SCHERRER, K. (1971) Europ. J. Biochem. 23,
    372.

43. SPOHR, G., IMAIZUMI, T. and SCHERRER, K. (1974) In Press.

44. IMAIZUMI, T., SPOHR, G. and SCHERRER, K. To be published.

45. GREENBERG, J.R. and PENMAN,S.(1966) J. Mol. Biol.21,527.

46. FAVRE, A., THOMA, G. and SCHERRER, K., to be published.

47. SCHERRER, K. (1971) FEBS Letters, 17, 68.

48. SHENKIN, A. and BURDON, R.H. (1972) FEBS Letters, 22, 157

49. WEINBERG, R.A. (1973) Ann. Rev. Biochem. 42, 329.

50. JELINEK, W., ADENSIK, M., SALDITT, M.,SHEINESS, D., WALL, R.,
    MOLLOY, G., PHILIPSON, L. and DARNELL, J.E. (1973), J.Mol.
    Biol. 75, 515.

51. MOLLOY, G.R., THOMAS, W.L. and DARNELL, J.E. (1972) Proc.Nat. Acad.Sci. USA, 69, 3684

52. DARNELL, J.E., PAGOULATOS, G.N., LINDBERG, U. and BALINT, R. (1970) Cold Spring Harbor Symp., Quant. Biol. 35, 555.

53. SAMARINA, O.P., LUKANIDIN, E.M., MOLNAR, J. and GEORGIEV, G.P. (1968) J.Mol.Biol. 33, 251

54. MOREL, C., KAYIBANDA, B. and SCHERRER, K. (1971) FEBS Letters 18, 84.

55. GEORGIEV, G.P. and SAMARINA, O.P. (1972) Advances in Cell Biology 2, 47.

56. LUKANIDIN, E.M., GEORGIEV, G.P. and WILLIAMSON, R. (1971) FEBS Letters, 19, 152.

57. GROSSBACH, U., (1973) Cold Spring Harbour Symp. Quant. Biol. 38, 000

58. PEMBERTON, R.E. and BAGLIONI, C. (1972) J. Mol. Biol. 65, 531

59. SPOHR, G.,GRANBOULAN, N., MOREL, C. and SCHERRER, K. (1970) Europ. J. Biochem. 17, 296.

60. SPOHR, G., IMAIZUMI, T., STEWART, A. and SCHERRER, K. (1972) FEBS Letters 28, 165.

61. MOREL, C., GANDER, E.S., HERZBERG, M., DUBOCHET, J. and SCHERRER, K. (1973) Europ. J. Biochem. 36, 455

62. GANDER, E., STEWART, A., MOREL, C. and SCHERRER, K. (1973) Europ. J. Biochem. 38, 443.

63. DARNELL, J.E., WALL, R., and TUSHINSKI, R.J. (1971) Proc. Natl. Acad. Sci. USA, 68, 1321.

64. MENDECKI, J., LEE, S.Y. and BRAWERMANN, G. (1972) Biochemistry, 11, 792.

65. EDMONDS, M.P., VAUGHAM, M.H. and NAKAZATO, H. (1971) Proc. Natl. Acad. Sci. USA 68, 1336.

66. MOLLOY, G.R., SPORN, M.B., KELLEY, D.E. and PERRY, R.P. (1972) Biochemistry, 11, 3256.

67. BLOBEL, G. (1973). Proc. Natl. Acad. Sci. USA, 70, 924.

68. ILAN, J. and ILAN, J. (1973) Proc. Natl. Acad. Sci. USA, 70, 1355.

69. DUBOCHET, J., MOREL, C., LEBLEU, B. and HERZBERG, M. (1973) Europ. J. Biochem. 36, 465

70. STEWART, A., GANDER, E., MOREL, C. LUPPIS, B. and SCHERRER, K. (1973) Europ. J. Biochem. 34, 205.

71. SHREIER, M.H., STAHELIN, T., STEWART, A., GANDER, E. and SCHERRER, K. (1973) Europ. J. Biochem. 34, 213.

72. AXEL, R., CEDAR, H. and FELSENFELD, G. (1973). Proc. Natl. Acad. Sci. USA, 70, 2029.

CONTROL OF GENE EXPRESSION DURING ERYTHROID CELL DIFFERENTIATION

Paul A. Marks, Richard A. Rifkind and Arthur Bank

Departments of Medicine and of Human Genetics
and Development, Columbia University, College of
Physicians and Surgeons, New York, U.S.A.

INTRODUCTION

Erythroid cell differentiation has proved to be a useful system for exploring several aspects of gene expression during mammalian cell differentiation (1,2). In particular, fetal mouse erythropoiesis has been employed as a system to study: (a) the basis of changes in types of globins formed during fetal development; (b) mitotic activity of differentiating erythroblasts in relation to the synthesis of globins; (c) the number of structural genes coding for globins; (d) the relation of mRNA synthesis to globin formation during erythroid cell differentiation and (e) the mechanism of the erythropoietin effect in stimulating hemoglobin synthesis.

Organ Sites of Erythropoiesis in Developing Mouse Fetuses

The mouse has a gestation period of 21 days. The first morphologically identifiable site of erythropoiesis in the developing fetal mouse occurs in the blood islands of the yolk sac at approximately the eighth day of gestation (2). Precursor cells of circulating nucleated erythroid cells proliferate in these yolk sac blood islands from about the 8th to the 10th day of gestation. Immature nucleated erythroblasts enter the fetal circulation on the 9th day (2,3). The yolk sac erythroid cells proliferate and continue to differentiate in the fetal circulation from the 10th day through, at least, the 13th day of gestation (2,4). Mitosis in these yolk-sac derived fetal erythroblasts may be observed through day 13 of gestation (5). In the early stages of differentiation of

221

these proerythroblasts, polyribosomes and mitochondria are abundant
in the cytoplasm. Cytoplasmic organelles progressively decrease in
concentration as these cells differentiate and as hemoglobin
accumulates. These cytoplasmic changes occur concomitantly with
progressive condensation of nuclear chromatin, disappearance of a
nucleolus and development of overall nuclear pycnosis and shrink-
age. The mature circulating erythrocyte of yolk sac blood island
origin is nucleated, but the cytoplasm contains no mitochondria or
ribosomes.

A second site of erythropoiesis in the fetal mouse becomes
morphologically detectable in the liver during the 10th day of
gestation (6). The erythroid cell precursors appear to be derived
from mesenchymal cells adjacent to the cords of hepatic epithelial
cells of ectodermal origin. These erythroid cell precursors,
referred to as hemocytoblasts, give rise to proerythroblasts which
differentiate through a series of morphologically identifiable
stages to non-nucleated reticulocytes. Unlike the terminal differentiation of yolk-sac-blood-island derived erythroid cells, the
differentiation of liver erythroid cells is characterized by nuclear expulsion prior to the loss of cytoplasmic ribosomes and mitochondria. It is of interest to note that the structural changes
associated with the differentiation of the yolk sac erythroid cells
are analogous to those characteristic of avian and amphibian erythropoiesis. Liver erythroid cell differentiation appears to involve structural changes characteristic of erythropoiesis in adult
mammalian bone marrow.

The development of the yolk sac erythroid cells from precursors in the blood islands appears to proceed as a cohort.
Morphologically, at each stage of gestation between days 9 and 15,
yolk sac erythroid cells differentiate in a relatively homogeneous
fashion (5). In contrast, the population of erythroid cells in
the fetal liver is heterogeneous with regard to cell stage. Liver
erythropoiesis, at least for a transient period, involves a self-
perpetuating precursor cell which yields differentiating erythroblasts over a period of time. From day 11 of gestation, the population of liver erythroid cells becomes increasingly more differentiated. On day 11, approximately 80 percent of the erythroid cells
present in the liver are at a very immature stage of differentiation, but by day 14, the proportion of these immature cells decreases sharply, to less than 5 percent. Concomitantly, there is
an increase in the proportion of orthochromic erythroblasts which
have synthesized hemoglobin. During this period, there is generally a greater than 10-fold increase in the total number of erythroid cells in the liver.

The data summarized above indicate that there are two distinct
populations of erythroid cells appearing at different times during

mouse fetal development, namely, the primitive cell line developing in yolk sac blood islands and the more definitive cell line
which appears initially in the liver.

Direct information on the morphological characteristics of
yolk sac and liver erythroid cells lines in the developing fetal
mouse is perhaps better than that available for any other species.
These findings of shifting sites of erythropoiesis with fetal
development are analogous to observations in other species, including man (7). The first erythroid cells in the human embryo
are morphologically detectable in yolk sac blood sinuses at about
18 days of gestation and the appearance of immature definitive
erythrocytes has been described in the liver of 12 mm human embryos
(5 to 6 weeks of gestation). Evidence for shifts from a primitive
to a definitive erythroid cell line have been described in the
chicken (8) and in the metamorphosis of the tadpole to the adult
frog (9). It is likely that similar changes occur in other species, but less definitive studies are available to document the
specific aspects of erythropoiesis during fetal development in the
rat (10), monkey (11), cattle, pig, sheep (12) and goat (13) (see
Table 1).

Patterns of Globin Synthesis During Fetal Development

Changes in the types of hemoglobin synthesized during fetal
development have been described not only for the mouse but for
several other mammalian as well as lower animal species (14).

Studies in the mouse have provided the most direct evidence
on the relationship between alterations in erythropoietic cell line
and types of hemoglobin formed. In the erythroid cells of the yolk
sac blood islands of strain C57B1/6J mice, three hemoglobins are
formed (15). These have been characterized as embryonic hemoglobin
E_I, composed of x and y chains, embryonic hemoglobin E_{II}, composed
of α and y chains and embryonic hemoglobin E_{III}, composed of α and
z chains. There is no detectable synthesis of β globin in yolk
sac erythroid cells.

Structural studies to date of the globin chains suggest that
α,β, x, y and z chains are controlled by separate genes (16,41).
Steinheider et al. (16) have analyzed the peptide digest of the z
chain. Their data suggest that about 20 of the 146 amino acids
are substituted in the z chain, as compared to the β chain. This
difference is less than that between human α and β globin chains.
The same authors have partially analyzed the structure of the mouse
x globin chain. They found that its amino acid composition matches
better the mouse α chain than mouse β chain. They estimate a minimum of 50 amino acid differences between the mouse α and mouse x
chain, yielding a maximum correspondence of 64 percent. It is of

P.A. MARKS, R.A. RIFKIND & A. BANK

TABLE 1

PATTERNS OF HEMOGLOBIN SYNTHESIS RELATED TO
CHANGES IN ERYTHROPOIETIC CELL LINES DURING FETAL DEVELOPMENT*

Species	Cell Line			
	Embryonic		Definitive	
	Site	Hemoglobin	Site	Hemoglobin
Mouse	Yolk Sac	E_I (xy)	Liver and Bone Marrow	A ($\alpha\beta$)
		E_{II} (αy)		
		E_{III} (αz)		
Man	? Yolk Sac	Gower I (ϵ)	Liver and Bone Marrow	F ($\alpha\gamma$)
		Gower II ($\alpha\epsilon$)		A ($\alpha\beta$)
		Portland I ($\zeta\gamma$)		A_2 ($\alpha\delta$)
Rabbit	? Yolk Sac	E_I (xϵ)	Liver and Bone Marrow	A ($\alpha\beta$)
		E_{II} ($\alpha\epsilon$)		
Chicken	Yolk Sac	E	Yolk Sac and Bone Marrow	A (α?)
		P (α^A?)		D (α?)
Frog	Liver	Type I	Liver and Bone Marrow	Frog I
		Type II		Frog II

*See text for references.

further interest that tryptic digest of mouse x chain yields two peptides which are identical to human Hbε peptides (16). The human ε chain appears to be more like mouse x chain than mouse α chain. This similarity suggests an interesting common evolutionary ancestry for mouse x and human embryonic globin chains.

Mouse fetal liver erythroid cells synthesize a single type of hemoglobin with a globin composition indistinguishable from that of the hemoglobin ($\alpha_2\beta_2$) present in the adult of this species (15). The change in pattern of hemoglobin synthesis from embryonic to adult type during mouse fetal development is associated with the substitution of liver erythropoiesis for yolk sac erythropoiesis. This cellular basis for changing patterns of hemoglobin synthesis during fetal development is a general phenomenon in the animal kingdom (Table 1) (14).

Evidence indicates that an analogous shift from a primitive to a definitive erythroid cell line is associated with the change in the types of hemoglobin synthesis in man (17), chick (9) and tadpole (9). An analogous progression from embryonic to adult hemoglobin has also been reported for rabbits (16), sheep and goats.

In addition to this pattern of changes in erythropoietic site and cell lines, which appears to determine changes in the hemoglobins formed, a further suggestion of pattern may be discerned in the structural alterations in the hemoglobins synthesized in primitive and definitive cell lines. In mouse, man, chicken, goat and sheep, conversion from embryonic to adult type hemoglobins includes the substitution of one globin chain. In certain species, such as man, in addition to embryonic and adult hemoglobin, so-called fetal hemoglobins occur. These are synthesized in cells in later stages of fetal development than those in which the embryonic hemoglobins are synthesized. In addition, the fetal hemoglobins are formed also in adult cells and, specifically in man, both adult hemoglobin HgA, and fetal hemoglobin HgF, can be formed in the same cell (12). In the mouse and man, and probably in rabbit, goat, sheep and chick, the substitution is in a beta-like chain. The alpha chain is constant in structure in the embryonic and adult hemoglobins, presumably reflecting continued activity for the structural gene for the alpha chain and shift in activity for the structural gene for the beta-type chain. This does not appear to be the case with the tadpole, frog hemoglobins which have no common peptide chain (9). It is of further ontogenetic interest that an embryonic hemoglobin has been characterized in mouse, hemoglobin E_I (15), in man, hemoglobin Portland (17), and in rabbit, hemoglobin E_I (16) which is composed of two different globin chains neither of which are structurally identical to the α or β globin of the adult of the species.

Rates of Synthesis of Globin Chains During Fetal Development

The earliest reported experiments are with day 9 yolk sacs of fetal mice in which the synthesis of α, x, y and z globin chains has been demonstrated (1). The syntheses of embryonic hemoglobin E_I and E_{III} cease by about day 11 of gestation. Embryonic hemoglobin E_{II} continues to be synthesized at a linear rate through at least day 13 (18). These data suggest that syntheses of embryonic globin chains x and z are terminated by day 11, while the syntheses of α chain and embryonic globin chain y continue for at least 1 to 2 subsequent days of yolk sac erythroid cell development. Similar but not identical data have been reported by Steinheider et al. (16). The main difference between these authors' data and those from our laboratory is that we have found that the rate of synthesis of z chain proceeds at about the same level as that of the y chain, while the x chain synthesis is terminated on day 10 to 11. By day 10 to 11, the onset of α and β globin chain synthesis in liver erythroid cells is first detectable. Thereafter, the synthesis of α and β continues at approximately equal rates (Fig. 1).

Primitive and Definitive Erythroid Cell Lines

The relationship between the primitive and definitive erythroid cell lines has not been elucidated. Two possibilities can be considered: (a) that the primitive erythroid cell line, the yolk sac erythroid cells, is the precursor of the definitive hemopoietic cell lines; (b) alternatively, the yolk sac erythroid cell lines and the definitive hemopoietic cell lines might diverge from a common pluripotential precursor cell at a stage of fetal development prior to the development of yolk sac blood islands (Fig. 2). The yolk sac blood island erythropoiesis in fetal mice proceeds as a cohort, while fetal liver erythropoiesis, and subsequent sites of definitive hemopoiesis, have a capacity for self-maintenance, as well as for the production of differentiated progeny. There is no definitive evidence in any species to indicate that the primitive erythroid cells are direct precursors of definitive erythroid cells. Moore and Metcalf (19) have demonstrated that fetal mouse yolk sacs contain pluripotential cells capable of producing erythroid, granulocytic and megakaryocytic colonies, assayed by the spleen colony method of Till and McCulloch, as well as *in vitro* colony-forming cells, granulocyte and macrophage precursors. Their observations are compatible with the hypothesis that the yolk sac serves as the primary source for colonization of subsequent sites of hematopoiesis. The data, however, fall short of direct evidence for this hypothesis.

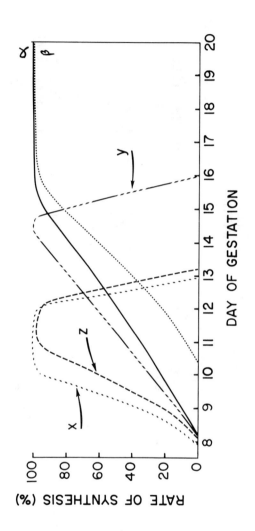

Fig. 1   Schematic representation of relative rates of synthesis of globins during fetal development. For representational purposes, 100 percent is set as the maximum rate of synthesis for each globin chain. This does not indicate rates of synthesis of a given globin chain relative to any other.

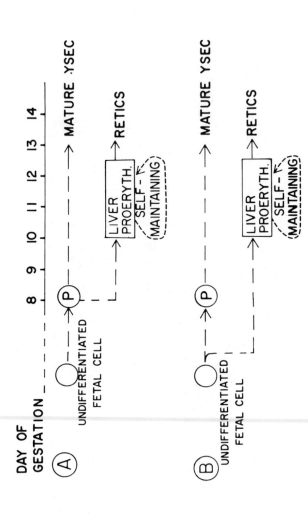

Fig. 2   Schematic representation of alternative relationships between primitive, yolk sac erythroid cell (ysec), line and definitive, fetal liver and adult bone marrow, erythroid cell lines.

Further, since the *in vitro* colony-forming assay employed to
determine the presence of precursor cells in explanted yolk sacs
yields only granulocytes and macrophages and no erythroid cells,
there are no data bearing on the question of the source of the
erythroid precursor cell or the pluripotential hematopoietic
cell. It is of interest that although pluripotential hemopoietic
cells are detectable by the spleen colony-forming assay of yolk
sacs *in vivo*, no demonstrable megakaryocytic or granulocytic cell
formation occurs in fetal mouse yolk sac blood islands *in situ*.
These findings suggest that in the yolk sac environment, differentiation is restricted to the erythropoietic cell lineage. The
relationship between primitive and definitive erythroid cell lines
are fundamental areas requiring intensive investigation.

DNA Synthesis, Mitosis and Hemoglobin Formation During Erythroid Cell Differentiation

As indicated above, yolk sac erythroid cells differentiate as
a cohort of cells *in vivo* (5). Globin synthesis occurs in cells
still capable of DNA synthesis and of cell division. This was
demonstrated in studies with yolk sac erythroid cells of 11 day
fetuses which were incubated with ^{3}H-thymidine to evaluate DNA
synthesis. Approximately 80 percent of these cells were labeled
with thymidine after 4 h of incubation. By day 11, yolk sac erythroid cells had synthesized approximately 45 percent of all the
hemoglobin to be formed by these cells. Between days 10 and 14 of
gestation, yolk sac erythroid cells undergo approximately two cell
divisions. With each succeeding division, there is a smaller
increment in hemoglobin content per cell (Table 2). Between day
10 and 11, the increase in content of hemoglobin per cell is 6
times greater than that which occurs in cells between days 12 and
13. While there may be hemoglobin synthesis following terminal
mitosis, it is at a considerably lower rate than that occurring
in earlier stages of yolk sac erythroid cell differentiation (18).

It has been suggested that the synthesis of specialized proteins does not occur in cells which are actively proliferating
(20). The above cited data indicate that this is not the case
for differentiation of erythroid cells derived from yolk sac blood
islands. Analogous data have been reported for differentiating
cells of the tadpole-frog erythroid line (21), Galea of the silk
moth (22), fibroblasts capable of collagen synthesis (23) and in
cells producing antibodies (24).

Erythroid cell differentiation may be a variation of the
theme of obligatory separation of mitotic activity and synthesis
of differentiated proteins, which does appear valid for differentiation of skeletal muscle (25). This hypothesis states that in

TABLE 2

NUMBER OF FETAL MOUSE YOLK SAC ERYTHROID CELLS,
CONTENT OF EMBRYONIC HEMOGLOBINS, AND MITOTIC INDEX
ON DAYS 10 TO 14 OF GESTATION
These data are derived from (5)

Day	No. of cells (x 10^6/ embryo)	Content of embryonic hemoglobins*		Increment in hemoglobin content per cell per day (μg/10^6 cells)	Mitotic Index**
		μg/embryo	μg/10^6cells		
10	0.31	3.5	11.3		3.2
				42.3	
11	0.70	37.5	53.6		3.8
				10.4	
12	1.22	78.0	64.0		3.4
				7.3	
13	1.41	102.0	72.3		0.4
				7.3	
14	1.50	121.0	80.6		0.0

*These values represent the average of at least three
separate experiments on each day. The values for micrograms
of hemoglobin per 10^6 cells were calculated as the quotient
of the average value for micrograms of hemoglobin per
embryo divided by the average number of cells.

**Based on counts of 2,000 cells from blood pooled from at
least 100 fetuses on each day.

differentiation there is a critical mitosis, following which the
definitive commitment to the synthesis of differentiated proteins
occurs. In case of the erythroid cell, the definitive mitosis
need not be the terminal division of a cell line. It differs from
divisions for self-renewal of the precursor cells by virtue of
initiation of expression of the program of differentiation. This
program determines the transition from precursor cell to erythroblast, including the number of divisions and the amount of hemo-

globin to be synthesized by the cell and its progeny (5,24). This hypothesis would further suggest that the definitive mitosis results in a process which, *in vivo*, is irreversible. The study summarized above in fetal mice from our laboratory (5) and those reported by Holtzer and his coworkers with chick erythropoiesis (25) are compatible with this hypothesis which would predict that the number of cell divisions and the amount of hemoglobin synthesis by these cells is programmed at the point of definitive mitosis and is basically independent of specific external influences thereafter.

mRNA for Globin - Control at the Level of DNA

A crucial question with respect to the regulation of gene expression during erythroid cell differentiation is the number of copies of the globin genes that exist in the genome. Approximately 95 percent of the total proteins synthesized during the course of erythroid cell differentiation are globins. Mechanisms regulating the rate of synthesis of differentiated proteins operate at the level of DNA or at the level of protein synthesis. At the level of DNA there are at least two models which could lead to synthesis of large amounts of a single protein. The first would involve multiple copies of the globin structural gene in the DNA of erythroid cells. This is referred to as gene reiteration. A second possibility is that in erythroid cells there occurs specific replication of the globin gene, referred to as gene amplification. In the synthesis of ribosomal RNA both gene reiteration and gene amplification seem to occur and serve as a precedent for suggesting these two models (26,27). Alternatively to these control models, the genetic locus determining the structure of globin may be unique and the large amount of globins synthesized during erythroid cell differentiation may reflect selective rates of transcription processing and/or translation of globin mRNA.

Earlier experimental approaches to determining the number of copies of globin genes in the genome employed techniques of DNA-RNA hybridization where partially purified globin mRNA was added in excess (28,29). In these studies with the mouse and chicken, it was estimated that globin mRNA hybridized with an amount of DNA corresponding to 30,000 to 60,000 copies of globin, respectively. More recently, in experiments performed under conditions where duck 9S RNA was hybridized with excess duck DNA, the results suggested that about five globin genes exist per genome (30).

Another approach involves the use of copy DNA. Reverse transcriptase from avian myeloblastosis virus has been used with purified globin mRNA to prepare partial DNA copies (cDNA) of the globin

mRNA. This cDNA provides a specific approach to measuring the
number of copies of globin genes in the genome by cDNA-DNA
hybridization (31,33). Using DNA prepared with globin mRNA of
duck (34) and of mouse (35), data have been obtained indicating
that the globin gene frequency is less than 5 times that of the
non-reiterated portion of the genome. In addition, Packman et al.
(34) demonstrated that the number of globin genes in duck reticulocytes does not differ substantially from those in duck liver.
These data indicate that the globin gene in the mouse and duck
genome is unique and that neither gene reiteration nor amplification accounts for the large amount of globin made as erythroid
cells differentiate. The much higher values for the number of
globin genes in the genome estimated from studies employing DNA-
RNA hybridization in the presence of RNA excess are misleading
and are possibly accountable to part of the globin mRNA being
hybridized with portions of many other genes. In other words, the
globin mRNA is transcribed from a single unique locus in the
genome, the nucleotide sequences of which are unique through a
predominant stretch that may have a portion which is related to
many other gene loci. Further, these data suggest that the globin
gene is present in non-erythroid cells, but not expressed.

Stability of Messenger RNA

There are several lines of evidence to indicate that the mRNA
for globin is relatively stable and may have a lifetime of several
days. Perhaps the most convincing is that globin synthesis proceeds in reticulocytes, non-nucleated cells which do not synthesize RNA (36,38). The question of when during the course of erythroid cell differentiation mRNA becomes stable has been more
difficult to answer. One approach has been to correlate the
capacityfor the new RNA synthesis with globin and non-globin
protein synthesis. Such studies have been done with fetal mouse
yolk sac erythroid cells. In these cells, between days 11 and 15 of
gestation there is a progressive decrease in the content of RNA.
The capacity for RNA synthesis falls sharply between days 11 and
13 of gestation. Paralleling this decrease in the rate of RNA
synthesis is a decrease in the formation of non-hemoglobin protein,
while the capacity for hemoglobin synthesis remains relatively
unchanged during this period. Over 90 percent of the non-hemoglobin proteins synthesized in yolk sac erythroid cells are nuclear
proteins (40), of which protein approximately 50 percent is insoluble in acid. These data suggest that globin mRNA is more stable
than non-globin mRNAs by day 11 of yolk sac erythroid cell differentiation. This interpretation assumes that the availability
of mRNA is the limiting factor in determining the rate of globin
and non-globin protein synthesis as yolk sac erythroid cells
differentiate. An alternative explanation is that mRNA for globin

is formed in excess of non-globin mRNA, relative to the level of
mRNA which is rate limiting in the synthesis of these proteins.

Another approach to estimating the stability of globin mRNA
during erythroid cell differentiation is to inhibit new RNA synthesis with actinomycin and measure the effect on protein formation (39). Incubation of 11-day yolk sac erythroid cells with
actinomycin D has little or no effect on the rate of synthesis of
hemoglobins, but inhibits non-globin protein synthesis by at least
90 percent.

This suggests that globin formation is directed by relatively
stable mRNA formed at some time prior to day 10 of gestation. On
the other hand, in 11-day yolk sac erythroid cells, the formation
of non-globin proteins may proceed on relatively short-lived
molecules of mRNA.

In contrast with yolk sac erythropoiesis, it has been possible
to demonstrate in liver erythroid cells a transition from hemoglobin synthesis sensitive to inhibition by actinomycin D on days
11 and 12 to insensitivity to the effects of this antibiotic by
day 13 of gestation (39). This development of resistance to
actinomycin D appears to reflect an alteration in the environment
in which erythropoiesis is proceeding. On both days 12 and 15,
actinomycin D inhibits RNA synthesis by more than 90 percent at
all stages of differentiation between proerythroblasts and orthochromic erythroblasts (41). On day 12, the antibiotic inhibits
the uptake of labeled iron or leucine employed as precursors of
hemoglobin synthesis, at all stages of erythroblasts. By day 15,
the antibiotic has little or no effect on the uptake of these
isotopes into polychromatophilic and orthochromic erythroblasts
which synthesize hemoblogin. These observations suggest that the
stabilization of the hemoglobin synthetic capacity in liver erythroid cells occurs at a specific stage of fetal development.

It must be emphasized that these interpretations of the
actinomycin studies are subject to verification by direct assay
of mRNA content. Singer and Penman (42) have shown that actinomycin inhibits RNA and, subsequently, protein synthesis in HeLa
cells, with little degradation of mRNA as measured by hybridization.

Patterns of mRNA Synthesis
During Yolk Sac Erythroid Cell Differentiation

At 11 days, only one-third of the total protein formed in
mouse yolk sac erythroid cells are hemoglobins, but by day 13
essentially all of the proteins synthesized in the cells are hemoglobins (39).

This alteration in the pattern of protein formation is associated with changes in the types of RNA synthesized at different stages of differentiation. RNA purified from polyribosomes of day 11 erythroid cells contain a major peak of rapidly synthesized RNA, corresponding to 9S (40). This 9S RNA is not recovered from 80S ribosomes and is not a degradation product of ribosomal RNA. Between days 11 and 13 of gestation, while there is a marked decrease in the overall rate of synthesis of RNA, the rate of synthesis of 9S RNA falls almost to nil, in parallel with the decrease in non-hemoglobin protein formation. It was further shown that the 9S RNA synthesized in 11-day cells is not identical, by the criteria of electrophoresis in agarose acrylamide gel, with the messenger RNA for hemoglobin isolated from polyribosomes of adult mouse reticulocytes (40). Because mouse yolk sac erythroid cells synthesize three types of embryonic hemoglobins, two of which contain α chains indistinguishable from the α chains of adult hemoglobin, one would anticipate that if the 9S RNA synthesized in these cells is mRNA for globin, it should be identical to the mRNA for globin found in adult mouse reticulocyte polyribosomes. It has also been found that agents such as actinomycin D or hydroxyurea, which block the synthesis of 9S RNA in yolk sac erythroid cells, inhibit nuclear protein formation but not hemoglobin synthesis (40). The characteristics of this 9S RNA, namely, that it has a rapid turnover, that it is electrophoreticaly distinct from adult reticulocyte mRNA for globin, and that it is not synthesized in the presence of actinomycin D or hydroxyurea, suggest it may be mRNA for one or more of the nuclear proteins. mRNA for globin in yolk sac erythroid cells appears to be synthesized prior to the tenth day of gestation and remains stable while these erythroblasts proliferate fourfold. The stable mRNAs for hemoglobins may be distributed to daughter cells through, on the average, two cell divisions.

Erythropoietin Induced Erythroid Cell Differentiation

Target cell of action. One of the most challenging problems in the molecular biology of eukaryote cell differentiation is the mechanism of action of hormones. These substances comprise a spectrum of chemical entities and exhibit remarkable cellular selectivity in inducing specific responses which may involve a sequence of events that effect genetic expression and require synthesis of new RNAs and proteins. Erythropoietin is the erythropoietic hormone. It has not been prepared in pure, biologically active form. Analysis of partially purified preparations (43) suggests that it has a molecular weight of 46,000 and is a glycoprotein.

Central to our understanding of the control of gene function during erythroid cell differentiation and the action of erythropoietin is identification and isolation of the immediate precursor of the hemoglobin-forming erythroid cell (erythropoietin responsive cell). Fetal mouse liver erythropoiesis is responsive to erythropoietin (44,45) and thus has proved to be a suitable tissue to approach the problem of identification of the erythropoietin responsive cell. On day 11 of gestation, when the fetal liver becomes a site of erythropoiesis, approximately 80 percent of the erythroid cells present are at a very immature stage, and morphologically classified as proerythroblasts (6). These cells are very active in incorporation of uridine into RNA and leucine into protein (14). This is indicated by a rate of uptake of ^{3}H-uridine and ^{3}H-leucine by these cells several fold higher than that in morphologically more differentiated cells in the same fetal livers and in morphologically comparable cells on subsequent days of gestation. Fetal liver is a transitional site of erythropoiesis (by birth, the liver is no longer a site of erythropoiesis) depending on a self-perpetuating precursor cell which yields differentiating erythroblasts, at least over a short period of time. The disappearance of metabolically active proerythroblasts may be the cellular basis for the loss in capacity for sustained erythropoiesis in the fetal liver, as these cells may be the erythropoietin responsive ones.

The identification and purification of the erythropoietin responsive cell from fetal liver was facilitated with the elucidation of certain aspects of erythropoietin action. In fetal liver erythroid cells, the hormone-induced increase in hemoglobin formation does not result from a direct effect on the rate of hemoglobin synthesis per cell (45,46). This is indicated by the observation that erythropoietin does not increase the uptake of ^{3}H-leucine per polychromatophilic or per orthochromatic erythroblast in cultures in which the hormone causes approximately a twofold increase in hemoglobin formation. The erythropoietin-stimulated increase in hemoglobin synthesis is caused by an increase in the number of cells synthesizing hemoglobin. The hormone acts to maintain the number of immature proerythroblasts and basophilic erythroblasts in the population, and to increase the total number of hemoglobin-forming cells. Erythropoietin is required for renewal of the immature population of erythroid cell precursors under these conditions *in vitro*. Studies from several laboratories (47) are consistent with this concept that erythropoietin stimulates erythroid cell differentiation.

In erythroid cells of fetal liver, the first detectable effect of erythropoietin is a selective stimulation of RNA synthesis in the most immature cells, the proerythroblasts (45,46). The hormone had no effect on RNA formation in more differentiated erythroid cells or in non-erythroid cells in fetal livers. The stimulation

of RNA synthesis by erythropoietin was used as a criterion for
identification of the erythropoietin-responsive cell. These erythropoietin-responsive cells are included in a class of precursor
cells designated proerythroblasts on the basis of cytological criteria. (It must be recognized that cytological criteria are inadequate to distinguish whether or not an erythroblast has initiated
the process of hemoglobin synthesis.) The cells in this population
are large and under light and electron microscopy display a high
ratio of nuclear to cytoplasmic material and an extended chromatin
pattern within the large nucleus. The cytoplasm contains abundant
polyribosomes, mitochondria and sparse elements of the endoplasmic
reticulum.

There is considerable evidence that the precursor cell
response to erythropoietin is distinct from that of the pluripotential hematopoietic stem cell. Stephenson and Axelrad (48), for
example, employing velocity sedimentation of mouse fetal liver
cells, obtained a partial separation of erythropoietin-responsive
cells from hematopoietic spleen colony-forming cells. Exploitation
of antigen differences between erythroid cell precursors and more
differentiated erythroid cells (49) provided an effective basis for
isolating a population of immature erythroid precursors. In the
presence of complement and antiserum to mature mouse erythroid
cells, polychromatophilic erythroblasts and more differentiated
cells are hemolyzed. Addition of erythropoietin to cultures of
the unlysed, purified erythroid cell precursors stimulated proliferation and differentiation to erythroblasts, with the initiation
of hemoglobin synthesis (50).

Erythropoietic effect on macromolecule synthesis. Erythropoietic stimulation of RNA synthesis occurs within one hour of
culture of fetal liver erythroid cells with the hormone (46). The
erythropoietin stimulation of RNA synthesis is not dependent on any
hormone-mediated effect on DNA synthesis (51,52). Inhibition of
DNA synthesis by hydroxyurea, cytosine arabinoside or 5-fluorode-
oxyuridine does not prevent the erythropoietin-stimulated RNA synthesis in proerythroblasts (51,53). While the effects of inhibition
of protein synthesis may depend on the nature of the inhibitor,
cycloheximide inhibition of protein formation does not prevent the
early hormone-stimulated RNA synthesis (54). Erythropoietin-stimulated synthesis of RNA in fetal liver proerythroblasts in culture
precedes detectable increase in cell number, the appearance of biologically active mRNA for globin, or hemoglobin synthesis (52,55).
An effect of erythropoietin on DNA formation was observed after 8
to 10 hours of culture (46). Inhibition of RNA or of protein synthesis eliminates the erythropoietin effect on DNA formation (56).
The early erythropoietin-stimulated RNA in rat marrow involves a
variety of species including 150S, 55S to 65S, 45S, 28S, 18S, 9S,
6S and 4S (57,58). Similarly, after 3 hours of culture with fetal

liver erythroblasts, erythropoietin stimulates several species of RNA, including ribosomal precursor RNA, Hn nuclear RNA and RNA sedimenting at greater than 60S (53).

With the preparation of purified populations of erythropoietin-responsive precursor cells, the effect of erythropoietin on RNA synthesis and, more specifically, mRNA for globin has been examined (55). Erythropoietin stimulates RNA synthesis in cultured erythroid precursor cells within one hour. The increase in RNA synthesis observed early involves Hn nuclear RNA, 45S, 32S, and 4S, and subsequently, 28S and 18S. No biologically active mRNA for globin was recoverable from these erythroid precursor cells prior to incubation with erythropoietin (55). After ten hours of culture with the hormone, there was a marked increase in globin mRNA activity. The appearance of globin mRNA activity correlated with the stimulation of globin synthesis in these cells, which occurred between five and ten hours of incubation (Table 3).

TABLE 3

ACTIVITY OF mRNA FOR GLOBIN
IN PRECURSOR CELLS CULTURE WITH ERYTHROPOIETIN

Source of RNA	Time of Culture	Total Proteins	Globin
	h	cpm	cpm
Total Cell	0	51,540	980
	10	35,360	6,940
Cytoplasmic Fraction	0	32,040	500
	10	39,920	7,420

RNA was extracted from precursor cells before and after culture with erythropoietin for 10 h. Two-fifths of the cells were used for extraction of total cell RNA and the remainder were used for extraction of RNA from the cytoplasmic fraction. The number of cells used were 7.5×10^7 and 6.2×10^7 for 0 time and 10 h preparations, respectively. The 6 to 16S fractions were prepared by sucrose gradient centrifugation and assayed in the Krebs ascites tumor cell-free system as described in Reference 55.

238 P.A. MARKS, R.A. RIFKIND & A. BANK

Hypothesis for erythropoietin action. The findings summarized
above suggest the following: Firstly, that the erythropoietin-
responsive precursor cell contains little or no globin mRNA in
biologically active form; that erythropoietin is necessary to
induce the transition from precursor stage to erythroblast stages
capable of hemoglobin synthesis; that this transition involves the
appearance of active globin mRNA, which could reflect either
initiation of transcription of globin genes or an increase in the
rate of processing of transcribed globin mRNA present in the precursor cells in an inactive form, such as a component of nuclear
HnRNA; that the erythropoietin-responsive cell is itself differentiated from a progenitor pluripotential stem cell.

This hormone responsive cell may have a receptor recognition
for erythropoietin, possibly on the cell membrane. The initial
effect of the hormone is to stimulate nuclear RNA synthesis. The
increase in RNA synthesis leads to an increase in protein forma-
tion-not specifically globin-and, as a consequence, increased DNA
synthesis and mitosis. Mitosis affords the opportunity for re-
programming the genes with consequent initiation of globin mRNA
synthesis and subsequent globin formation (Figure 3).

This reasoning is highly speculative, but is consistent with
the following known facts: erythropoietin acts selectively on
proerythroblasts, stimulation of a variety of RNAs being the
earliest detected effect on macromolecular synthesis. Erythropoietin stimulated DNA synthesis and mitosis is blocked by inhibitors of RNA formation. Globin mRNA is not present in an active
form in the erythropoietin responsive cell and appears only after
several hours of incubation with the hormone. Inhibition of RNA
or of DNA synthesis prevents erythropoietin stimulation of globin
formation. This hypothesis can be specifically tested with the
isolated erythropoietin-responsive cell. The critical issues of
the site of erythropoietin action and the mechanism of initiation
of globin mRNA transcription and its relation to mitosis remain to
be examined.

SUMMARY

Erythroid cell differentiation provides an important model to
investigate several aspects of the regulation of mammalian cell
differentiation.

1. Fetal development in many animal species is associated
with a change in the types of globins formed as gestation proceeds.
In mice, alteration in the type of hemoglobin synthesized during
fetal development is associated with the substitution of liver
erythropoiesis for yolk sac blood island erythropoiesis. There

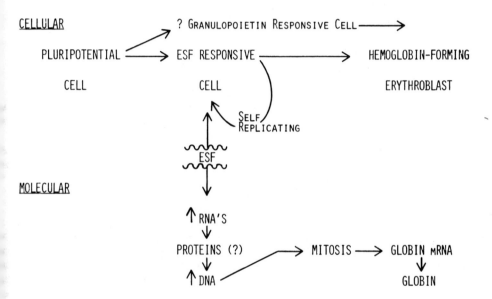

Figure 3. Schematic representation for hypothesis of mechanism
of action of erythropoietin induction of erythroid
cell differentiation and globin gene transcription.
ESF, erythropoietin.

appears to be a greater constancy in transcription of the α than β-type structural gene as sequential erythroid cell lines appear during gestation.

2. Mouse yolk sac erythroid cell differentiation proceeds as a cohort. There are at least two classes of proteins distinguishable with respect to relative dependence on continued mRNA synthesis. The major portion of nuclear proteins appear to be dependent on relatively short-lived mRNAs, while synthesis of the "differentiated" proteins, the globins, are dependent on relatively stable mRNA molecules.

3. During differentiation of yolk sac erythroid cells, DNA synthesis and cell division proceed in cells synthesizing hemoglobin.

4. Erythropoietin acts selectively on the most immature, morphologically identifiable erythroid cell precursor. This population of erythropoietin-responsive cells can be purified from fetal mouse livers and requires the hormone to proliferate and differentiate in culture.

5. The erythropoietin responsive precursor cell appears to contain no globin mRNA recoverable in a biologically active form. The initial effects of erythropoietin on macromolecular formation in these cells are to stimulate synthesis of RNA's of a variety of classes, but not specifically the appearance of biologically active globin mRNA. Only after 5 to 10 hours in culture with the hormone do these cells contain globin mRNA in a biologically active form. A hypothesis for the action of erythropoietin is presented.

ACKNOWLEDGEMENTS

Studies reviewed in this article which are from the laboratories of the authors were supported in part by grants from the National Institute of General Medical Sciences (GM-14552 and GM-18153) and National Science Foundation (GB-4631, GB-27388X).

Arthur Bank is a scholar of the American Cancer Society.

REFERENCES

1. MARKS, P. A. (1972) Harvey Lectures, Series 66, 43 (New York, Academic Press).
2. BANK, A., RIFKIND, R. A. & MARKS, P.A.; (1970) Regulation of Hematopoiesis, Vol. 1, 701 (A. S. Gordon, editor) New York, Appleton-Century-Crofts).
3. BARKER, J. E., KEENAN, M. A. & RAPHALS, L.; (1969) J. Cell. Physiol. 74, 51.
4. FANTONI, A., de la CHAPELLE, A., CHUI, D., RIFKIND, R. A. & MARKS, P. A.; (1969) Ann. N. Y. Acad. Sci. 165, 194.
5. de la CHAPELLE, A., FANTONI, A. & MARKS, P.A.; (1969) Proc. Nat. Acad. Sci. U.S. 63, 812.
6. RIFKIND, R. A., CHUI, D.H.K. & EPLER, H.; (1969) J. Cell. Biol. 40, 343.
7. BLOOM, W. & BARTELMEZ, G. W.; (1940) Amer. J. Anat. 67, 21.
8. WILT, F. H.; (1967) Advances in Morphol. 6, 89.
9. INGRAM, V. M.; (1972) Nature 235, 338.
10. HUNTER, J. A. & PAUL, J.; (1969) J. Embryol. Exp. Morphol. 21, 361.
11. KITCHEN, H., EATON, J. W. & STENGER, V. G.; (1968) Arch. Biochem. Biophys. 123, 227.
12. KLEIHAUER, E. & STOFFLER, G. (1968) Mol. Gen. Genet. 101, 59.
13. ADAMS, H. R., WRIGHTSTONE, R.N., MILLER, A. & HUISMAN, T. H. J.; (1969) Arch. Biochem. Biophys. 132, 223.
14. MARKS, P. A. & RIFKIND, R. A.; (1972) Science 175, 955.
15. FANTONI, A., BANK, A. & MARKS, P. A.; (1967) Science 157, 1327.
16. STEINHEIDER, G., MEDLERIS, H. & OSTERTAG, W.; (1971) Syntheses, Struktur und Funktion des Hamoglobins, 225 (Martin and Nowicki, editors) (J. F. Lehmanns, Verlag Munchen).
17. CAPP, G. L., RIGAS, D. A. & JONES, R. T.; (1970) Nature 228, 278.
18. FANTONI, A., de la CHAPELLE, A. & MARKS, P. A.; (1969) J. Biol. Chem. 244, 675.
19. MOORE, M. A. S. & METCALF, D.; (1970) Brit. J. Haematol. 18, 279.
20. EBERT, J. D. & KAIGHN, M. E.; (1966) Major Problems in Developmental Biology, 29 (M. Locke, editor) (New York, Academic Press).
21. MANIATIS, G. M. & INGRAM, V. M.; (1971) J. Cell. Biol. 49, 373.
22. KAFATOS, F. X. & FEDER, N.; (1968) Science 161, 470.
23. DAVIES, L. M., PRIEST, Z. H. & PRIEST, R. E.; (1968) Science 169, 91.
24. SZEINBERG, A. & CUNNINGHAM, A. J.; (1968) Nature 217, 747.
25. HOLTZER, H.; (1970) Symp. Internatl. Soc. Cell Biology, Gene Expression in Somatic Cells 9, 69 (H. Padykula, editor) (London, Academic Press).

26. BIRSTIEL, M. L., GRUNSTEIN, M., SPEIRS, J. & HENNIG, W.;
        (1969) *Nature 223*, 1265.
27. ATTARDI, J. & AMALDI, F.; (1970) *Ann. Rev. Biochem. 39*, 183.
28. WILLIAMSON, R., MORRISON, M. & PAUL, J.; (1970) *Biochem.
        Biophys. Res. Comm. 40*, 740.
29. FANCHES, Z., DE JIMENEZ, E., DOMINQUEZ, J.L., WEED, F. H., &
        BOCK, R.M.; (1971) *J. Mol. Biol. 61*, 59.
30. BISHOP, J. O., PEMBERTON, R. & BAGLIONI, C.; (1972) *Nature,
        New Biol. 235*, 231.
31. KACIAN, D. L., SPIEGELMAN, S., BANK, A., TERADA, M., METAFORA,
        S., DOW, L. & MARKS, P. A.; (1972) *Nature, New Biol. 235*,
        167.
32. VERMA, I. M., TEMPLE, G. H., MANN, H. & BALTIMORE, D.; (1972)
        Nature, New Biol. 235, 163.
33. ROSS, J., AVIV, H., SCOLNICK, E. & LEDER, P.; (1972) *Proc.
        Nat'l. Acad. Sci. USA 69*, 264.
34. PACKMAN, S., AVIV, H., ROSE, J. & LEDER, P.; (1972) *Biochem.
        Biophys. Res. Commun. 49*, 813.
35. HARRISON, P. R., HELL, A., BIRNIE, G. D. & PAUL, J.; (1972)
        Nature 239, 219.
36. MARKS, P.A., WILLSON, C., KRUH, J. & GROS , F.; (1962)
        Biochem. Biophys. Res. Commun. 8, 9.
37. KRUH, J., ROSS, J., DREYFUS, J. C. & SHAPIRA, G.; (1961)
        Biochim. Biophys. Acta 49, 509.
38. BISHOP, J., FAVELUKES, G., SCHWEET, R. & RUSSELL, E.; (1961)
        Nature 191, 1365.
39. FANTONI, A. de la CHAPELLE, A., & MARKS, P. A.; (1968) *J. Mol.
        Biol. 33*, 79.
40. TERADA, M., BANKS, J. & MARKS, P. A.; (1971) *J. Mol. Biol. 62*,
        347.
41. DJALDETTI, M., CHUI, D., MARKS, P. A. & RIFKIND, R. A.; (1970)
        J. Mol. Biol. 50, 345.
42. SINGER, R. H. & PENMAN, S.; (1972) *Nature 240*, 100.
43. GOLDWASSER, E. & KUNG, C.K.H.; (1972) *J. Biol. Chem. 247*, 5159.
44. COLE, R. J. & PAUL, J.; (1966) *J. Embryol. Exptl. Morph. 15*,
        245.
45. RIFKIND, R. A., CHUI, D., DJALDETTI, M. & MARKS, P.A.; (1969).
        Trans. Amer. Assoc. Phys. 82, 380.
46. CHUI, D., DJALDETTI, M., MARKS, P. A. & RIFKIND, R. A.; (1971)
        J. Cell Biol. 51, 585.
47. KRANTZ, S. B. & JACOBSON, L. O.; (1970) Erythropoietin and
        Regulation of Erythropoiesis, 118 (Chicago: University
        of Chicago Press)
48. STEPHENSON, J. R. & AXELRAD, A. A.; (1971) *Blood 37*, 417.
49. MINIO, F., HOWE, C., HSU, K. C. & RIFKIND, R. A.; (1972)
        Nature, New Biol. 237, 187.
50. CANTOR, L. N., MORRIS, A. J., MARKS, P. A. & RIFKIND, R. A.;
        (1972) *Proc. Nat. Acad. Sci. USA 69*, 1337.

51. GROSS, M. & GOLDWASSER, E.; (1970) *J. Biol. Chem. 245*, 1632.
52. DJALDETTI, M., PREISLER, H., MARKS, P. A. & RIFKIND, R. A.;
         (1972) *J. Biol. Chem. 247*, 731.
53. NICOL, A. G., CONKIE, D., LANYON, W. G., DREWIENKIEWICZ, C. E.,
         WILLIAMSON, R. & PAUL, J.; (1972) *Biochim. Biophys.
         Acta 277*, 342.
54. GROSS, M. & GOLDWASSER, E.; (1972) *Biochim. Biophys. Acta 287*,
         514.
55. TERADA, M., CANTOR, L., METAFORA, S., RIFKIND, R. A., BANK, A.
         & MARKS, P. A.; (1972) *Proc. Nat. Acad. Sci. USA 69*,
         3575.
56. MANIATIS ET AL.; In preparation.
57. GROSS, M. & GOLDWASSER, E.; (1969) *Biochemistry 8*, 1795.
58. GROSS, M. & GOLDWASSER, E.; (1971) *J. Biol. Chem. 246*, 2480.

REGULATION OF DEVELOPMENTAL PATHWAYS FOLLOWING INFECTION OF

ESCHERICHIA COLI BY BACTERIOPHAGE LAMBDA

Amos B. Oppenheim

Department of Microbiological Chemistry, The Hebrew
University-Hadassah Medical School, Jerusalem, Israel

The temperate bacteriophage lambda can be present in several
forms. On infection of the host, it can grow and multiply along
the lytic cycle, leading to the production of 100 progeny phages
in about 1 h. When conditions for this are unfavorable, alternatively the infected complex may follow the lysogenic pathway
(see Fig. 1). Following the establishment of the lysogenic condition, which requires phage repression and integration of phage
into the bacterial chromosome, the prophage multiplies passively
with the bacterial chromosome. Phage can occasionally be induced
spontaneously, or by appropriate treatment which destroys repression, such as UV irradiation or by heating cells harboring prophage
and a thermolabile repressor.

We have concentrated our studies on the point of decision
between lysis and lysogeny following infection, particularly on
the question which phage and host functions participate in the
decision between following along the lytic cycle or lysogenic
development.

The lambda phage genome carries the information for a large
set of genes, of which only some are known. A summary of the map
positions and functions of the relevant genes is shown in Fig. 2.

Synthesis of the cI repressor is essential for establishment
and maintenance of lysogeny, while the cro antirepressor seems to
be required for the lytic response. Surprisingly, several lines
of investigation showed that both the cI repressor and the cro

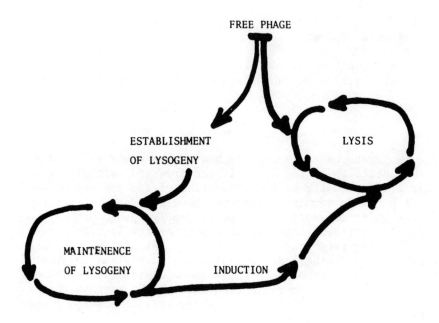

Fig.1. Developmental pathways in lambda bacteriophage

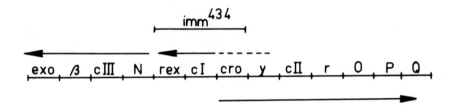

Fig. 2. Genetic map and transcription pattern of the regulatory region of λ bacteriophage. The arrows denote rightward and leftward transcription of the cro-cII-0-P operon, the cI-rex operon, and the N-cIII-exo operon. Cro probably acts in the shutoff of these three transcriptional units. cI repressor blocks the transcription of the N-cIII-exo and the cro-cII-0-P operons. cII and cIII activate repressor synthesis by acting at the y gene. The rex product is responsible for the inhibition of T4rII growth. N stimulates transcription to the left of N and to the right of cro, and activates Q. exo directs the production of exonuclease. 0 and P are necessary for the initiation of DNA replication at the r region. Q is a positive regulator for late gene transcription. The late genes responsible for the synthesis of the head and tail proteins and for lysis of the host (not shown) are located to the right of the Q gene. The genes responsible for the integration and excision are located to the left of exo (1).

antirepressor act as negative regulators at identical or closely
related operator sites (2) (Fig. 3). How then does the infected
complex select between lysis and lysogeny? Precise understanding
must await our further knowledge about the cro gene product and
its action. However, these findings led us to look for additional
elements that participate in the decision.

It has long been known that the physiological state of the
host cell also affects the decision between lysis and lysogeny.
Thus some components of the regulatory system must be present in
the host itself.

We found that in a mutant of E. coli defective in a membrane
protein, lambda infection is restricted in its decision and
follows only the lysogenic pathway. Thus λ wild type phage does
not form plaques, (3,4) and only clear mutants which are blocked
in the lysogenic pathway grow on this host. It appears as if the
cro gene is unable to express itself.

Polyacrylamide gel electrophoresis of cell envelopes extracted from the parent and mutant strains show that a protein component is practically absent in the mutant. This mutant strain is
unable to grow at 42°. We deemed it plausible, therefore, that
isolated revertants that can grow at 42° may have regained this
protein band. If the membrane mutation is indeed responsible for
the inability of λ⁺ phages to grow on this host, the revertants
would permit normal lambda development. Figure 4 shows that the
revertants do regain the protein band. Moreover, we found that
λ⁺ grows normally on the revertants (4). We conclude that probably a single mutation affects both λ expression and host membrane
structure. However, we cannot at present rule out the possibility
that the membrane modification is related to lambda development by
some indirect mechanism.

Figure 5 shows that the defective membrane permits the binding
of λ DNA to the host membrane, suggesting that the defect in normal λ regulation is not due to inability of the λ genome to bind
to the mutant's membrane.

We have studied several known functions of cro (4). Two of
these are depicted below: shutoff of exonuclease synthesis
(Fig. 6) and turnoff of repressor production (Fig. 7). It can be
seen that in both of these functions, the wild type phage behaves
differently when grown on the mutant host. The inability of
phages to shut off exonuclease synthesis and to turn off repressor
synthesis is typical of cro⁻ mutants when infecting wild type bacteria, leading to the conclusion that λ⁺ behaves as λcro⁻ in the
ER437 host.

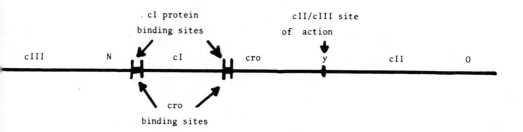

Fig. 3. Repressor and cro gene product binding sites. In binding to the right hand side of the cI gene, the repressor acts also to stimulate its own synthesis and cro may repress its own synthesis. Both the cI repressor and the cro antirepressor repress the N-cIII-exo operon and the cII-O-P operon.

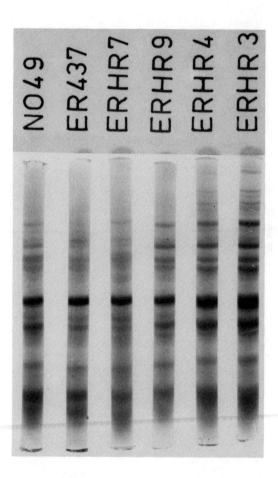

Fig. 4.   SDS polyacrylamide gel electrophoresis of cell envelopes.
NO49 is the parent strain; ER437 is the mutant, missing the upper
high molecular band (only traces of this protein can be seen;
ERHR 7,9,4, and 3 are heat resistant revertants that can grow at
42° (4).

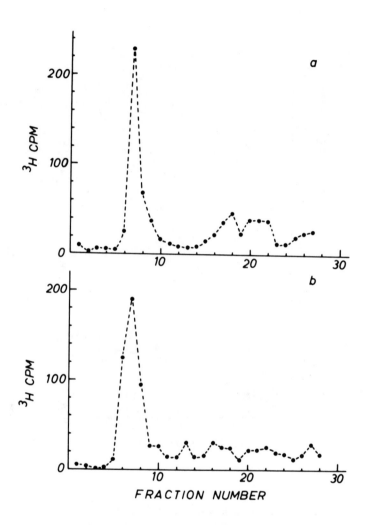

Fig. 5. Binding of λ DNA to the host membrane following infection.
Sucrose gradient analyses of gently lysed cells infected with
λcI$_{857}$.
a. infection of W3350; b. infection of ER437.

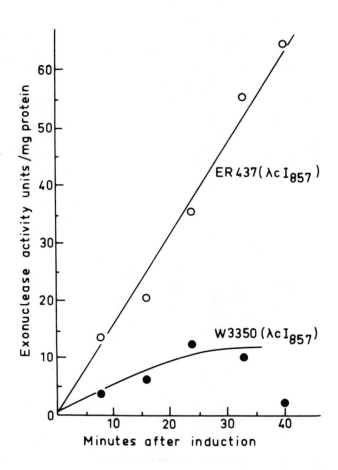

Fig. 6. Exonuclease synthesis following heat induction. Cells lysogenic for λcI857 were grown at 30° and transferred to 40° for heat induction. Samples were harvested and sonicated. The level of exonuclease was assayed by measuring the degradation of ^{3}H-thymidine-labelled E. coli DNA.

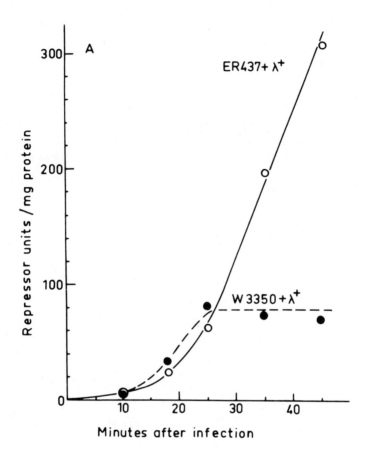

Fig. 7. Rate of repressor synthesis after infection. Cells infected at a multiplicity of 5 were diluted in prewarmed medium at
30° and aerated until harvesting. Repressor was assayed by ability
to facilitate the retention of ^{32}P λ DNA on millipore filters.
W3350 is a standard host; ER437 is a host mutated in its membrane
structure.

The ability of λ^+ to follow the lytic pathway in the ER437 host leads us to suggest that the host membrane participates in phage regulation (4). It is possible that the structure, allosteric state or the concentration of a membrane component takes part in the decision between lysis and lysogeny. Our working hypothesis is that the host membrane may act directly in the regulation of gene function.

ACKNOWLEDGMENTS

This work was supported by the Stiftung Volkswagenwerk, Germany.

REFERENCES

1. The Bacteriophage Lambda, ed. Hershey, A.D. (Cold Spring Harbor Laboratory) (1971).
2. ECHOLS, H., GREEN, L., OPPENHEIM, A.B., OPPENHEIM, A. & HONIGMAN, A. In preparation.
3. ROLFE, B., SCHELL, J., BECKER, A., HEIP, J., ONODERA, K. & SCHELL-FREDERICK, H. Molec.Gen.Genetics (In press).
4. OPPENHEIM, A., HONIGMAN, A. & OPPENHEIM, A.B. In preparation.

FAULTY PROTEINS: ALTERED GENE PRODUCTS IN SENESCENT CELLS AND ORGANISMS

H. Gershon[1], P. Zeelon[2] and D. Gershon[2]

Department of Immunology, Aba Khoushy School of
Medicine[1], and Department of Biology[2], Technion - Israel
Institute of Technology, Haifa, Israel

INTRODUCTION

The process of senescence is characterized by a progressive inability of the individual organism to defend itself against environmental insults. Superficially, the deterioration of the aging organism may appear to be composed of various degenerative processes occurring simultaneously. However, in attempting to formulate the simplest possible explanation for the many alterations observed in senescence, that is, to present a theory of aging, the initial causes of the modifications occurring at the subcellular level, whose effects are then expressed as the gross defects observed in the aging organism, should be considered.

Of the many theories which postulate basic processes responsible for age-related deterioration leading to senescence and death, few are amenable to direct experimental attack. In the last few years, we have been interested in the theories which propose that the synthesis and accumulation of faulty protein molecules in the cell with age cause deterioration of function and consequently cell death (1-3). The progressive production of defective protein molecules as a function of age may significantly contribute to the inability of the individual cell and, therefore, of the entire organism, to fulfil its various physiological and defensive functions. This postulated production of modified protein may be attributed to either stochastic events (somatic mutations or random modifications of RNA or other components of the

protein synthesizing machinery, rendering it less reliable) or to
programmed events dictated by specific genetic information. The
former of these two possible mechanisms of production of altered
protein molecules demands random alteration in protein primary
structure although the additional presence of random post-synthe-
tic alterations such as phosphorylation, acetylation, deamidation
etc. is not ruled out. A programmed modification of protein might
occur either during or subsequent to protein synthesis.

     In order to determine whether indeed, senescence involves the
production of faulty or modified proteins, we chose to study
various enzymes in two phylogenetically unrelated animal species.
The nematode, Turbatrix aceti and the C57B1 mouse. Initial experiments were performed to determine the levels of activity of
various enzymes as a function of age. It was found that all of
the nematode non-lysosomal enzymes studied demonstrated a marked
drop in detectable activity as a function of age (4). Two typical
nematode enzymes, isocitrate lyase and fructose-1,6-diphosphate
aldolase, were chosen for further study (5,6). Figure 1 depicts
the specific activity of aldolase as a function of nematode age.
Similar age-dependent drops in specific activity were detected in
the aldolases of mouse liver and mouse muscle (7,8). These age
related drops in specific enzyme activity might be attributed to
several possible causes. It might be that in the senescent organism there are simply less enzyme molecules present, due either to
a reduced level of synthesis or to an increased level of degradation. It might also be that the senescing organism produces
faulty enzyme molecules whose catalytic activity is reduced or
absent.   It is also possible that different isozymes may appear
with age. Isozymes could not be detected in the nematode aldolase
nor in the mouse liver aldolase systems (6,7). That is, the active
enzyme of senescent and young adults demonstrated the same electrophoretic mobility on cellulose acetate, the same affinity for
two different substrates (fructose 1-phosphate and fructose 1,6-
diphosphate) as attested by identical K_m, and the same temperature
stability. Thus the active enzyme of old animals appears to be
identical with that of young animals.

     To detect the possible presence of defective enzyme molecules
with reduced or absent catalytic activity, use was made of a
comparison between the level of enzyme activity and the presence
of enzyme antigen as detected by specific antibodies. Such a
technique has been used effectively in bacterial genetics studies
to detect the presence of catalytically inactive mutant enzyme
molecules (4). To this end, antisera were produced in rabbits to
a crude homogenate of 5 day old (young adult) T. aceti and to
C57B1 mouse live aldolase purified from young adult (3-4 month old)

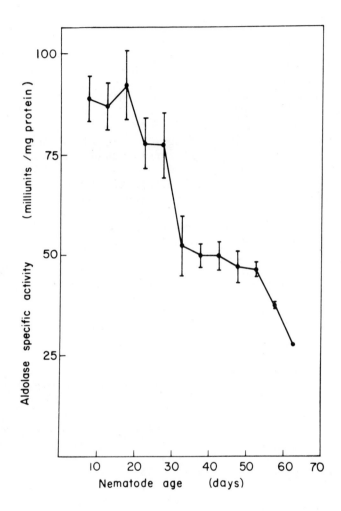

Fig. 1. Specific activity of aldolase in nematodes of various
ages. Synchronous populations of nematodes of various ages were
homogenized and crude preparations were assayed for aldolase
activity. The vertical lines denote the standard error of the
mean.

animals. The rabbit-anti-nematode homogenate contained precipi-
tating antibodies to the nematode aldolase. Titration of these
antibodies versus homogenates of age-synchronized populations of
nematodes of various ages demonstrated that the antibody was competent to precipitate 100 percent of the aldolase activity from
young as well as old populations. At maximal precipitation, no
residual antibody was detected in the supernate when assayed
against either young or old nematode homogenates. It was found
that increasing amounts of antibody were required to precipitate
equal amounts of initial enzyme activity from crude homogenates
of populations of increasing age (Figs. 2,3). In as much as it
has been demonstrated that this antiserum recognizes the aldolase
of young nematodes and senescent nematodes as identical (no residual antibody after 100 percent precipitation) and no isozymic
forms of the enzyme are detected, this requirement for increasing
amounts of antibody attests to the presence of catalytically defective enzyme molecules in the senescent nematode. This leads
to a progressive drop with age in the ratio of enzymatic units
to antigenic units.

The antiserum prepared against purified mouse live aldolase
is a monospecific antiserum which recognizes the purified enzyme
from young adult mice as identical with the enzyme present in
crude liver homogenates (Fig. 4). In this system, as in the nematode system, the ratio of enzyme to antigen decreases as a function of age. The 32 month old mouse has 1/2 the enzyme activity
per fixed amount of antigenic activity as does the 3 month old
mouse (Fig. 5). Thus catalytically inactive molecules have been
found to accumulate with age for several enzymes, in a number of
cell types, and in such phylogenetically varied organisms as
nematodes and mice (5-8). It is, therefore, suggested that this
is a universal phenomenon with regard to all proteins, cell types
and organisms.

Our estimate of the proportion of faulty molecules is probably minimal, for it can be assumed that drastically modified
proteins may lose much of their antigenic identity and will thus
not be identified as cross reacting material (CRM). It should
also be pointed out that the CRM values obtained are an average
for a large population of cells. It is conceivable that the proportion of CRM molecules may vary considerably from cell to cell
and thus a fraction of the cells in the population may contain
high levels of CRM while others have relatively low levels. It
seems plausible that there exists a certain threshold of CRM beyond which the physiological functions of a cell become insufficient for the maintenance of life.

Information is scarce regarding the amount of "noise", i.e.
the proportion of inactive or partially inactive protein molecules,

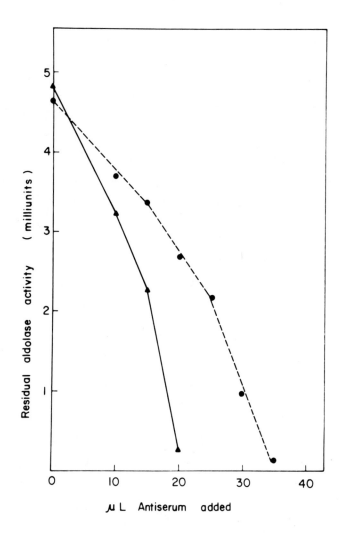

Fig. 2. Precipitation with antiserum of aldolase from young and old nematodes. Antiserum (60 µl) was added to 0.24 ml of homogenate containing 14.5 milliunits of aldolase activity. After 20 hours of incubation at 4° the preparations were centrifuged at 3,000 xg for 30 minutes. The supernatant was assayed for residual enzyme activity and the amount of aldolase precipitated was determined.

▲————▲ 6 day old nematodes
●————● 51 day old nematodes

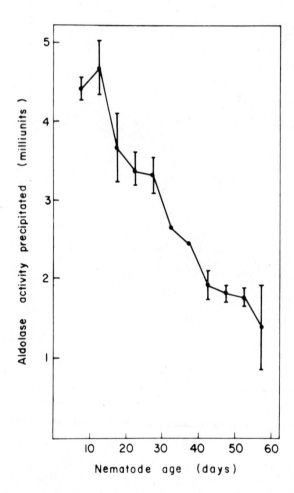

Fig. 3. Precipitation by a fixed amount of antibody of aldolase from nematodes of various ages. Precipitation was performed as described in the legend to Figure 2.

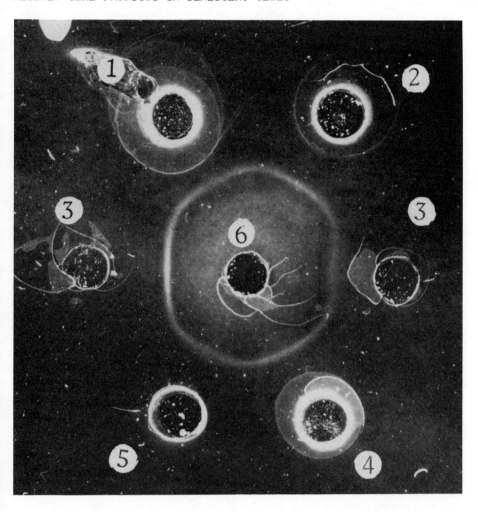

Fig. 4. Determination of monospecificity of antiserum
against liver aldolase serum by double diffusion in agar gel.
Immunological identity of pure mouse liver aldolase with aldolase
in whole homogenate from young adult and senescent mice is
demonstrated.
1 and 5 = liver homogenates of two young adult mice (2.5 months
old); 2 and 4 = liver homogenates of 2 senescent, 31 month old
mice; 3 = pure mouse liver aldolase; 6 = antiserum against
mouse liver aldolase.

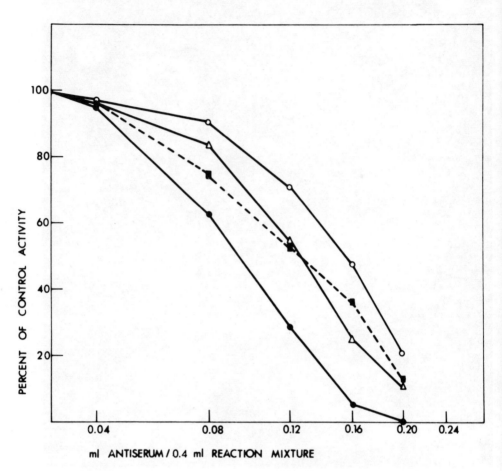

Fig. 5. Precipitation by antibody of aldolase of liver homogenates from 2-month-old and 31-month-old mice and the mixture of
both homogenates. Note lack of nonspecific inhibition or en-
hancement of precipitation in the mixture. Precipitation was
performed as previously described (7). The mixed homogenate of
old and young liver was prepared by mixing 0.015 units of enzyme
activity from each to give a final activity of 0.03 units. The
young and old liver preparations contained 0.03 units of activity.
●———●, young homogenate; o———o, old homogenate; Δ———Δ, mixture
of young and old homogenates; ■----■ , theoretical degree of
precipitation based on the assumption that the old homogenate
contains twice as much antigen per unit of enzyme activity as does
the young homogenate.

that causes a cell to lose its viability. This is particularly true for eukaryotic cells. There is very little data available concerning the rates at which the cells of various tissues reach this threshold. It thus appears that a study of the rate of CRM formation of the same enzyme in various tissues and its correlation to tissue function with age is of great importance.

Our results so far indicate that the population of enzyme molecules in aging organisms is composed of only two types of molecules: totally active and entirely inactive. The totally active molecules of old animals cannot be distinguished from molecules of young animals by any of the following criteria: kinetics of heat inactivation, electrophoretic mobility, affinity for the substrate and immunological identity. The entirely inactive molecules appearing as CRM in older animals are not the result of either specific inhibitors or inactivating proteolytic activity in old cells. These possibilities were ruled out by preincubating mixtures of preparations from old and young animals. No effect of this incubation could be detected on enzyme activity or its specific activity per antigenic unit (5,7 and Fig. 5). No indication of partial activity of a fraction of the molecules could be observed in our studies. Had inactivation been a random event, states of partial activity should have been detected by us.

The inactivation process that leads to CRM formation (and that is the only phenomenon of inactivation we are concerned with here) must be a minor one in chemical terms, in as much as the molecules fully retain their antigenic identity. This was shown by the double diffusion tests (7,8). It is suggested that there is an age-related, inherently directed program which leads to enzyme inactivation in the cell. It can be conceived that this inactivation is programmed as a continuation or a consequence of the normal development and differentiation program of the organism.

It should be mentioned that Holliday's results with Neurospora and cultured human cells (10,11) differ somewhat from our own. His results, based on either immunological studies and kinetics of heat inactivation (10) or solely on heat inactivation (11) seem to indicate random events in enzyme alteration. However, we have our doubts regarding the relevance of Neurospora and cultured cells as model systems for aging. Nonetheless the two mechanisms of random errors in proteins and a programmed process are not mutually exclusive.

The nature of enzyme inactivation will be resolved only by direct chemical analysis of purified enzymes from old and young

animals. This will be facilitated if CRM can be separated from
the active form of the enzyme. However, even if the separation
fails, the chemical analysis of purified enzyme from young and
old animals will provide direct evidence on whether the modifications in the protein which lead to inactivation are random or of
a uniform nature.

REFERENCES

1. MEDVEDEV, Z.A. (1966).   Protein Biosynthesis and Problems of
        Heredity and Aging.   Oliver and Boyd, Edinburgh and London.
2. ORGEL, L. (1963).   Proc.Natl.Acad.Sci.U.S. 49, 517.
3. ORGEL, L. (1970).   Proc.Natl.Acad.Sci.U.S. 67, 1476.
4. ERLANGER, M. & GERSHON, D. (1970).   Exp.Geront. 5, 13.
5. GERSHON, H. & GERSHON, D. (1970).   Nature, 227, 1214.
6. ZEELON, P., GERSHON, H. & GERSHON, D. (1973).   Biochemistry,
        12, 1743.
7. GERSHON, H. & GERSHON, D. (1973).   Proc.Natl.Acad.Sci.U.S.
        70, 909.
8. GERSHON, H. & GERSHON, D. (1973).   Mech.Aging and Develop. 2,
        in press.
9. YANOFSKY, C. & STADLER, J. (1958).   Proc.Natl.Acad.Sci.U.S.
        44, 245.
10. LEWIS, C.H. & HOLLIDAY, R. (1970).   Nature, 228, 877.
11. HOLLIDAY, R. & TARRANT, G.M. (1972).   Nature, 238, 26.

REGULATION OF THE EXPRESSION OF THE REOVIRUS GENOME

IN VIVO AND IN VITRO

George Acs, Daniel H. Levin, Michael Schonberg,
and Judith Christman

Institute for Muscle Disease, New York, New York;
Caroline Astell and Samuel C. Silverstein, Rockefeller
University, New York, New York

Animal viruses enter their host cells as nucleoprotein complexes. The role of the nucleic acid portion of these nucleoproteins has been understood for some time, but the importance of the proteins has been appreciated only recently with the discovery that many animal viruses contain DNA and RNA polymerizing activities. Recognition of an RNA transcriptase activity within vaccinia virus (1), for instance, resolved the theoretical problems surrounding the mechanism(s) whereby a double-stranded DNA virus initiates RNA transcription in the cytoplasm of a eukaryotic cell. The finding that RNA tumor viruses contain enzymes which catalyze the synthesis of DNA (2, 3) resolved, at least in part, one pathway by which those viruses may induce stable malignant transformation of animal cells. Similarly, the mechanism by which the double-stranded RNA containing reoviruses initiates genetic function in animal cells remained obscure until Borsa and Graham (4) and Shatkin and Sipe (5) demonstrated an RNA transcriptase activity within the virion.

Reovirus replicates in the cytoplasm of its host cell. The virus-directed synthesis of single-stranded and double-stranded RNA and of oligoadenylic acid occurs in discrete cytoplasmic factories (6, 7, 8, 9, 10). In contrast, viral protein synthesis takes place on polyribosomes which are located outside of the factory. The factory is not membrane-bounded and appears to be in direct contact with the cytoplasmic matrix.

These factories can be recovered in good yield and relatively high purity from the cytoplasm of reovirus-infected cells simply

265

by lysing the cells in detergent-containing buffers, and preparing a so-called "large granule fraction" by differential centrifugation (Fig. 1). The isolation of the factory fraction, which contains nascent and mature virions,has made it possible to study the synthesis of viral messenger RNA, and of the two RNA species -- dsRNA and oligo A which are present in the mature virion (Table 1). The synthesis of all three RNA species -- ssRNA, dsRNA, and oligo A, is catalyzed by the factory fraction. In this paper we present evidence supporting the hypothesis that maturing virions, in different stages of their development, are responsible for the synthesis of these three RNA species, and that the enzyme(s) responsible for the formation of single-stranded and double-stranded RNA and oligo A represents alternative activities of the same viral protein(s).

ssRNA

Synthesis. The RNA transcriptase activity contained in reovirus is latent and becomes manifest when the outer layer of viral capsomeres is removed by enzymatic digestion (7, 11). Removal of the outer capsomeres converts the virion (buoyant density 1.37 g/cm^3 in CsCl, diameter 750 Å) to a subviral particle (SVP) (buoyant density 1.40-1.43 g/cm^3 in CsCl and diameter 450-575 Å). Of the seven proteins recognized in the intact virion, only three are found in the SVP's. Although the SVP's do not contain oligo A, all 10 dsRNA genome segments are retained within them. The dsRNA presumably resides within the protein shell of the SVP since it is resistant to digestion with RNase or micrococcal nuclease (8).

SVP's catalyze the synthesis of ssRNA's which are of identical polarity to messenger RNA isolated from the polyribosomes of reovirus-infected cells (12). We have termed these ssRNA's "plus" strands to distinguish them from the complementary strands which we have termed "minus" strands.

The properties of the transcriptase activity (13) of the SVP can be summarized as follows:

1. RNA transcriptase activity requires all 4 ribonucleoside triphosphates, rATP, rGTP, rCTP, and rUTP; nucleoside diphosphates and deoxynucleoside triphosphates are ineffective as substrates.

2. For optimal synthesis, Mg^{++} and K^+ are the preferred cations.

3. The rate of RNA synthesis is proportional to the concentration of the particulate enzyme.

4. Due to the presence of nucleoside triphosphatases associated with the subviral particle, a nucleoside triphosphate

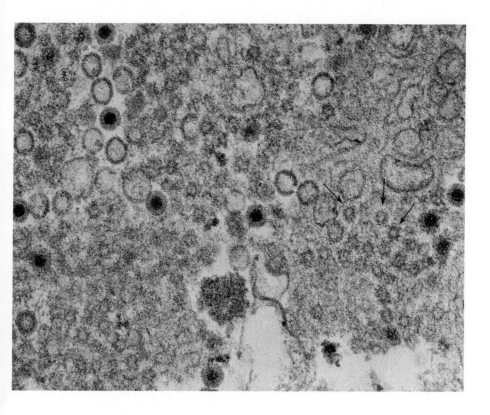

Fig. 1. Electron micrograph of the large granule fraction
(virus-producing factory) isolated from reovirus-infected mouse
fibroblasts 10 hr after infection. Shown here are mature and
incomplete virus particles as well as microtubules (arrows) which
we found characteristically in the viral factory.

TABLE 1

COMPARISON OF REOVIRUS dsRNA, OLIGO A, AND ssRNA SPECIES

RNA species	Molecular weight	Percent of RNA in virion
dsRNA:		
Large	2.3×10^6	
Medium	1.2×10^6	}80
Small	0.8×10^6	
Oligo A	$2\text{-}4 \times 10^3$	20
ssRNA:		
Large	1.2×10^6	--
Medium	0.6×10^6	--
Small	0.4×10^6	--

regenerating system is required to maintain RNA synthesis at a linear rate. We have obtained linear rates of RNA synthesis for up to 20 hours, yielding an approximately 40-fold excess of newly formed ssRNA over input dsRNA.

5. The RNA product, like messenger RNA synthesize in vivo, separates into three size classes (24S, 19S, and 14S) in sucrose density gradients.

6. All 10 of the ssRNA species of reovirus mRNA are synthesized in vitro by the subviral particles; only one strand of each dsRNA segment is transcribed.

7. The mechanism of synthesis is conservative with respect

to the two strands of the dsRNA genome; the parental double helix
remains intact in the subviral particle throughout RNA synthesis.

The large granule fraction catalyzes the in vitro synthesis
of "plus" or messenger RNA strands from the genome dsRNA. When
the large granule fraction is incubated with chymotrypsin, 10-20-
fold as much mRNA is synthesized as in the absence of this enzyme.
These results, in agreement with electron microscopic observations
and biological assays for infectious virus, confirm that there are
mature virions and subviral particles in the large granule fraction.
The subviral particles are responsible for the ssRNA synthesis
obtained in the absence of chymotrypsin, while the transcriptase
activity of the mature virions is activated by chymotrypsin (6).

Regulation of ssRNA Formation. Parental reovirions are
segregated into lysosomes where hydrolases digest the outer layer
of capsomeres(14). The resultant subviral particles can be quantitatively recovered from these organelles and are found to have
a buoyant density of 1.40 g/cm^3 in CsCl (Fig. 2). The protein
composition of the virion and of the in vivo uncoated subviral
particle are compared in Fig. 3. Proteins of the highest molecular
weight class (the lambda polypeptides) appear to be quantitatively
retained in the SVP. Proteins of the medium size class (the mu
polypeptides) are partially degraded; a cleavage product of the
mu-2 polypeptide, the δ polypeptide, is retained in the SVP. Of
the three proteins in the smallest size class (sigma) only one,
the polypeptide sigma-2, is retained in the SVP (15), (Fig. 3).
These in vivo uncoated particles are capable of transcribing the
whole viral genome. Analysis of the transcription product by
sucrose gradient centrifugation (Fig. 4) demonstrates three major
RNA species with sedimentation coefficients of 24, 19, and 14S,
corresponding to the three size classes of mRNA formed in reovirus
infected cells. When this RNA is annealed to dsRNA, the annealed
product displays the same distribution pattern on polyacrylamide
gel electrophoresis as the genome dsRNA (Fig. 5).

As indicated in Table 2, chymotrypsin has no effect on the
transcriptase activity of in vivo uncoated SVP's. Thus, functionally, these SVP's are completely uncoated. However, if the SVP's
are incubated with viral proteins, transcriptase activity becomes
latent once again. The density of the particle shifts from 1.39
to 1.375 g/cm^3 (Fig. 6), indicating the association of viral proteins with SVP's. Polyacrylamide gel electrophoresis of the proteins from these re-assembled particles (Fig. 7) demonstrates that
addition of the viral capsomere protein, σ_3 is principally responsible for these changes. Thus, σ_3 can be considered a regulatory
protein for transcription, converting SVP's from an enzymatically
active to an enzymatically inactive state. Chymotrypsin treatment
of the re-assembled particles again activates transcription

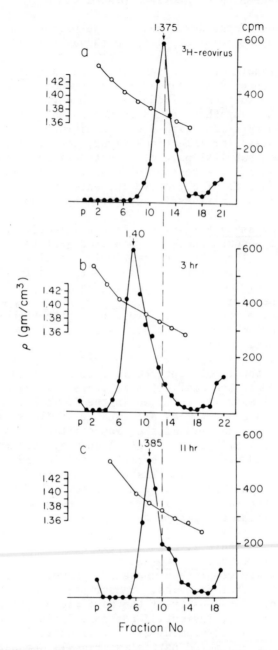

Fig. 2.   Comparison of buoyant densities in CsCl of mature reovirions and of particles uncoated in vivo. Mouse fibroblasts
were infected with (^{3}H) protein-labeled reovirus (panel a). At
3 hr (panel b) and 11 hr (panel c) after infection, cytoplasmic
extracts were prepared and the buoyant density of the labeled subviral particles was determined.

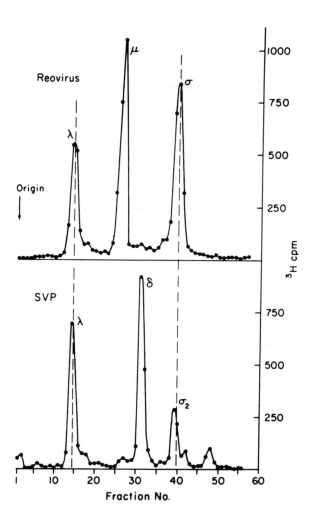

Fig. 3. Analysis by acrylamide gel electrophoresis of the protein composition of (^{3}H) protein-labeled reovirus (upper panel) and of subviral particles (lower panel) isolated 3 hr after infection.

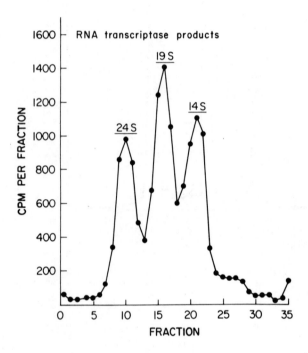

Fig. 4. Sucrose density gradient (5-20 percent) analysis of
labeled ssRNA synthesized in vitro by the RNA transcriptase of
subviral particles isolated from reovirus-infected mouse fibroblasts 10 hr after infection. Subviral particles were purified in
CsCl gradients, incubated with labeled nucleoside triphosphates in
the standard incubation system, and the RNA products of this incubation were analyzed in sucrose density gradients. All 3 size
classes of reovirus ssRNA were synthesized.

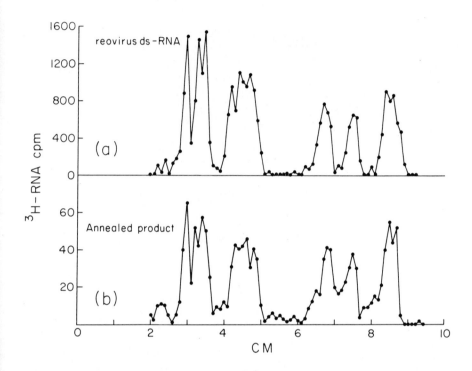

Fig. 5. Acrylamide gel electrophoretic analysis of reovirus (^{3}H)dsRNA(a) and the (^{3}H)dsRNA annealed product(b) obtained by annealing unlabeled denatured dsRNA with a large excess of the (^{3}H)ssRNA"plus"strands synthesized by the RNA transcriptase of the subviral particles isolated from reovirus-infected mouse fibroblasts. (See Fig.4). All 10"plus"strand species of reovirus mRNA were present in the reannealed dsRNA.

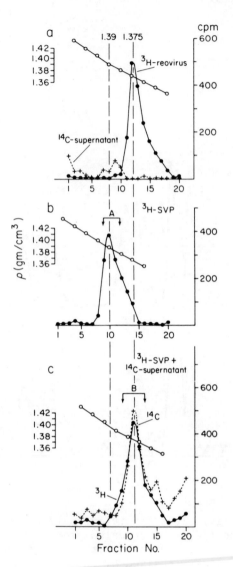

Fig. 6. Buoyant density analysis in CsCl of in vitro assembly of
(^{3}H)protein-labeled subviral particles and (^{14}C)-labeled supernatant proteins from reovirus-infected mouse fibroblasts. Cells
were infected with (^{3}H)-leucine-labeled reovirus (70 PFU/cell) in
the presence of 20 µg/ml cycloheximide for 10 hr. The (^{3}H) subviral particles were isolated (panel b) and incubated with (^{14}C)-
labeled proteins contained in the high speed supernatant of reovirus-infected cells; the reassembled particles (panel c) contained
both labels at the density of the mature virion. Mixing of the
(^{3}H) parental virion with the (^{14}C) protein supernatant produced
no change (panel a).

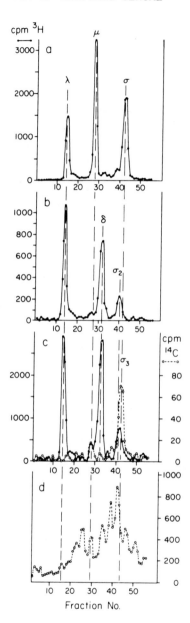

Fig. 7. Acrylamide gel electrophoresis of the proteins in the (^{3}H)protein-labeled subviral particles and the reassembled virions recovered from the CsCl gradients described in Fig. 6. (a) (^{3}H)-leucine labeled reovirus; (b) (^{3}H) subviral particles (Fig. 6b); (c) reassembled particles with both labels (Fig. 6c); and (d) (^{14}C)supernatant proteins.

TABLE 2

INCORPORATION OF (^{3}H)UTP INTO REOVIRUS RNA
CATALYZED BY IN VIVO UNCOATED SVP's INCUBATED
IN THE PRESENCE AND ABSENCE OF CHYMOTRYPSIN

Minutes of incubation	Acid-precipitable cpm:	
	-chymotr.	+chymotr.
0	510	550
30	2200	2150
60	3800	3900
90	6800	6900

SVP's were incubated for RNA synthesis in the presence of (^{3}H)UTP. One reaction mixture contained chymotrypsin (50 μg/ml). At the indicated time intervals,aliquots of each reaction mixture were analyzed for acid-precipitable radioactivity.

(Fig. 8), demonstrating that the RNA transcriptase has been masked and not inactivated (16).

Based on these observations, we feel justified in assuming that the transcriptase activity observed in the large granule fraction is due to progeny SVP's. These amplify the transcriptase activity of SVP's derived from parental virions. Completion of these SVP's by the addition of outer capsomere proteins terminates their role in messenger RNA synthesis.

dsRNA

Reovirus dsRNA is formed by sequential synthesis of its complementary strands (17). This has been determined by analyzing the distribution of ^{3}H-uridine in the complementary strands of in vivo synthesized dsRNA. Newly synthesized ^{3}H-uridine labeled dsRNA was isolated, thermally denatured, and reannealed in the presence of a large excess of unlabeled "plus" strands. These reannealed duplex molecules contain the original "minus" strands,

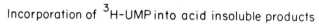

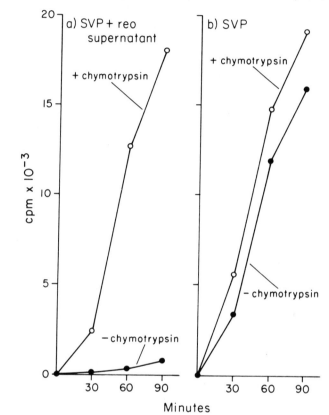

Fig. 8.   RNA transcriptase activity of subviral particles and reassembled particles.   L-cells were infected with 3,330 PFU/cell of reovirus in the presence of 20 µg/ml cycloheximide for 10 hr. The (^{3}H) subviral particles were isolated; a portion was reassembled with soluble viral proteins (see Fig. 6) and separated from subviral particles by centrifugation in CsCl.   The subviral particles (panel b) and the reassembled particles (panel a) were assayed for RNA transcriptase by the incorporation of labeled (^{3}H)UMP into ssRNA in the presence and absence of chymotrypsin.

but the original "plus" strands have been displaced. Subsequent
treatment of this mixture with RNase in 0.3 M NaCl results in
degradation of ssRNA but not of dsRNA. The amount of radiolabel
retained in the re-annealed dsRNA is a direct measure of the radiolabel present in the "minus" strand of the original duplex molecule. When infected cells are exposed to a 30 min pulse of ^{3}H-
uridine during the mid-logarithmic phase of viral replication and
the distribution of radiolabel in the complementary strands of
dsRNA is analyzed, over 95 percent of the uridine label is found
in "minus" strands (Table 3). In contrast, dsRNA obtained from
cells incubated continuously with ^{3}H-uridine is equally labeled in
its complementary strands (Table 3).

The in vitro synthesis of dsRNA is catalyzed by the large
granule fraction from reovirus-infected cells (8, 18, 19). Analysis of the in vitro-synthesized dsRNA by polyacrylamide gel
electrophoresis shows it to contain all ten species of reovirus
dsRNA in roughly the same proportion as in the mature virus
(Fig. 9). Annealing experiments demonstrate that the in vitro
synthesized dsRNA is labeled exclusively in the "minus" strands.
Hence, both in vivo and in vitro, dsRNA is formed by the sequential
synthesis of its complementary strands (Table 4).

Since there is no pool of "minus" strands in reovirus infected
cells, it seemed likely that "minus" strands are formed on preformed
"plus" strand templates.

To test whether dsRNA formation is dependent upon ssRNA templates, the large granule fraction was incubated for dsRNA synthesis in the presence of RNase. Addition of RNase to the reaction
mixture at the beginning of the reaction abolished dsRNA synthesis
completely. However, addition of RNase to the reaction mixture
after the synthesis of dsRNA was completed had no effect on the
newly synthesized dsRNA (Table 5). Decreasing the salt concentration of the reaction mixture to a level which permitted the complete RNase digestion of exogenously added reovirus dsRNA did not
alter this result. Several conclusions may be drawn from these
results:

1) dsRNA is formed by the synthesis of "minus" strands on
   ssRNA templates.

2) The "plus" strands, which are precursors of and templates for
   dsRNA formation, reside within a structure which is per-
   meable to ribonuclease.

3) Newly synthesized dsRNA resides within a structure which is
   impermeable to ribonuclease.

Double-stranded RNA contained within SVP's derived from chy-
motrypsin-treated virions is also nuclease resistant. Moreover,

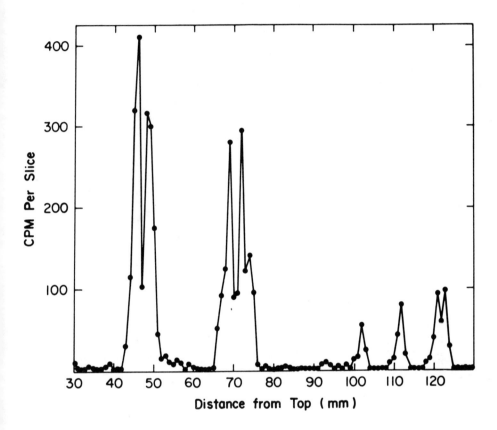

Fig. 9. Acrylamide gel electrophoresis of reovirus dsRNA synthesized in vitro. The large granule fraction of reovirus-infected
L-cells was extracted 10 hr after infection. RNA synthesis was
allowed to proceed in vitro in the presence of labeled precursors.
The dsRNA was isolated and analyzed. Its profile is similar to
viral dsRNA (see Fig. 5), indicating that all 10"minus"strands of
reovirus dsRNA were synthesized proportionately.

TABLE 3

DISTRIBUTION OF (^{3}H)URIDINE IN COMPLEMENTARY STRANDS OF dsRNA AFTER
CONTINUOUS- AND PULSE-LABELING

Expt. No.	Period of (^{3}H)uridine labeling (hr)	Acid-insoluble, RNase-resistant radioactivity(cpm)[*]			
		(a)	(b) After denaturation	(c) After reannealing with excess[**] unlabeled "plus"-strands	Ratio (c)/(a)
1	0-9	50,500	437	28,500	0.55
1	8-8.5	5,450	245	5,440	1.00
2	0-11	52,000	60	28,800	0.56
2	11-11.5	12,400	75	12,400	1.01

L-cell-reovirus complexes were formed at a multiplicity of 100 PFU/cell. The infected cells were resuspended in warmed medium containing 0.5 μg/ml of actinomycin D at a concentration of 3 x 10⁶ cells/ml, divided into two portions, and incubated at 37°C. (^{3}H)uridine (10 μCi/ml) was added to one aliquot of cells at the end of the adsorption period (time = 0) and was present throughout the experiment. The second aliquot of cells was labeled with (^{3}H)uridine (10 μCi/ml) for the half-hour preceding termination of the experiment (time = 8-8.5 or 11-11.5 hr). Incorporation of (^{3}H)uridine was stopped by the addition of an equal volume of frozen isotonic saline and the cells were harvested by centrifugation. The conditions used for RNA extraction, denaturation, and annealing are described in the text.

[*] Samples were digested with 8 μg/ml of pancreatic RNase in 0.3 M NaCl-0.02 M Tris·HCl (pH 7.4) for 30 min and assayed for acid-insoluble radioactivity (12). The aliquots used for analysis in Expt.2 were proportionately smaller. [**] Eight-fold (A260) excess.

TABLE 4

IN VITRO SYNTHESIS OF THE "MINUS" STRAND OF
REOVIRUS dsRNA

Treatment of dsRNA synthesized in vitro	Acid-precipitable cpm in dsRNA	
	Expt. 1	Expt. 2
Untreated	4,550	4,125
RNase (in 0.3 M NaCl)	4,350	3,950
RNase (in 0.03 M NaCl)	200	110
Denatured, reannealed with excess "plus" strands, RNase (in 0.3 M NaCl)	4,310	3,760

A large granule fraction was prepared from reovirus-infected L-cells 9 hr after infection. The fraction was incubated for RNA synthesis for 30 min in the presence of radiolabeled precursors; dsRNA was isolated and the amount of label in the "minus" strand was determined as described in the text. For the two experiments shown, the percent of total label incorporated into the "minus" strand was 99 and 95, respectively.

TABLE   5

EFFECT OF RIBONUCLEASE ON dsRNA
SYNTHESIS IN VITRO

RNase addition	Acid-precipitable cpm in dsRNA
Not added	7,931
15-30 min	6,904
0-30 min	1,012

At the indicated time intervals, ribonuclease
(10 μg/ml) was added to the reaction mixtures
containing the large granule fraction. Total
RNA was extracted with phenol and the acid-
precipitable radioactivity in the isolated
dsRNA determined.

these SVP's and the RNA transcriptase they contain are resistant
to digestion by chymotrypsin. Chymotrypsin treatment of the large
particle fraction has no effect on the rate or extent of dsRNA
synthesis. Hence, SVP's in the process of maturation appear to be
responsible for the formation of dsRNA. Recently, Zweerink et al.
(18) and Wantanabe et al. (19) have presented data in agreement
with this hypothesis.

The similarities in location and chymotrypsin resistance of
both the dsRNA synthetase and RNA transcriptase prompted us to
search for other properties of these enzymes which might confirm
their identity. Reovirus RNA transcriptase exhibits a temperature optimum of 45°C; the dsRNA synthetase is also maximally
active at this temperature. These data suggest that the dsRNA
synthetase and the ssRNA transcriptase are alternative activities
of the same proteins, and that these proteins form the SVP.

OLIGO A SYNTHESIS

Approximately 20 percent of the RNA molecules contained within reovirus are single-stranded oligomers, 6-12 nucleotides in length, composed principally of adenylic acid. The large granule or virus-factory-containing fraction of reovirus-infected cells synthesize oligo A which migrates in polyacrylamide gel together with or slightly faster than oligo A extracted from purified virions (Fig. 10). The enzyme is specific for ATP. It is not inhibited by pre-treatment of the large granule fraction with RNase or DNase (Fig. 11).

Incubation of the large granule fraction with chymotrypsin, which stimulates ssRNA synthesis and does not affect dsRNA synthesis, completely inhibits oligo A synthesis (20). Polyacrylamide gel analysis of the proteins remaining in the large granule fraction after chymotrypsin digestion shows that the proteins which compose the viral core (λ_1, λ_2, and σ_3) have been conserved, while the outer capsomere proteins have either been lost (σ_1 and σ_3)or altered (μ_2 cleaved to δ) (20).

The precise location of oligo A within the reovirion has not been identified. Digestion of reovirus with chymotrypsin removes the outer capsomeres and the oligo A. To test whether the in vitro synthesized oligo A behaves similarly, a large granule fraction was incubated with ^{3}H-ATP and then digested with chymotrypsin. The in vitro synthesized oligo A is released from the particulate fraction following this treatment (Fig. 12), indicating that it resides within a structure which is similar to reovirus in its sensitivity to proteolysis by chymotrypsin.

The chymotrypsin sensitivity of the oligo A synthetase seemed to distinguish this enzymatic activity from the SVP-associated dsRNA synthetase and ssRNA transcriptase. We therefore examined the temperature dependence of the oligo A synthetase. The temperature optimum of the oligo A synthetase is 45°C, a value identical to that of the single and double-strand polymerizing enzyme(s). The nearly parallel temperature dependence of these three activities suggests that the oligo A synthetase is yet another activity of the enzyme(s) within the SVP (Fig. 13).

DISCUSSION

Based on findings from several laboratories, as well as those outlined here, the replicative cycle of reovirus has been established in some detail. Shortly after infection, the intact virion is segregated within lysosomes where cellular hydrolases selectively degrade the outer capsomeres. The resultant subviral particle

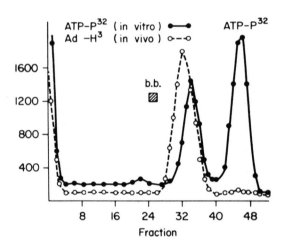

Fig. 10. Analysis by acrylamide gel electrophoresis of reovirus
oligo A synthesized in vivo and in vitro. (^{3}H)Adenosine-labeled
oligo A was isolated from purified reovirus. For the in vitro
oligo A, the large granule fraction, isolated from reovirus-
infected L-cells 10 hr after infection, was incubated with (^{32}P)
ATP for 30 min. The (^{32}P)oligo A was isolated and co-electro-
phoresed with the in vivo (^{3}H)oligo A and a marker of bromphenol
blue (bb).

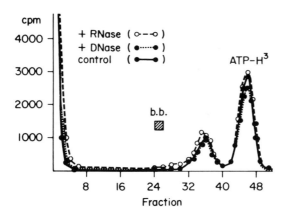

Fig. 11. Effect of ribonuclease and deoxyribonuclease on the in vitro synthesis of reovirus oligo A. The large granule fraction was isolated from reovirus-infected L-cells 10 hr after infection. In separate reaction mixtures, oligo A synthesis from (^{3}H)ATP was allowed to proceed in the presence of RNase (8 µg/ml) or DNase (10 µg/ml). The labeled oligo A products were compared with (^{3}H) oligo A from a control incubation mixture by electrophoresis on parallel acrylamide gels. (bb) = bromophenol blue dye marker.

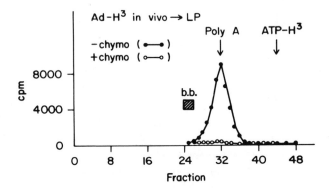

Fig. 12.   Effect of chymotrypsin on the retention of oligo A by
reovirions.   (^{3}H)Adenosine-labeled large granule fractions were
isolated from reovirus-infected cultures grown in the presence
of the label for 10 hr.   One portion was treated with chymotrypsin
(100 μg/ml) for 30 min and precipitated with 8 percent trichloroacetic acid.   An untreated portion was similarly precipitated.
The precipitates were dissolved and electrophoresed on separate
acrylamide gels with bromphenol blue markers.   Only the untreated
fraction retained (^{3}H)oligo A in the precipitate.

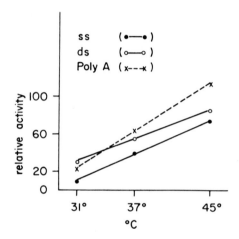

Fig. 13. Temperature optima for the synthesis of reovirus dsRNA, ssRNA, and oligo A.

is the functional unit of infection and is preserved intact throughout the replication cycle. This SVP contains its own RNA transcriptase in association with the dsRNA genome and synthesizes all 10 ssRNA species by transcribing one strand of each dsRNA segment. Neither strand of the genome template is displaced during transcription, indicating a conservative transcription mechanism.

The "plus" strands synthesized by these SVP's have dual functions: they serve as messengers for viral protein synthesis, and they form templates for dsRNA synthesis. At early times in the viral replicative cycle, it is possible that some "plus" strands function first as messenger RNAs, and subsequently combine with the proteins for which they coded to form SVP's. Subviral particles, containing ssRNAs, are responsible for the synthesis of complementary "minus" strands, thereby forming dsRNA. After dsRNA is formed, these SVP's become impermeable to nucleases and synthesize new "plus" strands. The final steps in the formation of the virus are the synthesis of oligo A and the addition of outer capsomere proteins.

The chymotrypsin resistance, temperature optimum, particulate location, and effect of nucleases upon the activities of reovirus dsRNA synthetase and ssRNA transcriptase, lead us to the conclusion that these two polymerases are alternative activities of the same protein(s), and that these protein(s) are the structural units of the SVP. Reagents which destroy the structural integrity of the SVP inactivate the ssRNA transcriptase to the same extent that they release dsRNA from it.

It seems likely that the oligo A synthetase is a third activity of the core polymerase(s), and that this activity, like that of the ssRNA transcriptase, is governed by outer capsomere proteins. Since oligo A is formed after dsRNA in the sequence of viral maturation, we suggest that addition of outer capsomere proteins to the maturing SVP alters the conformation and/or enzymatic activity of the RNA transcriptase, converting it to an oligo A synthetase. The function of oligo A in the viral replicative cycle remains obscure. Perhaps its synthesis governs the rate of maturation of SVP's to virions. In any case, it is important to note that some outer capsomere proteins are required for the expression of the oligo A synthetase, while the presence of another outer capsomere protein, σ_3, inhibits the expression of the RNA transcriptase.

REFERENCES

1. KATES, J.R., AND MACAUSLAN, B.R. (1967). Proc.Nat.Acad.Sci.
    U.S.A., 58, 134-141.
2. TEMIN, H.M. & MIZUTANI, S. (1970). Nature, 226, 1211-1213.
3. BALTIMORE, D. (1970). Nature, 226, 1209-1211.
4. BORSA, Y. & GRAHAM, A.F. (1968). Biochem.Biophys.Res.Commun.
    33, 895-901.
5. SHATKIN, A.Y. & SIPE, J.D. (1968). Proc.Nat.Acad.Sci. U.S.A.,
    61, 1462-1469.
6. GOMATOS, P.J. (1970). J. of Virology, 6, 610-620.
7. SKEHEL, J.J. & JOKLIK, W.K. (1969). Virology, 39, 822-831.
8. ACS, G., KLETT, H., SCHONBERG, M., CHRISTMAN, J., LEVIN, D.H.,
    & SILVERSTEIN, S. (1971). J. of Virology, 8, 684-689.
9. SAKUMA, S. & WATANABE, Y. (1972). J. of Virology, 10, 943-950.
10. BELLAMY, A.R. & JOKLIK, W.K. (1967). Proc.Nat.Acad.Sci.
    U.S.A., 58, 1389-1395.
11. BANERJEE, A.K. & SHATKIN, A.J. (1970). J. of Virology, 6,
    1-11.
12. HAY, A.J. & JOKLIK, W.K. (1971). Virology, 44, 450-453.
13. LEVIN, D., MENDELSOHN, N., SCHONBERG, M., KLETT, H., ACS, G.,
    SILVERSTEIN, S., & KAPULER, A. (1970). Proc.Nat.Acad.Sci.
    U.S.A., 66, 890-897.
14. SILVERSTEIN, S.C. & DALES, S. (1968). J.Cell.Biol. 36,
    197-230.
15. SILVERSTEIN, S., ASTELL, C., LEVIN, D.H., SCHONBERG, M. &
    ACS, G. (1972). Virology, 47, 797-806.
16. ASTELL, C., SILVERSTEIN, S.C., LEVIN, D.H. & ACS, G. (1972).
    Virology, 48, 648-654.
17. SCHONBERG, M., SILVERSTEIN, S.C., LEVIN, D.H. & ACS, G.
    (1971). Proc.Nat.Acad.Sci. U.S.A., 68, 505-508.
18. ZWEERINK, H.J., ITO, Y. & MATSUHISA, T. (1972). Virology,
    50, 349-358.
19. WATANABE, Y., PREVEC, L. & GRAHAM, A.F. (1967). Proc.Nat.
    Acad.Sci. U.S.A., 58, 1040-1046.
20. SILVERSTEIN, S., KLETT, H., CHRISTMAN, J. & ACS, G.
    (In preparation).

SV40 DNA MOLECULES WHICH CONTAIN HOST CELL DNA

Ernest Winocour, Niza Frenkel, Sara Lavi and
Shmuel Rozenblatt

Department of Genetics, Weizmann Institute of Science
Rehovot, Israel

Closed-circular SV40 DNA molecules, in which parts of the viral genome are deleted and replaced by covalently-linked cell DNA (called substituted SV40 DNA) are produced in monkey BS-C-1 cells infected under certain conditions (1,2). The proportions of such substituted molecules in the yield depend upon the multiplicity of infection and the passage history of the inoculum (2). Although substituted SV40 DNA molecules are defective with respect to plaque formation, they nevertheless replicate in cells infected at high multiplicity (3), presumably by complementation with non-substituted virus. The proportion and types of host sequences in the substituted viral genome have been found to vary in different populations. In one population examined, the host sequences comprised as much as 60 percent of the substituted viral genome (4). By hybridization analysis, these host sequences were found to be both of the reiterated and non-reiterated type (4,5). In other populations, the host sequences were almost exclusively of the non-reiterated type (4). We have compared, by homology tests, the host sequences in three independently-derived populations of substituted SV40 DNA molecules (4). Populations A and B were derived by independent sets of high-multiplicity serial passages, starting from the same plaque purified virus stock; population C arose during the serial passage of non-plaque purified virus. No detectable cross-homology was found between the host sequences of populations A and B; on the other hand, population C contained a significant fraction of host sequences which was homologous to those in both the A and B populations. Hence, the host sequences in substituted SV40 cannot represent a random sample of the total sequences present in the mammalian genome. The number of different families of host sequences that can be incorporated into the SV40 genome is clearly limited.

The primary recombination events which give rise to the sub-stituted viral genome have yet to be clarified. It appears highly likely, however, that the recombination process involves the chro-mosomal integration of virus DNA followed by the excision of linked viral and cellular sequences. Evidence supporting the con-cept of viral integration during the lytic infection of monkey cells by SV40 has been obtained from studies on the RNA metabolism of infected cells (6,7) which demonstrate the presence of "giant" RNA molecules containing covalently-linked cell-specific and virus-specific sequences (7). Thus, the types of host sequences in sub-stituted SV40 most probably reflect the number and nature of the viral integration sites on the host genome. On this basis, our results to date suggest (a) that the integration of SV40 DNA into the monkey cell genome occurs at a limited number of sites, and (b) that the integration sites are closer to the non-reiterated families of cell sequences rather than to reiterated families.

Although defective with respect to plaque-formation, sub-stituted SV40 may possess other biological activities. Our attempts to assess the biological properties of the substituted virus have been hindered by the fact that we have not so far suc-ceeded in obtaining populations which are completely free of "wild type" non-substituted virus. If substituted SV40 integrates and transforms cells, we may be faced with the difficult task of deciding which of the genes introduced by the virus is responsible for the transformation - the truly viral genes or the cellular genes which are linked to the viral genes. The amount of non-reiterated host DNA (1000-2000 base pairs) is certainly sufficient to code for a few gene products. Closed-circular viral DNA mole-cules containing covalently-linked host DNA sequences have also recently been found in serially-passaged isolates of polyoma virus (S. Lavi and E. Winocour, in preparation). Thus, the phenomenon of recombination between viral and host genomes during lytic infec-tion may be a general feature of the DNA tumor viruses. It is an exciting, but at the same time a rather sobering thought, that these viruses may be responsible for the transfer and stable inte-gration of cellular genetic information.

REFERENCES

1. ALONI, Y., WINOCOUR, E., SACHS, L. & TORTEN, J.; 1969. *J. Mol. Biol. 44*, 333.
2. LAVI, S. & WINOCOUR, E.; 1972. *J. Virol. 9*, 309.
3. LAVI, S., ROZENBLATT, S., SINGER, M.F. & WINOCOUR, E.; 1973. *J. Virol.* (In press).
4. FRENKEL, N. & WINOCOUR, E.; 1973. Submitted for publication.
5. ROZENBLATT, S., LAVI, S., SINGER, F.M. & WINOCOUR, E.; 1973. *J. Virol.* (In press).
6. WEINBERG, R.A., WARNAAR, S.O. & WINOCOUR, E.; 1972. *J. Virol. 10*, 193.
7. ROZENBLATT, S. & WINOCOUR, E.; 1972. *Virology 50*, 558.

STUDIES ON THE REPLICASE OF ENCEPHALOMYOCARDITIS VIRUS

B. Diskin, H. Rosenberg and A. Traub

Biochemistry Department, Israel Institute for
Biological Research, Ness Ziona, Israel

The RNA-dependent RNA polymerases (replicases) of the small RNA animal viruses which belong to the picornavirus group (polio, mengo, encephalomyocarditis, etc.) were discovered about ten years ago (1). They were found in the cytoplasm of infected cells, bound to relatively large structures, sedimenting between 200 to 300 S. The enzyme is associated with a double-stranded RNA template - a duplex made of a parental viral RNA strand and its complementary strand. It is the complementary (-) strand of the duplex which serves as template for the transcription of molecules of progeny viral RNA which are then incorporated into virions.

Quite a few attempts were made to isolate a soluble, RNA-dependent replicase from cells infected with a picornavirus, but until now without success. As is well-known, the main progress in this field was made with the replicases of the RNA bacteriophages, mainly with that of bacteriophage Qβ. The new information gained on the structure of Qβ replicase, and particularly on the mode whereby it is assembled, mostly from preexisting E.coli proteins, has led to the impression that we are dealing here not only with formation of a new viral enzyme, but also with a mechanism involved in regulation of host and viral functions, and therefore of general interest for the understanding of the process of infection with an RNA virus, including infection with animal RNA viruses.

I would like, therefore, first to review very briefly the recent work on Qβ replicase. The current picture of Qβ replicase

295

is that of a complex protein composed of four polypeptide subunits
of approximate molecular weights (I) 70,000; (II) 65,000; (III)
45,000; and (IV) 35,000 daltons, respectively. Of the four subunits, the formation of only one, polypeptide (II), is coded by the
viral genome. The other three are pre-existing E.coli proteins
which have been incorporated into the structure of the new replicase after infection. This is the core enzyme. It uses a double
stranded RNA template and transcribes the complementary viral RNA
strand of the duplex. The same enzyme can also function as a poly
C-dependent poly G polymerase when provided with a poly C template.
This property proved to be of utmost importance for the isolation
of the core enzyme, since poly C could be used as template for the
assay of enzyme activity (2-7).

When infection is first initiated by penetration of a molecule of parental viral RNA strand, early synthesis of complementary
strands upon the parental RNA template occurs. This function requires, in addition to the core enzyme, two additional E.coli proteins. This is the holoenzyme, composed of a single virus-coded
protein and five E.coli proteins. Recent work (8,9) aimed at
identifying the E.coli proteins of Qβ core replicase has shown
that subunits III and IV are identical to E.coli elongation factors Tu and Ts, and subunit I to interference factor i, found to
stimulate initiation of translation of the replicase cistron and
inhibit translation of coat protein cistron from mRNA and Qβ
bacteriophages.

Currently there is no information on whether a similar mode
of assembly of replicase occurs also in animal cells infected with
an RNA virus of the picornavirus group. This is due to the fact
that the replicases of these viruses have not yet been isolated
in pure form and analysis of their subunit composition could not
be carried out.

Our present studies have been concerned with the isolation of
the replicase of EMC virus.

As enzyme source we use BHK 21 cells infected for 7 h with
EMC virus. When the cells are homogenized in a hypotonic medium
and fractionated by centrifugation, most of the replicase activity
is found in the post-mitochondrial fraction. Replicase is taken
to mean a complex of enzyme and an endogenous viral RNA template.
It has been shown by Caliguiri and Tamm (10) that in HeLa cells
infected with poliovirus, incorporation of labeled uridine occurs
into viral RNA which is found associated with a smooth membrane
fraction. This fraction was shown to manifest activity of polio
replicase. We have therefore separated the post-mitochondrial
fraction by isopycnic gradient centrifugation in a 20-60 percent

discontinuous sucrose gradient and analyzed the different fractions, for replicase, protein and lipid phosphorus. (Table 1).
The greater part of the enzyme is found in the second fraction
from the top (Fraction 2), at a sucrose density of 1.080 g/cm^3.
(When uninfected cells are fractionated by this method, Fraction 2
is found to contain the smooth membranes of the endoplasmic reticulum.) Fraction 2 from infected cells contains 30 percent of the
total lipid P, but only 1.5 percent of the protein. The ratio
between protein and lipid P is typical for the composition of
membrane material. The isopycnic gradient isolation step achieves
about a 40-fold enzyme purification with retention of about 50
percent of the original activity. It was clearly revealed that we
were dealing with an enzyme that is tightly bound to membrane.
The enzyme could be sedimented, after dilution of the sucrose, and
obtained in a membraneous pellet. An electron-micrograph of the
membrane pellet, taken after negative staining, is shown in Fig.1.
The membranes have a unique structure which is not found in uninfected BHK cells. They are arranged in multi-layers and form
closed concentric circles. Similar structures were first described
by Amako and Dales (11) in L cells infected with mengo virus. It
should be pointed out that the amount of smooth membranes found in
Fraction 2 obtained from infected cells is about five-fold greater
than that obtained from a similar preparation of uninfected cells.
This reflects the extensive synthesis of new membranes that take
place during infection.

Rapid proliferation of smooth membranes in cells infected
with picornaviruses was described before by Penman (12), Amako and
Dales (11), and Caliguiri and Tamm (10). By following the distribution of radioactive choline, added before or after infection,
these authors showed that the membranes formed after infection are
composed of a mixture of old and new membrane material. It is not
yet known whether this is a result of degradation of the old cellular membranes to the molecular level, followed by incorporation
of the precursors into new membranes, together with newly-synthe-
sized precursors, formed after infection; or whether the new
membranes are in fact a mosaic made of stretches of old and new
membranes. The molecular mechanism that triggers such an extensive membrane synthesis during infection is not known. However,
it should be pointed out that it is in striking contrast to the
almost complete inhibition of synthesis of other major cell components such as RNA, protein and DNA - all occurring at an early
stage of infection. The viruses of the picornavirus group are
composed of RNA and protein, and are not enveloped by a lipopro-
tein membrane. The synthesis of new membranes after infection was
considered as an aberrant event, a "cytopathic effect" with no
functional relationship to virus replication. However, the

TABLE 1

DISTRIBUTION OF EMC REPLICASE, PROTEIN AND LIPID P IN THE ISOPYCNIC SUCROSE GRADIENT FRACTIONS*

Fraction	Percent Sucrose in Fraction	Replicase (units)**	Protein (mg)	Specific Activity (units/mg protein)	Lipid P (μmoles)
Cytoplasmi extract	-	5200	81.60	63.7	13.86
Fraction 1	10.2	120	0.75	160.0	0.69
Fraction 2	18.0	2640	1.20	2203.0	5.10
Fraction 3	26.0	450	6.48	69.0	4.14
Fraction 4	28.0	165	20.00	8.2	0.83
Fraction 5	32.0	172	23.10	7.4	0.96
Fraction 6	40.0	185	13.50	13.6	0.82
Fraction 7	46.5	160	7.80	20.0	0.86
Fraction 8	51.0	158	6.46	26.8	0.045
Pellet	-	86	0.65	14.3	-

* Prepared from 3x10^9 infected cells.

** 10 μl aliquots were assayed for replicase activity as described in (14).

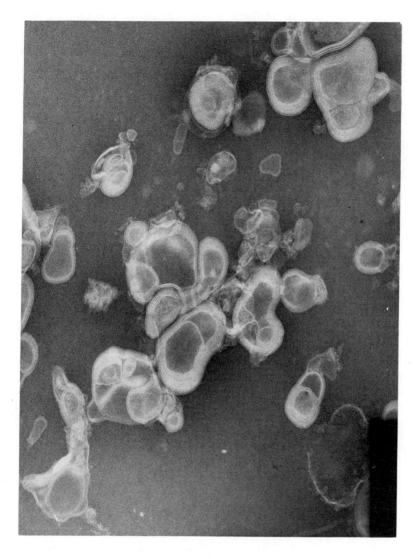

Fig. 1. Electron microscopy of pellet of Fraction 2. A negative
stained preparation was made with 2 percent phosphotungstic acid
(x 165,000).

finding that EMC replicase and its RNA template are bound to newly-
formed smooth membranes suggest that these membranes probably ful-
fill an essential function in the synthesis of viral RNA.

Up to this stage we were dealing with a complex of enzyme and
template RNA bound to a smooth membrane; the next step was to extract the enzyme from the membrane and separate it from its template RNA. This was dependent on the availability of an alternative RNA or other polynucleotide template with which to assay the
activity of the extracted enzyme. Indeed, the rapid advance in
the purification of Qβ replicase was made possible only after the
finding that core replicase functions also as a poly C-dependent
poly G polymerase, and thus could be assayed with a poly C template.

Our approach, therefore, was to examine if EMC replicase acts
also as a poly C-dependent poly G polymerase after removal of the
associated RNA template. Removal of RNA was carried out by digestion with micrococcal nuclease. However, degradation of the RNA
could be performed only after a prior separation of the replicase-
RNA complex from most of the membrane material. Only then did the
RNA become susceptible to nuclease action. This was done in the
following way: Fraction 2 membranes were preincubated with 0.02 M
dithiothreitol and 0.05 percent Triton X-100, and then centrifuged
at 50,000 rpm (Spinco rotor SW50) through a 4.5 ml, 5-20 percent
sucrose gradient containing 0.02 M dithiothreitol and 0.05 percent
Triton X-100 (Fig. 2). The pellet, containing about 50 percent of
the replicase activity and only 2 percent of the lipid P, was then
digested with micrococcal nuclease. Activity of the nuclease was
terminated by chelating the Ca^{++} ions with ethyleneglycol-bis-
(aminoethyl ether)-N, N-tetraacetic acid (EGTA), and the treated
pellet was assayed for activity of poly C-dependent poly G polymerase (Fig. 3). We observed a definite response to poly C. This
was taken as an indication that when once solubilized and separated
from its RNA template, EMC replicase may also be assayed during
further purification steps for an assay for activity of poly G
polymerase.

Various attempts were now made to extract the enzyme from the
membranes: extraction with high salt, non-ionic detergents, digestion with phospholipase C, etc. - all with negative results. This
led to the use of the ultimate weapon of membrane chemistry: sodium
dodecyl sulfate (SDS): Fraction 2 membranes were preincubated with
0.02 M dithiothreitol and 0.05 percent Triton X-100 and then
treated with 0.3 percent SDS. The clarified solution was passed
rapidly through a small Dowex column in 0.05 M sodium phosphate
buffer pH 7.0 for rapid removal of SDS and viral RNA (13). The
protein was eluted first with TMG buffer (0.01 M Tris HCl pH 7.0,

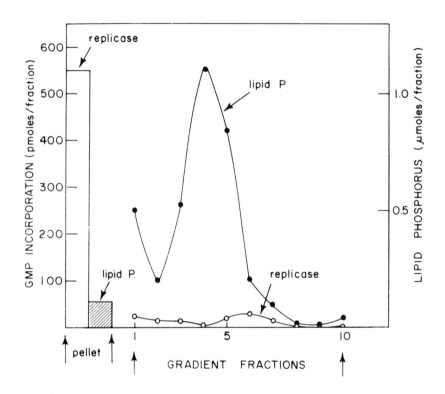

Fig. 2. Separation of EMC replicase from Fraction 2 membranes.
Fraction 2 pellet was treated with 0.02 M dithiothreitol and 0.05
percent Triton X-100 and sedimented for 16 h at 50,000 rpm through
a 4.5 ml 5-20 percent sucrose gradient containing 0.02 M dithiothreitol and 0.05 percent Triton X-100. Lipid P (●——●) and
replicase activity (o——o) were determined in the pellet and
gradient fractions. For details see (14).

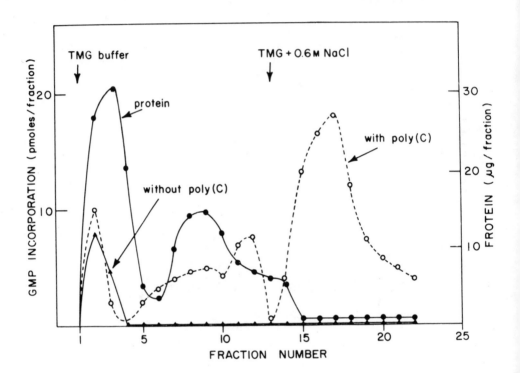

Fig. 3. Dowex-1 chromatography of poly (C)-dependent replicase. The enzyme was extracted from a Fraction 2 pellet by a mixture of dithiothreitol, Triton X-100 and SDS and chromatographed on a 0.5x4 cm Dowex-1 column as detailed in (14). (●——●) protein; (o——o) poly (C)-dependent activity; (▲——▲) endogenous template RNA-dependent activity.

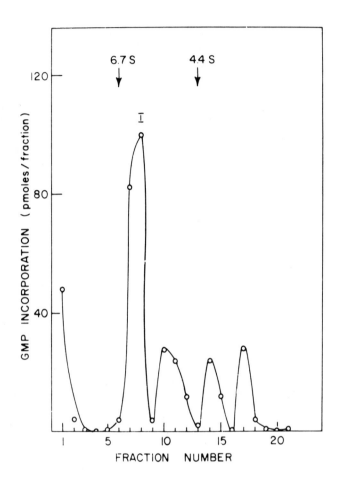

Fig. 4. Glycerol gradient centrifugation of poly (C)-dependent replicase. Pooled active fractions of the 0.6 M NaCl eluate from the Dowex-1 column were loaded on a 5-20 percent glycerol gradient, centrifuged and assayed for activity as described in (14). Alcohol dehydrogenase (6.7 S) and bovine serum albumin (4.4 S) were used as sedimentation markers. (o——o) poly (C)-dependent replicase activity.

0.01 M MgCl$_2$, 5 percent glycerol),and then with TMG buffer containing 0.6 M NaCl (Fig. 4). The fractions were assayed for
endogenous RNA-dependent replicase and for poly C dependent poly G
polymerase. The first portion of the eluting TMG buffer contained
most of the protein, some endogenous RNA-dependent replicase, and
some poly G polymerase. Elution with salt released a barely detectable amount of protein, but a significant amount of poly G
polymerase.

     SDS is of course a very strong medicine with unpleasant
side effects. It results in about a 90 percent loss of enzyme
activity, but at the present time this is the only means we have
to release the enzyme from association with RNA and membrane. It
should be mentioned that also in the case of the Qβ replicase,
separation between template RNA and protein constituted a major
difficulty in the purification of the enzyme. In the mammalian
system, there is the additional need to separate the enzyme from
membrane.

     The enzyme in the 0.6 M NaCl eluate was further purified by
centrifugation through a 5-20 percent glycerol gradient
(20 h/25,000 rpm;Spinco rotor SW25.1)(Fig.4). We found a peak of
activity at a region corresponding to a sedimentation coefficient
of about 6 S, but there is also some tailing of activity at upper
regions of the gradient. We do not yet know whether the heavy
peak is due to aggregation of a lighter protein or whether the
lighter peaks indicate a certain change in the conformation of the
enzyme as a result of the SDS treatment. It may also be due to
loss of subunits. A summary of the purification procedure is
presented in Table 2. It should be noted that although there is
an 850-fold purification, we obtain in the end only a few micrograms of protein. Indeed, at this stage the enzyme is extremely
labile, with a half-life of between 2-4 h.

     The enzyme found in the 6S peak was further analyzed by SDS-
polyacrylamide-gel electrophoresis (Fig. 5). The bands correspond   to approximate molecular weights of (I) 72,000; (II)
65,000; (III) 57,000; (IV) 45,000 and (V) 35,000 daltons, respectively. With different preparations, there are differences in
stain retention by the polypeptide bands, indicating a quantitative difference in the proportions of the polypeptides. At the
present state of enzyme purification it is not clear whether all
the polypeptides found in the gel are true subunits of EMC poly G
polymerase. This will be clarified only after the isolation of a
larger amount of a homogenous enzyme. However, there seems to be
a remarkable similarity between the molecular weights of the four
subunits of core Qβ replicase (70,000, 65,000, 45,000, 35,000) and

TABLE   2

APPEARANCE OF POLY(C)-DEPENDENT POLY (G) POLYMERASE ACTIVITY AFTER
DIGESTION OF MEMBRANE-FREE PELLET WITH MICROCOCCAL NUCLEASE

Exp. No.	Additions	[^{3}H] GMP incorporation	
		Before Nuclease	After Nuclease
		CPM	CPM
1	None	3,980	96
2	80 µg poly (C)	3,965	780
3	80 µg ribosomal RNA (BHK 21)	3,943	102

The procedure for obtaining the membrane-free pellet and the
digestion with micrococcal nuclease are described in (14).
Twenty-five µl aliquots were assayed for enzyme activity,
using a reaction mixture containing all 4-ribonucleoside
triphosphates, as described in (14).   Omission of ATP, CTP and
UTP in the assay of Exp. 2 did not change the activity.   BHK 21
ribosomal RNA was isolated from purified ribosomes of uninfected
BHK 21 cells.

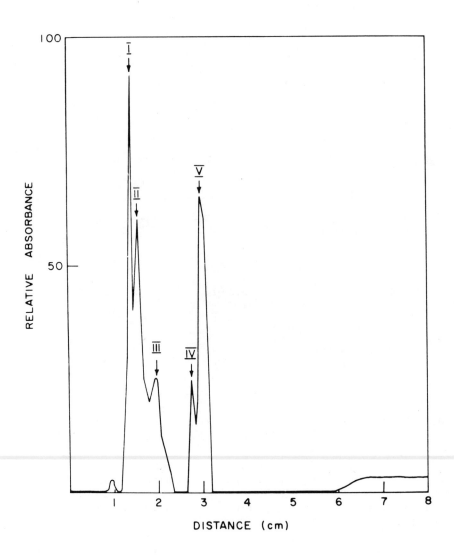

Fig. 5. SDS-polyacrylamide gel electrophoresis of poly (C)-dependent replicase in peak I of glycerol gradient. The SDS-polyacrylamide gels (10 percent) were prepared and run as described by Weber and Osborn (15).

that found for polypeptides I, II, IV and V of the EMC poly G polymerase. This may of course be just fortuitous, but on the other hand, it may indicate that we are dealing with a group of proteins similar in both structure and function, which are present both in E.coli and BHK cells. It may be conceived that during infection with an RNA virus they associate with the virus-coded polypeptide, and together form the core replicase.

This is how far we have come with the isolation procedure. The main difficulty is to separate the enzyme from its RNA template and from association with membrane. So far this could be done by extraction with SDS and at the price of a very substantial loss of enzyme activity. Further progress will largely depend on the successful scaling-up of the isolation procedure, and on finding means whereby to stabilize the activity of the isolated enzyme. It should also be emphasized that, so far, the soluble enzyme that we have isolated shows only an activity of a poly C-dependent poly G polymerase. Although smooth membranes isolated from uninfected cells did not manifest such an activity it still remains to be shown that the poly G polymerase can use also an EMC viral RNA as template. Up till now the addition of EMC RNA did not elicit any response. The isolated enzyme may still lack a subunit essential for the transcription of viral RNA.

REFERENCES

1. BALTIMORE, D. & FRANKLIN, R.M. (1963). J.Biol.Chem 238, 3395-3400.
2. HARUNA, J. & SPIEGELMAN, S. (1965). Proc.Nat.Acad.Sci.USA, 54, 579-587.
3. EIKHOM, T.S. & SPIEGELMAN, S. (1967). Proc.Nat.Acad.Sci.USA, 57, 1833-1840.
4. SHAPIRO, L., FRANZE de FERNANDEX, M.T. & AUGUST, J.T. (1968). Nature, 220, 478-480.
5. KONDO, M., GALLERANI, R. & WEISSMAN, C. (1970). Nature, 228, 525-527.
6. KAMEN, R. (1970). Nature, 228, 527-533.
7. KAMEN, R. (1972). Biochim.Biophys.Acta, 262, 88-100.
8. BLUMENTHAL, T., LANDERS, T.A. & WEBER, K. (1972). Proc.Nat. Acad.Sci.USA, 69, 1313-1317.
9. GRONER, Y., SCHEPS, R., KAMEN, R., KOLAKOFSKY, D. & REVEL, M. (1972). Nature New Biology, 239, 19-20.
10. CALIGUIRI, L.A. & TAMM, I. (1970). Virology, 42, 100-111.
11. AMAKO, K. & DALES, S. (1967). Virology, 32, 201-215.
12. PENMAN, S. (1965). Virology, 25, 148-152.
13. LENARD, J. (1971). Biochem.Biophys.Res.Commun. 45, 662-668.

14.   ROSENBERG, H., DISKIN, B., ORON, L. & TRAUB, A. (1972). <u>Proc</u>.
      <u>Nat.Acad.Sci. USA</u>, <u>69</u>, 3815-3819.

15.   WEBER, K. & OSBORN, M. (1969). <u>J.Biol.Chem</u>. <u>244</u>, 4406-4412.

INDUCTION OF C-TYPE PARTICLES IN MAMMALIAN CANCER CELLS

Y. Becker, Genia Balabanova, Eynat Weinberg and M.Kotler

Laboratory for Molecular Virology, Hebrew University-
Hadassah Medical School, Jerusalem, Israel

INTRODUCTION

Temin postulated (1,2) that the viral DNA synthesized by the oncorna virion-associated reverse transcriptase (3,4) integrates into the host cell DNA as an essential step in the cellular transformation process. The studies of Hill and Hillova, who demonstrated that permissive cells were transformed by purified DNA molecules from transformed cells (5), confirmed Temin's hypothesis. Thus, the oncorna virus-transformed cell contains viral DNA sequences in the cellular genome. The mechanism which leads to the integration of the viral DNA molecules into the cellular DNA is not yet known. Also, the cellular mechanisms which control the expression of the viral DNA are not yet understood. In permissive cells, transformation is accompanied by virus production, while in nonpermissive cells transformation occurs but without virus production. These findings suggest that in nonpermissive cells, the transcription of the viral DNA is controlled by the host cell process. Although the viral DNA is repressed in the nonpermissive cells, it was demonstrated (6) that virus synthesis could be induced by fusion of transformed cells with permissive cells. Treatment with 5-bromodeoxyuridine (BUdR) also induced virus replication (7), similar to the effect of arginine deprivation on nonpermissive cells (8). Although the mechanism of virus induction is not understood, the induction of virus replication was used to study the presence of oncorna viruses in cancer cells.

309

EXPERIMENTAL RESULTS

A. ROUS SARCOMA VIRUS TRANSFORMED RAT CELLS - A MODEL FOR C-TYPE VIRUS INDUCTION

1. RSV-transformed rat cells.

Rous sarcoma virus (RSV)-transformed rat cells (designated R (B77) contain viral genomes but do not produce virions (6,9,10). It is possible to activate a C-type virus from these cells by: a) co-cultivation of the R(B77) cells with permissive cells (6), b) treatment of the transformed cells with 5-bromodeoxyuridine (BUdR) (7), and c) incubation of the cells in an arginine-deficient medium (8). The present study extends our previous results on the induction of C-type virus in R(B77) cells and deals with the time course of virus release from arginine-deprived and BUdR-treated cells.

The R(B77) cell-line of Rous sarcoma virus-transformed rat cells (7,9) was used. The cells were grown in Eagle's minimal essential medium (GIBCO,Grand Island,New York) with 5% tryptose phosphate broth (DIFCO Laboratory, Detroit, Michigan) and 5% calf serum. Cells were grown in Rous bottles at a concentration of 6-8 x 10^7 cells per bottle.

2. Isolation of C-type virus particles.

Two techniques were used to induce C-type particles: a) the cells in Rous bottles were incubated in Eagle's medium deficient in arginine, serum and tryptose phosphate and b) the cells were treated with BUdR, added to the complete Eagle's medium at a concentration of 30 µg/ml, followed by incubation for 24 h. The BUdR-containing medium was removed and the cells were reincubated in fresh medium.

The treated cultures were labeled with uridine-5-T (1 µCi/ml, specific activity 13.8 Ci/mM; obtained from the Nuclear Research Center, Negev, Israel) for 6 hour periods starting at 0, 6, 12, and 18 h after arginine deprivation or BUdR treatment.

Three criteria were used to characterize the C-type particles released from R(B77) cells after treatment with arginine-deficient medium and BUdR: a) sedimentation in sucrose gradients (15-65% w/v) determine the density of the particles, as previously described (8), b) assay for reverse transcriptase activity in purified virions, according to Temin and Mizutani (3) and Baltimore (4). To further characterize the enzymatic activity present in the isolated particles, the response to the polymers poly (rA). oligo (dT) and poly dA.dT (0.05 OD units per reaction mixture;

Collaborative Research, Waltham, Massachusetts) (11) was studied
c) characterization of the viral RNA isolated from the labeled
virions.

The labeled particles were treated with 5% sarcosyl in
the presence of HeLa cell RNA (0.6 absorbancy units) and 0.4%
diethyl pyrocarbonate (Baycovin, Bayer, Leverkusen, Germany). The
labeled RNA and virus debris were loaded on a sucrose gradient
(15-30% w/v; in 0.01 M Tris. HCl, 0.001 M EDTA and 0.2 M NaCl,
pH 7.4) together with ^{14}C-uridine labeled RSV RNA which served as
a marker for 60-70S RNA. The gradients were centrifuged in the
50.1 rotor of the preparative Beckman Ultracentrifuge for 180 min
at 45,000 rpm at 4°. Fractions were collected dropwise and the
radioactivity in each fraction determined.

3. Time course of C-type virus induction by arginine deprivation
   and BUdR treatment.

To compare the kinetics of release of C-type particles
into the culture medium on incubation of R(B77) cells in an arginine-deficient medium with the effect of BUdR, which is known to
induce the synthesis of C-type particles in different cells (12-15),
cultures of R (B77) cells were incubated in arginine-deficient medium or treated with BUdR, labeled with radioactive uridine and
the release of uridine labeled particles into the medium followed.
It was found that labeled particles, which sediment to the bottom
of the centrifuge tubes, were gradually released from the arginine-
deprived cells during the initial 24 h. Similarly, radioactive
particles were released from BUdR-treated cells but the yield of
virions was 1/3 that obtained from the arginine-deprived R (B77)
cells (Fig. 1A). It was also demonstrated that these particles
are resistant to RNase treatment (not shown) and band at a density
of 1.16 g/ml (Fig.1B).   It is not yet known if virus particles
are released from the BUdR treated cells during the 24 h of incubation with the drug.

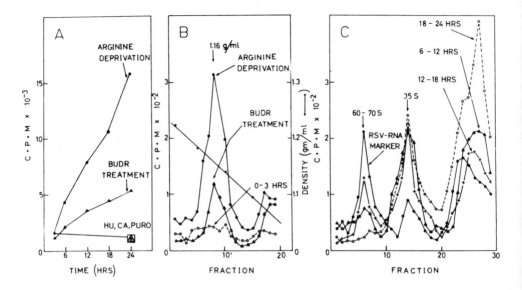

FIGURE 1. Kinetics of C-type virus release from arginine-deprived
and BUdR-treated R (B77) cells during the initial twenty-
four hours after virus induction.

A) A series of R (B77) cell cultures in Roux bottles
(80 x 10^6 cells/bottle) were incubated in arginine deficient medium and labeled with ^{3}H-uridine (1 µCi/ml) for 6 hour periods
starting at times zero, 3, 6, 12, and 18 hours after arginine deprivation. Zero time of BUdR treatment is considered the time when
fresh medium was added after the removal of the drug from cultures
treated with 30 µg/ml BUdR for 24 hours. At various time intervals
the medium was collected from each culture bottle and centrifuged
at 2,000 rpm at 15 minutes and the supernatants centrifuged at
27,000 rpm for 60 minutes in a No.30 rotor of the Beckman preparative ultracentrifuge. Each pellet was resuspended in 1 ml of
0.01 $\underline{M}$ Tris buffer HCl - 0.001 $\underline{M}$ EDTA, pH 8.4, and the TCA precipitable radioactivity was determined. Cultures of R(B77) cells de-
prived of arginine were treated with hydroxyurea (HU) (5 x 10^{-2} $\underline{M}$),
cytosine arabinoside (CA) (50 µg/ml) or puromycin (PURO) (50 µg/ml),
added to the cultures at zero time. The treated cells were labeled
with ^{3}H-uridine for 24 hours. The medium of these cultures was
collected, treated as described above and the TCA precipitable radioactivity determined.

Symbols:

●——● ^{3}H-uridine labeled particles released from arginine deprived cells.

▲_____▲ ^{3}H-uridine labeled particles released from BUdR treated cells.

▢   radioactivity in the medium of hydroxyurea treated, arginine deprived cells.

△   as above, but for cytosine arabinoside treated, arginine deprived cells.

+   as above, but for puromycin treated, arginine deprived cells.

B) Characterization of C-type particles released from arginine-deprived and BUdR-treated cells. The particles present in the medium of arginine-deprived cells labeled during the periods 0 to 3 hours (O---O) and 18 to 24 hours (●---●)and of BUdR-treated cells labeled during 18 to 24 hours (▲---▲) were centrifuged in sucrose gradients (15-65% w/v); the gradients were collected and the radioactivity in each fraction determined.

C) Analysis of RNA species present in the isolated C-type particles. Virions present in the medium of arginine deprived cells at the end of 6 hours of labeling with ^{3}H-uridine, starting at 12 h (△---△), 18 h (+ --- +), and 24 h (O --- O) after arginine deprivation, were banded in sucrose gradients: The RNA was extracted from virus-containing fractions with sarcosyl and centrifuged in sucrose gradients under conditions which permitted isolation of 70S RNA species. The distribution of the radioactivity in each fraction of the gradient was determined. RSV RNA labeled with ^{3}H-uridine was used as a marker for 60-70S RNA (●---●).

To characterize the RNA present in the C-type particles, the cells were labeled for 6 h periods during the initial 24 h incubation in the arginine-deficient medium and the particles in the medium were purified by centrifugation in sucrose gradients. The labeled viral RNA species were extracted and analyzed in sucrose gradients. It was found (Fig.1C) that the C-type particles released from the arginine-deprived cells after 6, 12, and 18 h contained both 60-70S and 35S RNA species. The virions labeled and released during the period 18-24 h contained 35S RNA species only. This finding is taken to indicate that the C-type particles released shortly after induction contain the 60-70S RNA genomes. It is possible that later on the larger genomes are dissociated to 35S RNA molecules. This finding explains our previous observation that the C-type particles released from arginine-deprived cells and harvested after 4-5 days contain 35S RNA species only.

         The virus particles released from the arginine-deprived
or BUdR treated cells also contain a reverse transcriptase activity
which is markedly stimulated to incorporate ^{3}H-TMP into DNA in the
presence of poly (rA). oligo (dT) but not of poly dA.dT (Table 1),
in agreement with the findings of Goodman and Spiegelman (11).
From the results presented in Figure 1 and Table 1, it is possible
to conclude that the synthesis of C-type virions was induced in
the R(B77) cells as a result of arginine deprivation and BUdR
treatment.

TABLE 1. EFFECTS OF POLY (rA). OLIGO (dT) AND POLY dA.dT ON THE
         REVERSE TRANSCRIPTASE ACTIVITY IN THE INDUCED C-TYPE
                              PARTICLES.

Source of Enzymatic Activity	Endogenous Reaction	Enzymatic Reaction	
		Plus Poly (rA).oligo (dT)	Plus Poly dA.dT
		^{3}H-TMP INCORPORATED (cpm)	
RSV (8E strain)	853	18,194 (x21)*	2555 (x2.2)
Particles released from BUdR treated cells **	442	5,917 (x12)	1026 (x2.3)
Particles released from arginine de- prived cells **	666	10,342 (x15)	4099 (x6)

*   In parentheses, the extent of stimulation as compared to
    endogenous incorporation.

** Harvest from the medium of one culture (6-8x10^7 cells) at
   48 hours after virus induction.

         To determine how long after treatment the induced cells
are able to synthesize and release the C-type particles, R(B77)
cultures were labeled with ^{3}H-uridine for 24 h intervals during
a four day period. It was found that the rate of particle release
from arginine-deprived (Fig. 2A) and BUdR-treated (Fig.2C) cells
increased during 48 h and later decreased. Most of the radioactivity released from the treated cells (Fig.2A and 2C) was found in
C-type particles which banded in sucrose gradients at a density of
1.16 g/ml (Fig.2B and 2D). The yield of particles in each gradient
is from the same number (6-8 x 10^6) of cells. These results are
taken to indicate that although less C-type particles are released
from BUdR treated cells as compared to the arginine deficient cells,
the kinetics of virus release is the same in both systems. The

number of cells in each culture which are induced and the synthesized virions are still to be studied.

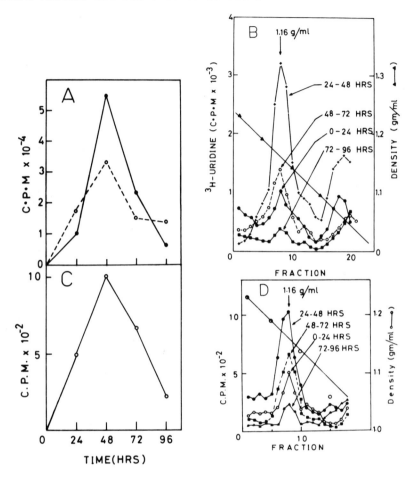

FIGURE 2. Kinetics of virus release from R(B77) cells deprived of arginine and treated with BUdR.

     A. R(B77) cells in a series of Roux bottles were incubated in an arginine deficient medium. Cell cultures were labeled with ^{3}H-uridine for periods of 24 hours, starting at the time of arginine deprivation and every 24 hours during the subsequent four days. Fresh cultures were labeled and harvested, and the radioactive particles released to the culture medium collected by centrifugation. The TCA precipitable radioactivity was determined.

     Symbols:

     ●---● Experiment 1
     O---O Experiment 2

B. The particles present in the pellets obtained from the medium removed from the labeled arginine-deprived cells were analyzed by centrifugation in sucrose gradients. The gradients were collected dropwise and the radioactivity in each fraction was determined. The density of several fractions was determined in a refractometer.

Symbols:

Particles from arginine deficient cells labeled during the periods: 0 to 24 hours ● ---●; 24 to 48 hours + --- +; 48 to 72 hours 0 --- 0; 72 to 96 hours ■ --- ■.

C. A series of R(B77) cell cultures in Roux bottles was treated with BUdR (30 µg/ml) for 24 hours. The BUdR was then washed, fresh Eagle's medium was added and the cells were reincubated at 37°. Every 24 hours a different culture was labeled with ^{3}H-uridine and the medium was harvested at the end of the labeling period. The particles present in the medium were centrifuged to the bottom of the centrifuge tubes, resuspended in buffer and radioactivity was determined (0 --- 0).

D. The particles released from BUdR treated cells to the medium in the experiment presented in B were analyzed by centrifugation in sucrose gradients.

Legend: 0 to 24 hours 0 --- 0; 24 to 48 hours ● --- ●; 48 to 72 hours ■---■; 72 to 96 hours ▲----▲.

4. Effect of inhibitors on the induction of C-type virions.

To study the effect of inhibitors of DNA and protein synthesis on virus release, cell cultures were labeled with radioactive uridine immediately after arginine deprivation for a 24 h period in the presence of hydroxyurea (HU; 5 x 10^{-2} M ref.12), cytosine arabinoside (CA; 50 µg/ml, ref.4) or puromycin (PURO; 50 µg/ml). Hydroxyurea and cytosine arabinoside were obtained from Sigma, St. Louis, Missouri and puromycin from Calbiochem, Switzerland. The particles in the media of the inhibited cells were collected by centrifugation and their radioactivity determined. To study the kinetics of virus release from arginine-deficient or BUdR-treated cells during a 4 day period, replicate R (B77) cultures were labeled with ^{3}H-uridine for 24 h intervals starting at 0 time, 24, 48, and 72 h. The radioactive particles present in the culture media at the different time intervals were collected and analyzed by centrifugation in sucrose gradients. The synthesis and release of virions from arginine deficient cells was prevented when the cultures were treated with hydroxyurea or cytosine arabinoside inhibitors of DNA synthesis (16,17). Inhibition of protein synthesis by puromycin also prevented virus release (Fig.1A). C-type particles were found in the medium of arginine‑deprived cells at 6 h after treatment; some radioactive particles may have been released from the cells after 3 h. This result is taken to indicate that a period of 3 to 6 h treatment with the inducers is required before virus particles can be detected in the culture media.

5.Conclusions

       The results of the present study extend our previous findings (8) on the induction of C-type particles in R(B77) cells. We have demonstrated that a) C-type particles are induced in R (B77) cells by BUdR treatment; b) virus particles are released from arginine deprived or BUdR treated cells as early as 6 h after arginine deprivation or the removal of BUdR; c) inhibition of cellular DNA synthesis by hydroxyurea or cytosine arabinoside prevents virus synthesis; d) virus particles released during the initial 18 h after arginine deprivation contain 60-70S and 35S RNA genomes and the release of C-type virions from the cells declines 48 h after induction. This suggests that DNA synthesis in the induced cells is essential for the induction of the synthesis of C-type particles (18). It was also found that treatment of arginine deprived R(B77) cells with hydroxyurea (5×10^{-2}M) during the initial 6 h after arginine deprivation, followed by removal of the inhibitor by washing and reincubation of the cells in the absence of the drug for 24 h, prevented virus formation. Shlomai & Becker, (unpublished results) also showed that arginine deprivation or BUdR treatment of the cells causes a gradual inhibition of DNA synthesis. During the initial 6 h, cellular DNA synthesis was detected in the induced cells but its level was very low at 12 h. A similar effect of arginine deprivation on cell DNA synthesis was described in Burkitt's lymphoblasts (19).

       A mixture of 35S and 60-70S RNA species was extracted from the C-type particles released from arginine deprived cells shortly (6 to 18 h) after treatment. It is of interest that the relative amount of 60-70S RNA species gradually decreased in these particles until only 35S RNA molecules were found in particles which were labeled more than 18 h after experimental treatment. The presence of 35S RNA species indicates that monomeric forms of the RNA genomes can exist in C-type particles. Further studies are in progress to characterize the C-type virions released from the cells after induction by BUdR treatment and arginine deprivation and to elucidate the mechanisms of this phenomenon.

B. INDUCTION OF C-TYPE PARTICLES IN HUMAN LEUKEMIC CELLS

The successful induction of C-type particles in rat cells transformed by Rous sarcoma virus, which contain the viral DNA genomes as a provirus (20) but do not produce virus particles, led us to study human leukemic cells. The aim was to induce the synthesis of C-type virus replication in the leukemic cells by arginine deprivation. Recent studies on human leukemic cells have revealed the presence in the cell cytoplasm of an RNase sensitive DNA polymerase (21) complexed with 70S RNA (22), as well as virus-specific polysomal RNA (23). The DNA synthesized by the cytoplasmic enzyme hybridizes specifically to nuclear DNA from leukemic cells (24). It was therefore of interest to find if C-type particles can be induced in human leukemic cells.

1. Induction of C-type particles in human leukemic cells.

Blood samples were obtained from patients with acute, lymphoblastic and chronic leukemias. The white blood cells were separated and resuspended in arginine deficient Eagle's medium. White blood cells from healthy donors were used as controls. The cells were labeled with ^{3}H-uridine, incubated for 5 days and the medium assayed for the presence of particles. The cytoplasmic fractions were assayed for the presence of RNA dependent DNA polymerase activity.

The results presented in Fig.3 demonstrate that particles which sedimented in sucrose gradients at the same position as Rous sarcoma virions were obtained from white blood cells from a patient with chronic lymphocytic leukemia (Fig. 3A). These particles contained a DNA polymerase activity (Fig. 3B) which is RNase sensitive (not shown). Particles were also obtained from white blood cells from a patient with an acute lymphocytic leukemia (Fig. 3C); these cells were found to contain an RNase sensitive DNA polymerase (Fig.3D). Similar results were obtained from a number of other leukemic patients.

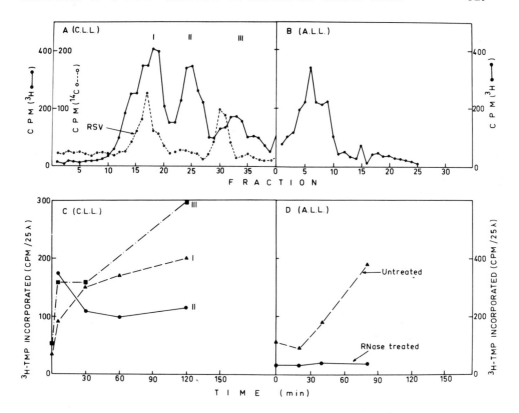

FIGURE 3. Isolation of particles from white blood cells of chronic
          leukemic patients after arginine deprivation.

        A) A 30 ml sample of heparinized blood was taken from
patients with CLL and 300 ml of blood was obtained from healthy
donors. The blood samples were distributed into tubes and were
left for 2 hours at room temperature. The upper parts of each
blood sample which contained the white blood cells were pooled,
the cells were washed in buffer and the number of cells in each
preparation was determined. About 60 x 10^6 cells were seeded into
each bottle containing 50 ml of Eagle's medium with or without
arginine. Some of the culture bottles were labeled with 1.5 μCi/ml
of ^{3}H-uridine (19 Ci/mM, Nuclear Research Center, Negev, Israel).
Five days later, the cells and debris were deposited by centrifugation for 25 min at 2,500 rpm. The supernatants were pooled and
recentrifuged for 60 min at 25,000 rpm in the Beckman No. 30 rotor.
The pellets were resuspended with Eagle's medium containing 5%
calf serum to approximately 1/200 of the starting volume. The

concentrated preparations were loaded on continuous sucrose gradients (15-65% w/v) in 0.01 M Tris HCl buffer, pH 8.0, 0.001 M
EDTA) and centrifuged for 180 min at 45,000 rpm in the Beckman
SW 50.1 rotor. The gradient was scanned for the presence of visible bands and the sucrose gradients collected dropwise. The
radioactivity in the particles isolated from the ^{3}H-uridine labeled
CLL cells was determined (● --- ●).

        B) The same sucrose gradient analysis was performed as
described in A) but on white blood cells obtained from a blood
sample taken from a patient with acute lymphocytic leukemia (ALL).

        C) A similar sucrose gradient analysis was carried out
with unlabeled particles released to the medium of arginine deprived CLL cells. The bands were removed by inserting a syringe into
each of the three bands present in the sucrose gradient. To each
sample from the various bands, an equivalent amount of Tris-EDTA
buffer, pH 8.1, containing 0.1% dithiothreitol and 0.25% Nonidet
P-40 was added. The preparations were incubated with the four
nucleoside triphosphates (including 3H-TTP) under conditions of
the reverse transcriptase assay as described by Temin & Mizutani
and Baltimore (3,4). At different time intervals, samples were
removed from each reaction mixture and the radioactivity labeled
DNA determined.

        D) Cytoplasmic RNase sensitive DNA polymerase in white
blood cells from an ALL patient. The arginine-deprived cells were
harvested and the cytoplasmic fraction divided into two portions:
one was incubated with RNase and the other was untreated. The
two preparations were incubated under conditions of DNA synthesis
and the TCA precipitable radioactivity was determined at different
time intervals.

2. Characterization of the isolated particles.

        Four criteria were used to determine if C-type particles
were obtained from the medium of arginine deprived leukemic cells:
a) banding in sucrose gradients at a density similar to Rous sarcoma virions; b) the presence of a reverse transcriptase in the
particles; c) the synthesis of DNA on 70S RNA template and d)
morphology of particles.

        Preliminary studies (23) indicated that particles resem-
bling C-type particles were obtained from arginine deprived leukemic cells. It was also demonstrated that the particles contain
a reverse transcriptase which synthesizes DNA on a 70S RNA template.
The isolated particles banded at a density of 1.17 g/ml. Such
particles were not induced in normal white blood cells by arginine
deprivation. Further studies on a larger group of leukemic patients

are needed to confirm these findings and to determine the role of a virus in human leukemia.

C. VIRUS PARTICLES FROM HUMAN CARCINOMA CELLS

1. Human carcinoma cell-line

A biopsy specimen was taken from an abdominal carcinoma tumor of a 63 year old male patient. A cell suspension was prepared by mincing and washing with Hank's salt solution. The cells were sedimented by centrifugation at 1500 rpm, resuspended in medium at a concentration 10^6 cells/ml and seeded in bottles, which were incubated at 37°. The medium consisted of 60% Basal Eagle's medium supplemented with 15% 199 medium, 15% of a 0.5% solution of lactalbumin hydrolysate in Hank's buffer and 10% fetal calf serum. The cell monolayers were treated with a solution of trypsin - versene, the cells were resuspended in fresh medium and then subcultured at 4 to 7 day intervals. In one of the cultures which was kept for 4 weeks at 32° in the incubator without change of medium, foci of round epitheloid cells were seen. The epitheloid cells grew well and were propagated as a cell line designated HCCL (human carcinoma cell line).

2. Particles isolated from the medium of HCCL.

Labeling of HCCL with ^{3}H-uridine resulted in the appearance in the culture medium of labeled particles which banded in the sucrose gradients (15-65% w/v) at a density of 1.17 g/ml. This density is slightly higher than that of Rous sarcoma virions (1.16 g/ml) (Fig.4).

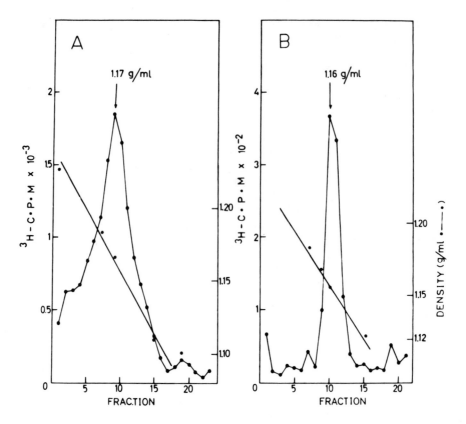

FIGURE 4. Isolation of RNA-containing particles released from CCL.

A) CCL cells were incubated in the presence of ^{3}H-uridine, and particles present in the medium were collected and analyzed by centrifugation in a linear sucrose gradient (15-65% w/v) in a Spinco SW 50.1 rotor for 180 min at 45,000 rpm and 4°.

Fractions were collected from the bottom of each tube and the density (measured in a refractometer) and radioactivity of each fraction determined.

B) External marker of RSV ^{3}H-uridine labeled virions to density gradient centrifugation of CCL released particles. Marker was prepared by the same method as described in the Legend to A.

The particles obtained from the sucrose gradient were tested for the presence of RNA directed DNA polymerase; in some preparations, RNase sensitive DNA polymerase activity was detected (Fig.5A). The particles were incubated for 5 min under conditions favorable for DNA synthesis by the endogenous RNase sensitive DNA polymerase and the RNA was isolated and analyzed by centrifugation

in a sucrose gradient to determine if the DNA is synthesized on a
70S RNA template. It was found (Fig.5B) that indeed nascent DNA
chains were attached to 70S molecules. An additional band of
radioactive DNA which sedimented faster in the gradient was also
found (Fig.5B). The nature of the template for this DNA species
is not yet known.

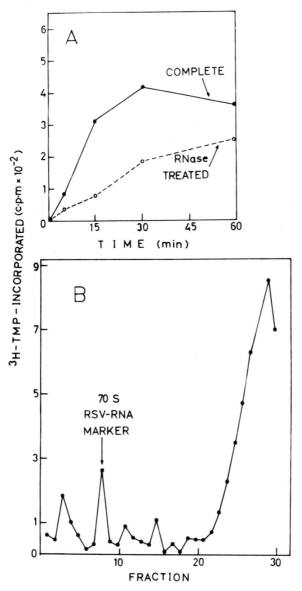

FIGURE 5. 70S RNA-DNA hybrid synthesized by RNA-directed DNA
          polymerase associated with the particles released in the
          medium by CCL cells.

Y. BECKER ET AL

A) Kinetics of DNA synthesis by the RNA-directed DNA polymerase present in the particles released from the medium of CCL cells. The particles were disrupted with Nonidet P-40 (10 min at 4°). One half (O --- O) was incubated with ribonuclease (50 µg/ml) and the rest was untreated (● --- ●).

A standard reaction mixture was added to the disrupted virions. After incubation for one hour, samples were taken at different time intervals to determine the extent of DNA synthesis.

B.) The particles isolated from the medium after treatment by Nonidet P-40 were subject to the standard polymerase assay according to Temin and Mizutani (3). The product of a 10 min reaction at 37° were extracted and analyzed by centrifugation in a linear sucrose gradient (15-30% w/v) in a Spinco SW 50.1 rotor at 45,000 rpm for 100 min to isolate the 70S RNA. The TCA precipitable radioactivity in each fraction was determined.

3. Biological activity of the isolated particles.

Preliminary experiments showed that cell-free medium from HCCL (prepared by filtration) caused cellular transformation in human embryo muscle-cell cultures. Cell lines obtained from the foci of transformed cells are now being investigated.

CONCLUSIONS

The studies on the induction of C-type viruses in cancer cells demonstrated that virus replication can be induced in transformed cells which carry viral DNA. The exact mechanisms of the virus induction process is not yet known, mainly because of the lack of knowledge concerning the processes which regulate transcription and replication of nucleic acids in mammalian cells. It is assumed that BUdR treatment and arginine deprivation have the same effect on the host cell, resulting in the exposure of the viral DNA to transcription which yields viral RNA molecules to serve as messenger RNA and as genomes for virion formation. With arginine deprivation, it was possible to demonstrate that leukemic cells could be induced to synthesize particles with properties resembling those of oncorna viruses. Further studies to induce the formation of virus-like particles in cells from human tumors are in progress.

The isolation of virus-like particles from cancer cells does not provide sufficient evidence to conclude that these particles are the cause of the disease. Tumor cells from mammalian hosts were recently demonstrated to contain proviruses (26) which can be induced to synthesize virus particles. Further experiments with human cancer cells should provide essential information on human C-type viruses. The preliminary results with human carcinoma cells support our belief that human tumors might indeed contain proviruses. Further studies on human oncorna viruses and their role, if any, in transformation in vivo represent a main direction in the present phase of human cancer research.

ACKNOWLEDGEMENTS

This study was supported by grants from the Leukemia Research Foundation, Inc., Chicago, Illinois and the Israel Cancer Association.

The studies on C-type particles in human cells is part of a Ph.D. thesis to be submitted by G. Balabanova to the Senate of the Hebrew University, Jerusalem.

REFERENCES

1. TEMIN, H.M. (1964). Nat. Cancer Res.Monog. 17, 557-570.

2. TEMIN, H.M. (1971). J. Nat. Cancer Inst. 46, III-VII.

3. TEMIN, H.M. & MIZUTANI, S. (1970). Nature, 266, 1211-1213.

4. BALTIMORE, D. (1970). Nature, 226, 1209-1211.

5. HILL, M. & HILLOVA, J. (1972). Nature N B, 237, 35-39.

6. KOTLER, M. (1971). J. Gen. Virol. 12, 199-206

7. KLEMENT, V., NICOLSON, M.O. & HEUBNER, R.J. (1971). Nature N B
    234, 12-14.

8. KOTLER, M., WEINBERG, E., HASPEL, O. & BECKER, Y. (1972).
    J. Virol. 10, 439-446

9. ALTANER, C. & TEMIN, H.M. (1970) Virology, 40, 113-134.

10. GELDERBLOM, H., BAUER, H. & FRANK, F. (1970). J. Gen. Virol. 7,
    33-45.

11. GOODMAN, M.C. & SPIEGELMAN, S. (1971). Proc. Nat. Acad. Sci. USA,
    68, 2203-2206

12. AARONSON, S.A., TODARO, G.J. & SCOLNICK, E.M. (1971). Science,
    174, 157-159

13. HSIUNG, G.D. (1972). J. Nat. Cancer Inst. 49, 567-570.

14. LOWY, D.R., ROWE, W.P., TEICH,N. & HARTLEY, J.A. (1971),Science,
    174, 155-156

15. STEWARD, S.E., KASNIC, G., DRAYCOTT, C., FELLER, W., GOLDEN, A.,
    MITCHELL, E. & BEN, T. (1972). J. Nat. Cancer Inst. 48,
    273-277.

16. CHU, M.Y. & FISCHER, G.A. (1962). Biochem. Pharmacol. 11,
    423-430.

17. ROSENKRANZ, H.S. & LEVY, J.A. (1965). Biochem. Biophys.Acta,
    95, 181-183

18. TEMIN, H.M. (1964). Virology, 23, 486-494.

19. WEINBERG, A. & BECKER, Y. (1970). Exptl. Cell Res. 60, 470-474.

20. TEMIN, H.M. (1971). Ann. Rev. Microbiol. 25, 609-648.

21. SARNGADHARAN, M.G., SARIN, P.S., REITZ, M.S. & GALLO, R.C. (1972). Nature N B, 240, 67-72.

22. BAXT, W., HEHLMANN, R. & SPIEGELMAN, S. (1972). Nature N B, 240 72-75.

23. HEHLMAN, R., KUFE, D. & SPIEGELMAN, S. (1972). Proc. Nat. Acad. Sci. USA, 69, 435-439.

24. BAXT, W.G. & SPIEGELMAN, S. (1972). Proc. Nat. Acad. Sci.USA, 69, 3737-3741.

25. KOTLER, M., WEINBERG, E., HASPEL, O., OLSHEVSKY, U. & BECKER,Y. Nature, in press.

26. RUPRECHT, R.M., GOODMAN, N.C. & SPIEGELMAN, S. (1973). Proc. Nat. Acad. Sci. USA, 70, 1437-1441.

RNA DIRECTED DNA POLYMERASE IN C-TYPE PARTICLES FROM NORMAL

RAT THYMUS CULTURES AND MOLONEY LEUKEMIA VIRUS

Yael Teitz

Israel Institute for Biological Research, Ness-Ziona
and University of Tel-Aviv Medical School

INTRODUCTION

For the last few years we have been studying the metabolic
process involved in the morphogenesis of the Moloney leukemia
virus (MLV) and, particularly, in identifying and characterizing
the enzymic system responsible for the synthesis of the RNA
moiety (the genetic material) of this murine leukemia virus.
Hopefully, such metabolic studies will throw light on how onco-
genic viruses transform the cells they infect; however, it should
be emphasized that different viral genes may be involved in viral
reproduction in contrast to viral transformation.

1. STRUCTURE AND COMPOSITION OF THE MLV PARTICLE

The morphology of the mature MLV particle, illustrated
diagramatically in Fig. 1 is complex; it consists of a large,
roughly spherical, particle about 1,000 Å in diameter, containing
the genetic material as a single-stranded ribonucleic acid with a
molecular weight of about 10 million daltons. Thus it is one of
the largest natural strands of ribonucleotides known in nature,
and is capable of providing information for at least 50 new proteins in the infected cells. The RNA is probably arranged in a
ring-shaped complex with the capsid protein, which is the internal

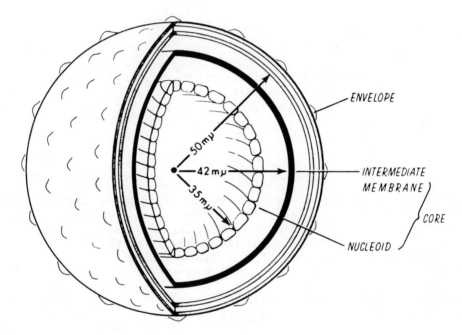

Fig. 1.   Diagramatic illustration of the morphological structure
of the mature MLV particle.

group-specific antigen, common to all the murine tumor viruses. The RNA with the capsid protein forms the nucleoid which is surrounded by a membrane, presumably of a protein nature, with which the RNA-directed DNA polymerase enzymes are associated. An additional membrane, the outer envelope-membrane, is acquired by the viral particle when it is released from the cell by a process known as "budding", in which the viral particle is literally enveloped by the host cell membrane. Several modifications in the chemical constitution or structure of the cellular membrane occur on introduction of viral induced antigens. These viral surface antigens (located in the viral outer envelope) are type-specific and are different for the various strains or types of the murine leukemia viruses.

In order to demonstrate in vitro the RNA-directed DNA polymerase activity, commonly known as reverse transcriptase activity, the viral particles are treated with a non-ionic detergent (Nonidet-P_{40} or Triton X^{100}) to dissolve the outer envelope of the virus particles, thereby permitting the introduction of the metabolites required for DNA synthesis.

2. VIRAL INFECTION OF RAT THYMUS CELL CULTURES

Injecting MLV into a newborn mouse or rat, their natural hosts, will produce a typical lymphatic leukemia in the animal with the formation of a lymphoma in the thymus (1).

For metabolic studies with MLV, we have prepared cell cultures from the thymus of newborn rats and succeeded in establishing several cell lines, of which a few have been grown in our laboratory for more than five years (2). Most of the experimental results reported in the present work are concerned with the cell line T_{21} (Fig. 2). We infected this cell line with MLV and established a chronically MLV infected cell line $T_{21}M$ (2). As cán be seen from Fig. 3, the virus does not have any cytopathic effect on the cells. The viral infection is productive and complete viral particles are released into the culture medium by the "budding" process.

Very little is known concerning the stages or the metabolic pathways involved in the biosynthesis of different viral components and the stages of viral replication. Even the cellular location of the synthesis of the various viral components is obscure; we have not yet identified the enzyme or enzymes responsible for the synthesis of the viral RNA.

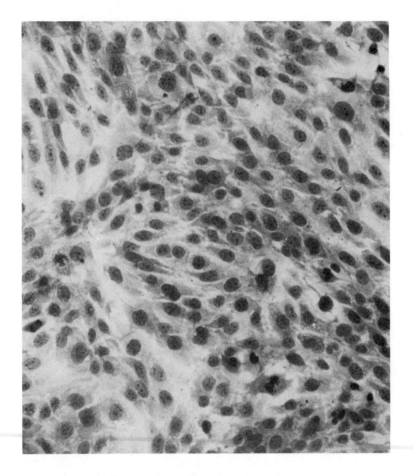

Fig. 2. Control cell line ($T_{21}C$) passage 234. Cells from a
monolayer of fibroblastic cells with several mitotic figures
Giemsa x 183.

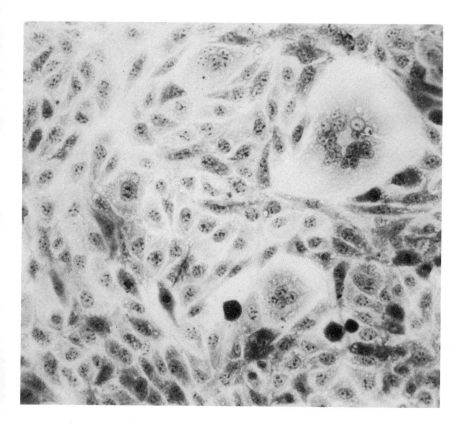

Fig. 3. MLV infected cell line ($T_{21}M$) passage 263 Giemsa x 183.

The first viral component that can be detected in the virus
infected cells is the group-specific antigen (capsid protein).
Using the fluorescent antibody staining technique we were able to
show that almost all of the cells in chronically MLV infected $T_{21}M$
were infected (2). (See Fig. 4). Using electron microscopy, the
budding process whereby the virus particles are released into the
medium can be visualized (Fig. 5). An immature virus particle
nearing completion of bud formation is seen in Fig. 6, with its
typical three layers -hence the designation C-type particle.

Mature virus particles found in the culture medium often
showed dense nucleoids, indicating some denaturation of the viral
RNA which is quite labile and undergoes fragmentation. When RNA
is extracted from such mature viral particles, a low yield of 70S
RNA is obtained with relatively high yields of low molecular weight
viral RNA of 35S, 20S and 4 to 9S RNA.

We have fractionated the cells chronically infected with MLV
($T_{21}M$) to obtain the various cytoplasmic membranes[x] and have
characterized them chemically. The enzyme, RNA directed DNA polymerase, was found to be associated mainly with the rough membrane
(endoplasmic reticulum) and with the plasma membranes (3) (Table
1).

3.   CHARACTERIZATION OF MLV PARTICLES FROM RAT THYMUS CELLS

Since no cytopathic effect appears in the MLV-infected cells,
we have assayed the amount of virus particles released into the
medium by measurement of ^{3}H-uridine radioactivity incorporated into
virus particles, which have a typical density of 1.16-1.18 g/ml
when isolated in a sucrose gradient (4). Curve A, Fig. 7, shows
a single absorption peak corresponding to a single peak of radioactivity in a density gradient purification of uridine ^{3}H-labeled
virus from 200 ml of cell culture fluid. Electron microscopic
examination of the peak fractions at a sucrose density of 1.16-1.18
g/ml revealed many typical C-type particles, but the preparation
was not free of cellular debris. Recentrifugation and separation
on a second sucrose gradient resulted in a relatively pure preparation of the C-type particles; all of the ultraviolet (UV) absorbancy and radioactivity were found in a single fraction at a density
of 1.17 g/ml (Curve B, Fig. 7).

---

[x]In this part of the work, D. Dekel and A. Keysary of the Israel
Institute for Biological Research participated.

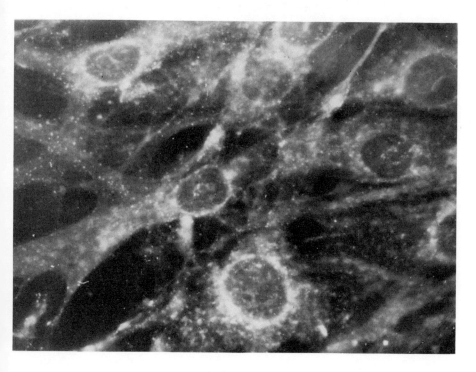

Fig. 4. Cell line $T_{21}M$ passage 259 stain appears as cytoplasmic
fine flecks, concentrated along the nuclear and cytoplasmic
membranes.

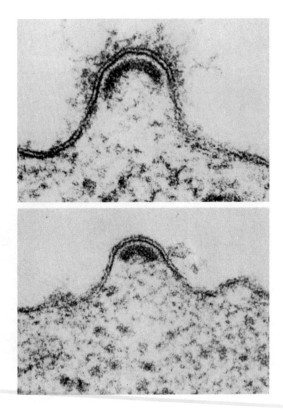

Fig. 5.   Immature MLV particle observed at the early stages of
bud formation in rat thymus cells chronically infected with MLV
x 75000

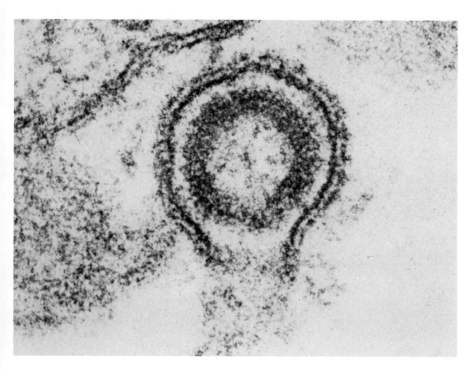

Fig. 6.   Immature C-type MLV particle nearing completion of bud
formation observed in rat thymus cells chronically infected with
MLV.   x 80,000

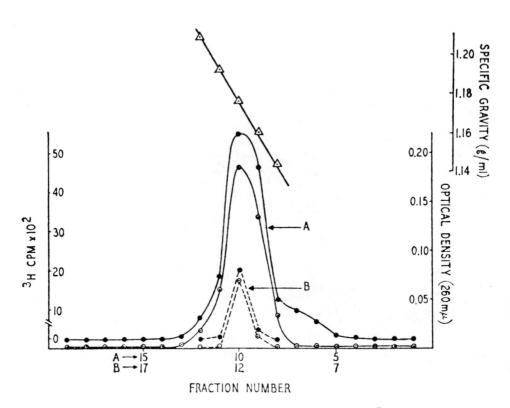

Fig. 7. Sucrose gradient purification of uridine ^{3}H-labeled
particles from MLV-infected rat cell cultures $T_{21}M$ (passage 212).
Growth medium (10 ml) containing uridine-^{3}H(3μCi/ml) was added to
each of 3 days old confluent monolayer of cells in 8 ounce bottles. After 24 hours at 37°C the culture fluid was concentrated
in presence of 100 ml cold carrier and the viral band purified.
A - first sucrose gradient (1/6 of each fraction), B - second
sucrose gradient (1/4 of each fraction), ● - counts per minute
(cpm); o - OD 260 mµ; A - sucrose density.

TABLE   1

CHARACTERISTICS OF THE DIFFERENT CELL FRACTIONS

F r a c t i o n		Enzymic Activity	
Density g/ml	Phospholipid μg/50 μg protein	mμ mole/50 μg protein/30'	
		Endogenous	+DNA
1.11	5.5	0.4	5
1.14	11.1	2.5	25
1.18	18.4	4.0-5.0	40-50

The MLV particles released from the rat thymus cells showed
leukomogenic activity in mice. The virus was also characterized
by an electron microscopic co-precipitation test elaborated by us
(4). In a positive reaction, rat anti-MLV gamma-globulin co-pre-
cipitated with rabbit anti-rat gamma-globulin contained aggregates
of viral particles surrounded by a dense layer, the antibody
protein (Fig. 8).

4. C-TYPE PARTICLES (NCV) FROM NON-INFECTED RAT THYMUS CELLS

Surprisingly, the non-infected rat thymus cell cultures,
which were intended to serve as controls for the MLV-infected
cells, were found also to release C-type particles, which sedimented at a density of 1.14-1.18 g/ml. Figure 9 shows absorbancy and
radioactivity curves for particles released into 800 ml of culture
media. The peak represents about 20 percent of the radioactivity
and about 15 percent of the ultraviolet absorbance, compared to
the values obtained for the MLV infected cells. Examination of
the surface of non-infected rat thymus cultures revealed budding
particles (4). These virus-like particles did not produce lymphoma on injection into mice or rats, nor did they reveal the
presence of any MLV antigen as indicated by fluorescent antibody
staining or by a complement fixation test with anti-MLV sera. A
negative reaction was obtained in the electron microscopic co-
precipitation test. Immunologically, we could not detect any
antigen common to any other known RNA tumor virus (murine, avian
or feline). We conclude that these particles appearing in non-
infected cultures (NCV) whose nature is unknown at present, may
be a new type of virus. These particles, naturally present in the
rat thymus in a latent or abortive form, presumably become evident
on passage in culture. No C-type particles were observed in
tissues taken directly from normal living rats, although the presence of such particles, even in germ-free mice, is common.

5. RNA DIRECTED DNA POLYMERASE IN MLV AND NCV TYPE PARTICLES

The discovery of RNA directed DNA polymerase activity in the
disrupted virions of the RNA tumor viruses (5), prompted us to
examine the MLV and the virus appearing in non-infected cultures
(NCV) for the presence of RNA directed DNA polymerase activity.
The enzymic activity of samples of purified C-type particles was
assayed in a reaction mixture similar to that described by Temin
(5) and Table 2. The RNA directed DNA polymerase catalyzes the
synthesis of polydeoxyribonucleotide chains by the formation of

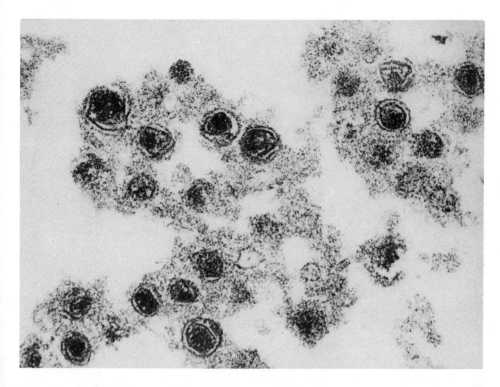

Fig. 8. Positive reaction in co-precipitation test.
Thin section of pellet of precipitates of MLV rat anti-MLV serum,
and rabbit anti-rat gamma-globulin. Viral particles coated with
layer of antibody-anti gamma-globulin complex.   x 100,000

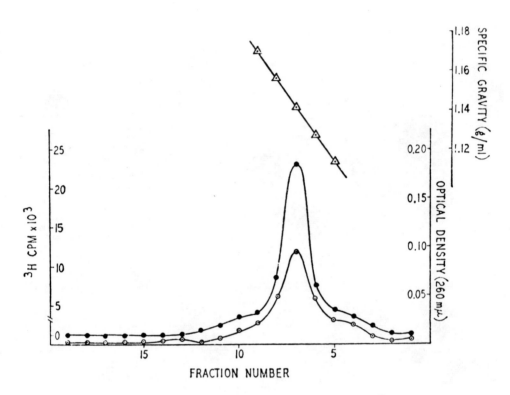

Fig. 9.   Sucrose gradient purification of uridine ^{3}H-labeled
particles from control cell cultures (T$_{21}$C) passage 221.
Growth medium (10 ml) containing uridine [3]H (3μCi/ml) was added
to each of thirty 8-ounce bottles immediately after plating.
After 3 days the medium was harvested and replaced with fresh
medium. The second harvest was after 2 days. The culture fluid
(780 ml) from the 30 cultures after labeling for 5 days was purified. o - OD 260 mμ (1/20th of each fraction); ●-CPM (1/20th of
each fraction)   Δ - sucrose density.

TABLE   2

EMZYMATIC ASSAY OF VIRAL C-TYPE PARTICLES FOR RNA
DIRECTED DNA POLYMERASE ACTIVITY

Temperature	$40°$
Time	$60'$
Protein in sample	50 μg
0.1 M Tris buffer	pH = 8.3
1 mM Mn-acetate	
0.1 M NaCl	
0.04 M Dithiothreitol	
0.1 mM each of dATP, dGTP, dCTP	
1.56 μCi H^3-TTP (Specific activity 9.6 Ci/m mole)	
0.05 percent "Nonidet - P_{40}"	

3'5' phosphodiester bonds. Apart from its substrate, the 5'-tri-
phosphates of deoxythymidine, guanosine, adenosine and cytidine,
the enzyme requires an RNA template and a divalent ion, Mn^{++}; the
optimal pH is 8.3. The product is hydrolysed by DNase. The characterization and the kinetics of incorporation of ^3H TMP by both
types of virus particles are shown in Table 3 and Fig. 10. Initially, the reaction proceeded linearly and the rate of incorporation then declined. The rate of synthesis of both viral
particles is similar; both preparations were inhibited to the same
degree by rifamycin (see Table 4). However, a difference in the
inhibitory effect of actinomycin D on the incorporation of ^3H-TTP
was found between the MLV and NCV (6) (Table 5). While 0.5 μg of
actinomycin D inhibited 50 percent of the incorporation of ^3H-TMP
by MLV, 5 μg of actinomycin D was required to cause a 50 percent
reduction in the incorporation into NCV. This difference in
response to actinomycin D might serve to distinguish the DNA polymerase of MLV from that of the NCV. McDonnell et al. (7) have
pointed out that DNA polymerase has two or more distinct enzymic
activities. The steps in the overall reaction can be differentiated by actinomycin D as shown schematically in Fig. 11. The
first reaction on the RNA template forms the hybrid product RNA-
DNA and is inhibited by rifamycin. The second reaction forms DNA
on the hybrid template. Actinomycin D inhibits only the second
reaction i.e. the formation of the double stranded DNA. Only the
determination of the efficiency and specificity of the isolated
enzymes acting on various templates and their sensitivity to inhibitors might confirm the suggestion that the DNA polymerases
from MLV and NCV are different.

6.   PURIFICATION OF RNA DIRECTED DNA POLYMERASE FROM
              MLV AND NCV PARTICLES

     Solubilizing the enzymes was effected by treatment of the
viral particles with detergents (7). From the lysate of the
virus particles, the insoluble material was removed by centrifugation (16,000 x g for 10 minutes) and the supernatant was applied
to a sucrose gradient. A single peak of enzymic activity sedimented (Fig. 12). Using as external markers BSA and LDH[*] with known
sedimentation coefficients (S_{20w} of 4.4s and 6.7s respectively)
gave an estimate of about 9s for the enzyme, and thus an estimated
molecular weight of about 200,000 daltons. Most of the soluble
viral protein sedimented in the range 1-3s (see Fig. 12).

_____
[*] BSA - Bovine serum albumin
   LDH - Lactic dehydrogenase

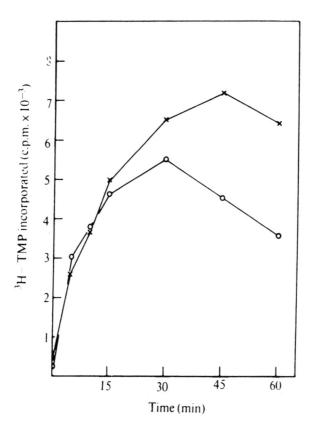

Fig. 10. Kinetics of incorporation.
Standard complete assay mixture was used as described in Table 2.
At various times 0.2 ml aliquots were withdrawn and the incorporation terminated.
x - MLV, o - NCV viral C-type particles.

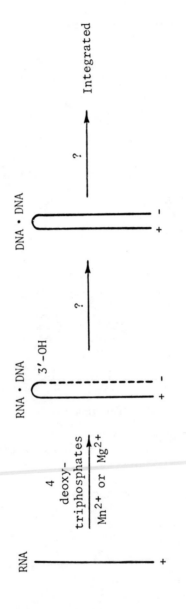

Fig. 11. Schematic steps in the RNA directed DNA polymerase enzymic reaction.

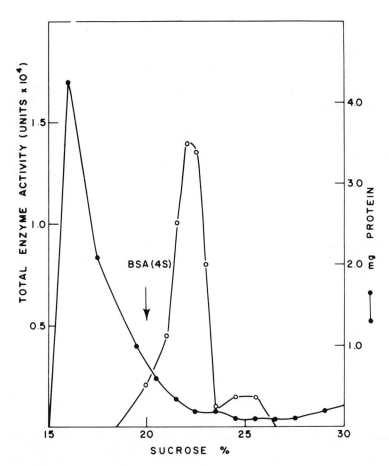

Fig. 12.   Sucrose gradient centrifugation of RNA directed DNA
polymerase.
Enzyme preparations were loaded on 15-30 percent sucrose gradient
and centrifuged for 17 h at 200,000 xg.   Fractions (0.2 ml) were
collected and assayed for activity.   Alcohol dehydrogenase (6.7S)
and bovine serum albumin (4.45) were used as sedimentation markers.
o - RNA directed DNA polymerase activity;   ● - protein content was
assayed according to Lowry's method (11).

TABLE   3

COMPARISON OF INCORPORATION OF ^{3}H-TMP BY MLV AND
NCV C-TYPE PARTICLES

Condition of assay	^{3}H-TMP (cpm)	
	"normal"	MLV
Complete	3,990	4,700
At 4°C	180	250
Without Mn^{2+}	300	400
Without Mn^{2+} but with Mg^{2+}	2,000	2,500
Without nucleotides	1,700	1,900
Without 'Nonidet P_{40}'	1,100	1,300
With post-DNase	150	200
With pre-RNase	220	270

TABLE   4

RIFAMYCIN INHIBITION OF INCORPORATION OF ^{3}H-TTP BY NCV AND MLV
C-TYPE PARTICLES

Source of C-type particles	Antibiotic (µg)	^{3}H-TMP (cpm)	Inhibition percent
NCV rat thymus cells	none	3,000	
	10	2,480	33
	40	380	90
MLV-infected rat thymus cells	none	4,100	-
	10	2,940	28
	40	470	89

To each 0.22 ml of complete assay mixture (described in
Table 3) 0.01 ml antibiotic was added. The reaction was
terminated after 30 min.

TABLE   5

ACTINOMYCIN D INHIBITION OF INCORPORATION OF ^{3}H-TTP BY MLV
AND NCV C-TYPE PARTICLES

Source of C-type particles	Antibiotic (μg)	^{3}H-TMP (cpm)	Inhibition percent
NCV rat thymus cells	none	3,400	-
	0.5	3,300	none
	1	3,500	none
	5	1,700	50
	10	1,050	70
MLV-infected rat thymus cells	none	3,200	-
	0.5	1,600	50
	1	830	74
	5	320	90
	10	220	93

To each 0.22 ml complete assay mixture (described in Table 2),
0.01 ml antibiotics was added. The reaction was terminated
after 30 min.

Usually 1-2 percent of the viral protein sedimented as the 9s fraction. The positional peak of enzyme activity was similar for the MLV and NCV.

The soluble enzyme fraction from the peak fractions of the sucrose gradients was analyzed by SDS-polyacrylamide gel electrophoresis. For determining the molecular weight of the polypeptide chains consisting of the subunits of the enzyme protein, the stained bands were scanned by a densitometer; the results are shown in Fig. 13. There is a striking similarity between the patterns of the enzymes from MLV and MCV (see M and C, respectively in Fig. 13). The MLV enzyme consists of five bands; 30,000, 40,000, 70,000 and 2 bands in the range of 90,000-110,000 daltons. The NCV enzyme showed only four bands; 30,000, 40,000, 70,000 (exactly the same as in the MLV) and a single band in the range 90-110,000 daltons; therefore, one band is missing as compared to MLV, suggesting that in this range of molecular weight one subunit is depleted or completely lacking. It is still doubtful whether the two low molecular weight bands, of 30,000 and 40,000 daltons are an integral part of the enzyme or represent some viral protein contaminant, as enzyme preparations which we obtained using electrofocusing did not show bands of molecular weight lower than 70,000 daltons. This point is presently being clarified in our laboratory.

The enzyme preparation obtained from the peak fractions of the sucrose gradients (Fig. 12) showed an absolute requirement for external templates. Fractions sedimenting at higher densities usually had some endogenous activity. The enzyme preparations were examined for their specific activity towards various synthetic templates (Table 6). These synthetic templates are valuable in monitoring the purification steps of the enzyme. As can be seen from Table 6, the synthetic polymer poly $rA-dT_{12-16}$ is the most efficient template. The specific activity obtained with the MLV enzyme preparation is in the same range as reported for the avian meoblastosis virus (AMV) and Rauscher Leukemia Virus enzyme (8).

The fact that poly $dA-dT_{12-16}$ is a poor template is also in accord with the findings of other laboratories for the viral DNA polymerase (8).Table 7 shows the results obtained when natural templates were employed. RNA extracted from the C-type particles of MLV and NCV seems to provide the best templates for the enzyme.

The lower molecular weight fractions, 4s-9s viral RNA, seemed as good templates as the higher molecular weight, 37s-70s viral RNA fractions. These preliminary results are in accord with the findings of Bishop's group (9) that natural 4s RNA serves as an initiator for the templates of this enzyme.

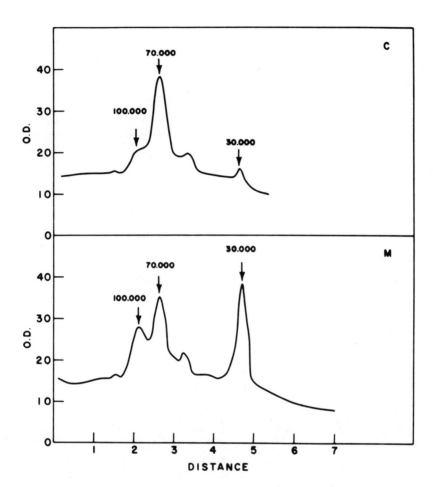

Fig. 13. SDS-polyacrylamide gel electrophoresis of RNA dependent
DNA polymerase.
Enzyme protein samples from peak fractions of the sucrose gradients
were precipitated at 0° by 5 percent trichloroacetic acid. The
sediments obtained by centrifugation at 16,000 xg were dissolved in
0.01 M sodium phosphate, pH 7.8 and dissociated by heating at 100°
at 15 min with 0.1 M sodium phosphate pH 7.8, 1 percent SDS and 1
percent 2-mercaptoethanol. They were separated by SDS polyacrylamide gel electrophoresis. The SDS-polyacrylamide gels (7.5 percent) were prepared and run as described by Weber and Osborn (12).

TABLE   6

EFFICIENCY OF VARIOUS SYNTHETIC TEMPLATES FOR THE MLV POLYMERASE

Template	Unit Enzyme p mole d TMP/10 min/µg protein
poly rA	2
poly rA-dT$_{(12-16)}$	400
poly dA	0.2
poly dA-dT$_{(12-16)}$	0.3
poly rA-poly dT	130
poly dA-poly dT	100
poly d(A-T) - poly d(A-T)	100
oligo dT$_{(12-16)}$	0.3
WITHOUT TEMPLATE	0.3

The complete assay mixture consisted of the following in 0.2 ml: 100 mM Tris-HCl (pH 8.3), 40 mM dithiothreitol, 1 mM Mn-acetate, 0.1 M NaCl, 0.1 mM each of d ATP, d GTP, d CTP and 1 µM ^{3}H d TTP, 2.5 µC ^{3}H d TTP (Schwartz 17.4 Ci/m mole), about 1000 counts per min per p mole, 0.01 percent Nonidet 1-40, 1 µg synthetic template and 1 µg MLV polymerase (sucrose gradient peak fractions, Fig.12). Incubated for 10 min at 40°C. The reaction was terminated by chilling the tubes and adding 0.1 ml of 0.1 M sodium pyrophosphate (pH 7.0) 0.1 ml of 0.2 M EDTA, 50 µg yeast RNA and 3 ml cold 10 percent TCA. The precipitate was collected by filtration through Whatman glass fiber paper GF/B (2.5 cm) washed ten times with 5 ml 5 percent TCA containing 10^{-3} M sodium pyrophosphate and twice with 5 ml of ethanol. The glass fiber papers were dried and the radioactivity was determined in a liquid scintillation counter.

One unit of enzyme activity is the amount which catalyzes the incorporation of 1 p mole of d TMP in 10 min at 40° by 1 µg enzyme protein into an acid insoluble product.

TABLE   7

TEMPLATE EFFICIENCY OF NATURAL RNAs AND REQUIREMENT OF OLIGO d T
AS PRIMER UNIT FOR THE MLV POLYMERASE

Source RNA		Unit Enzyme p mole d TMP/10 min/µg protein	
		Template	Primer
		RNA	RNA+oligo dT$_{(12-16)}$
MLV	(70-35S)	165	100
	(9- 4S)	280	150
NCV	(70-35S)	100	80
	(9- 4S)	290	140
Globin mRNA	(9S)	3	30
Mengo Virus	(37S)	14	110
Ribosomal RNA	(28S & 16S)	2	2
Yeast RNA		2	2
WITHOUT TEMPLATE		0.2	0.2

To each 0.2 ml complete assay mixture as described in Table 6
1 µg of natural template RNA, 1 µg oligo d T or 0.1 µg viral
RNA was added to the reaction mixture. The reaction was terminated after 30 min.

Addition of oligo dT did not improve the ability of viral RNA to serve as a template, although its addition improved the template activity of globin mRNA and mengo 37s RNA[*]. The beneficial addition of oligo dT for globin mRNA was originally reported by Verma et al. (10) for the AMV enzyme.

Using the different templates, a comparison was made between the enzyme preparations from MLV and NCV with regard to their specificity toward different templates. It can be seen from Table 8 that the NCV enzyme shows only 10 percent activity with the synthetic templates as compared with the MLV enzyme. The MLV enzyme incorporates two or three times, respectively, the amount of ^{3}H-TMP when thymus DNA or activated thymus DNA was used. For both enzymic preparations, ribosomal RNA or yeast RNA were poor templates. The most important finding was that both enzyme preparations showed the greatest activity with homologous RNA (extracted from homologous viral particles).

The MLV enzyme seemed to work as well on NCV RNA as on MLV RNA. However, as the MLV were grown originally on the same rat thymus cell cultures, one cannot preclude the possibility that MLV is contaminated with the NCV particles. Therefore, it can be concluded that the RNA of a particular virus seems to be the most specific and efficient template for its specific enzyme.

Summarizing, MLV-and NCV-directed DNA polymerases, solubilized and purified from C-type particles, have been characterized by their primary requirements, template specificity and subunit composition. Although the two enzymes differed in their subunit composition, and in the efficiency of their use of non-specific natural or synthetic templates, showed equal specificity and efficiency on their endogenous RNA templates.

---

[*] Both RNA preparations were generously supplied by Dr. M. Ravel, Weizmann Institute of Science.

TABLE   8

COMPARISON OF RNA DIRECTED DNA POLYMERASE ACTIVITY OF MLV
AND NCV WITH VARIOUS TEMPLATES

| | Unit Enzyme p mole d TMP/10 min/μg protein | |
| Natural Templates | Source of Enzyme | |
Source	MLV	NCV
MLV RNA	300	18
NCV RNA	300	290
Thymus DNA	20	7
Thymus DNA (activated)	40	20
Synthetic Templates		
poly rA-dT$_{(12-16)}$	350	35
poly dA-dT$_{(12-16)}$	1	0.3
poly rA-poly dT	120	18
poly dA-poly dT	100	10
poly d(A-T) - poly d(A-T)	100	10
poly rA-poly rU	0.3	0.1
WITHOUT TEMPLATE	0.2	0.1

One μg MLV polymerase of 3 μg NCV polymerase protein peak
fractions from the sucrose gradients (Fig. 12) were assayed.
Reaction mixture and conditions were as described in Tables
6 and 7.

ACKNOWLEDGMENTS

This study was partially financed by a grant from the Israel
Cancer Association.

The first part of this work was done in the Viral and
Rickettsial Disease Laboratory, California State Department of
Public Health, Berkeley, California in collaboration with
Drs. N.E. Cremer, L.S. Oshiro and E.H. Lennette.

REFERENCES

1. Moloney, J.B. (1960). J.Nat.Cancer Inst. 24, 933.
2. Cremer, N.E., Taylor, O.N., Oshiro, L.S. & Teitz, Y. (1970).
      J.Nat.Cancer Inst. 45, 37.
3. DEKEL, D. & TEITZ, Y. (1972). Harefuah, 83, No.12, 540.
4. TEITZ, Y., LENNETTE, E.H., OSHIRO, L.S. & CREMER, N.E.
      (1971). J.Nat.Cancer Inst. 46, 11.
5. TEMIN, H.M. & MIZUTANI, S. (1970). Nature, 226, 1211.
6. TEITZ, Y. (1971). Nature New Biol. 232, 34, 250.
7. McDONNELL, J.P., GARAPIN, A.C., LEVINSON, W.E., QUINTRELL, N.,
      FANSHIER, L. & BISHOP, J.M. (1970). Nature, 228, 433.
8. TEMIN, H.M. & BALTIMORE, D. (1972). Adv. in Virus Research,
      17, 129.
9. TAYLOR, J.M., FARAS, A.J., VARMUS H.E., GOODMAN, H.M.,
      LEVINSON, W.E. & BISHOP, J.M. (1973). Biochemistry, 12,
      (3) 460.
10. VERMA, J.M., TEMPLE, G.F., FAN, H. & BALTIMORE, D. (1972).
      Nature New Biol. 235 (58), 163.
11. LOWRY, O.H., ROSEBROUGH, N.J., FARR, A.L. & RANDALL, R.J.
      (1951). J.Biol.Chem. 193, 265.
12. WEBER, K. & OSBORN, M. (1969). J.Biol.Chem. 244, 4406.

THE MOLECULAR BIOLOGY OF THE STEROID HORMONES

Gordon M. Tomkins

Department of Biochemistry and Biophysics, University
of California, San Francisco, San Francisco, California

In man and the other vertebrates, hormones are produced in
small quantity in specialized endocrine cells in response to
physiological or developmental stimuli, reach their target tissues
through the circulation, and induce specific cellular reactions
tending either to restore metabolic balance or promote differentiation. Our work has primarily been concerned with the mechanism
of glucocorticoid action. Before beginning a discussion of the
specific molecular details however, I should like to make some
general remarks about the evolution and biology of the hormones,
since important clues on fundamental mechanisms in present-day
organisms might be found by considering their evolutionary
history.

In this context, hormones should be regarded as a subclass
of the wide variety of chemical effectors which mediate intercellular communication. I imagine that the first step in the
evolution of a cellular communication network was the development
of appropriate biological "symbols", that is, primitive unicellu-
lar organisms began to generate specific regulatory molecules
which denoted particular physiological states. Examples of this
can be seen in present-day bacteria which, when subjected to
carbon-source starvation accumulate cyclic AMP (1) and when deprived of an essential amino acid, produce guanosine 3'5'-tetra-
phosphate (2). These molecules coordinate complicated cellular
responses suited to a particular nutritional stress and, in terms
of the present discussion, act as "symbols" for the specific
deprivation state. The correspondence between a given physiological condition and a particular mediator might be conceived of

as a kind of "metabolic code" in which each biological state requiring adaptation (for example, glucose starvation) is represented by its unique "symbol" (3).

It seems obvious that a necessary later step in the evolution
of hormonal communication was the development of the capacity for
the transmission of such symbols to other cells and of the
ability of the recipient cells to respond. At first, this coupling very likely occurred at random between two mutant organisms.
As a result, a mutual symbiotic relationship between them would
have been established. For such a coupling to have survival
value, it must be assumed that the recipient cell responded by
alleviating the metabolic distress of the sender and that this
response conferred a selective advantage upon both sender and
responder. Therefore, the ability to transmit, receive, and
respond to metabolic information would have been coded in the
genes of both the primitive sender and responder cells. If a
process like this actually did take place, then the two linked
cells might have evolved together as a simple multicellular system. Considerations like this, and our knowledge of the integrative actions of the hormones in higher organisms, suggest that
the evolutionary development of chemical intercellular communication preceded and promoted the appearance of multicellular forms
of life.

The existence of hormonal communication among relatively
primitive modern organisms such as the fungi is consistent with
a long evolutionary history. In this regard, it is interesting
to note that the Neurospora contain a hormone-sensitive membrane-
bound adenyl cyclase (4), that slime mold cells employ cyclic AMP
to coordinate their differentiation (5) and, particularly relevant to our present concern, that the water fungus Achlya, uses
steroids to control sexual differentiation (6).

I should also like to consider another aspect of the general
biology of hormonal responses--their kinetics. It seems to me
that the cellular responses to hormones can be described by one
of three basic time courses. The most rapid, a "spike", analogous
to the action potentials which travel along nerve cell membranes
on stimulation, consists of a rapid response followed by a prompt
return to the basal state and a variable period during which the
cell cannot be restimulated. Kinetics of this type occur when
cyclic AMP concentrations respond to epinephrine stimulation of
the adenyl cyclase of fat cell membranes.

A second class of responses can be described as "square
waves". Reactions of this type usually occur over a longer time
scale (hours or days) than spikes, begin with the application of

the hormone and continue as long as the hormone is present, but
not beyond. Thus, removing the hormone terminates the response,
allowing the cell to return to its basal state. Kinetics like
this are frequently produced by the steroids.

A third characteristic response, the genesis of which is more
mysterious than those of the other two, might be called a "step".
In this case the hormone triggers a response which continues even
after the hormone is no longer present. Such kinetics are characteristic of developing systems, and are probably elicited by a
variety of hormonally active substances.

Although our work has been concentrated on the adrenal glucocorticoids, there are strong indications that, at the molecular
level, general principles underlie the action of all the steroid
hormones, so that a detailed understanding of one of these
effectors might explain the actions of the other hormones as well.
Nevertheless, at the cellular level, the physiology of the glucocorticoids is highly specific and remarkably complex. Virtually
every organ in fetal and adult animals contains specific cytoplasmic receptor molecules for these hormones, consistent with the
observations that almost all tissues respond physiologically to
them (7). A mass of data indicates that there are several distinct
physiological modes of glucocorticoid action. The two which are
generally recognized are the so-called "anabolic" and "catabolic"
effects. The former refers primarily to the liver, where these
hormones promote the synthesis of macromolecules including glycogen, proteins, and nucleic acids. Catabolic effects are exerted
on peripheral organs such as muscle, and in lymphoid and connective
tissue. This response promotes tissue breakdown with degradation
of cellular proteins to free amino acids, which, when they reach
the liver via the circulation, are converted to glycogen.

In addition to these "classical" responses, there is a third
type of glucocorticoid effect which is not generally appreciated:
stimulation of embryonic development. The glucocorticoids promote
the development of many organ systems, including the nervous system (8), blood forming organs (9), liver (10), pancreas (11), gas-
trointestinal tract (12), and lungs (13). Of particular interest
for the present discussion is the fact that glucocorticoids speed
up the attainment of sexual maturity (14).

Our studies lead us to believe that most, if not all, of
these physiological responses are based on a single underlying
molecular mechanism. To investigate this mechanism we have established several systems of cultured mammalian cells which possess
functions responsive to physiological concentrations of the glucocorticoids. Most of our work has been carried out using cultured

rat hepatoma cells in which the adrenal steroids stimulate the synthesis of a specific intracellular enzyme, tyrosine amino-transferase (15). By and large, neither cell growth nor mor-phology are affected by these hormones, although several other more subtle changes in cell physiology occur because of exposure to these steroids. These changes include alterations in the cell surface (16); a decrease in the activity of cyclic AMP phospho-diesterase (17); an increase in the acceptor activity of phenyl-alanine transfer RNA in certain clones (18); and, in other clones, an increase in the level of glutamine synthetase (19). Glucocor-ticoid action in these cells is therefore very specific, making the system very useful for studies of hormonal mechanisms.

Unlike the interactions between cells and non-steroid hor-mones, the first specific contact between hepatoma cells and the corticosteroids takes place in the cytoplasm, rather than at the membrane. Our studies show that the steroids penetrate the cell membrane readily (20) and associate with specific allosteric pro-tein receptors in the cell cytosol (21). These receptors have high affinity for physiologically active glucocorticoids, and the biological potency of a particular steroid correlates almost per-fectly with its receptor-binding activity (22). Certain steroids, such as progesterone, block the hormonal activity of the gluco-corticoids (23). These hormone antagonists also associate with the receptors (22), but as we shall see presently, the consequences of this interaction are different from those of a receptor-inducer combination.

The binding of an active glucocorticoid, for example, dexa-methasone, with the receptor appears to promote conformational changes in the latter which permit the receptor-steroid complex to associate reversibly with high affinity to specific "acceptor" sites in the nucleus (24). A number of arguments lead to the con-clusion that it is this combination of the receptor with the nuclear acceptor sites which is responsible for the biological action of the steroid. In this view, the hormone itself is an allosteric effector which enhances the formation of a particular receptor conformation (23), allowing the latter to associate with its specific nuclear acceptor sites. Conversely, the combination of the receptors with glucocorticoid antagonists prevents the attainment of the nuclear binding conformation of the receptors (25). Receptor-progesterone complexes therefore, remain in the cytoplasm rather than migrating to the nucleus. These conclusions have been derived from a large number of experiments in which the association of the steroid with its receptor and the subsequent binding of the receptor-steroid complex to the nucleus have been studied in intact hepatoma cells and in cell-free extracts derived from them.

More dramatic illustrations of the biological role of receptors in steroid action come from studies showing that a deficiency in the normal complement of these molecules results in
complete loss of control over the affected tissue. For example,
we have shown that the X-linked genetic androgen-insensitivity
syndrome in mouse (which is analogous to testicular feminization
in humans) is associated with a deficiency of cytoplasmic dihydro-
testosterone receptor activity (26). Further, we have found that
cultured mouse lymphoma cells, which are normally killed by the
glucocorticoids, can become steroid-resistant and that a class of
the steroid-resistant cells lacks cytoplasmic glucocorticoid
binding activity (27).

A question of obvious interest relates to the nature of the
nuclear acceptor sites since they appear to be the immediate locus
of steroid action. Studies carried out using cell-free media have
shown that glucocorticoid-receptor binding activity is destroyed
on treatment of the nuclei with pancreatic deoxyribonuclease, suggesting that these sites contain DNA (24). Other in vitro experiments have shown that dexamethasone-receptor complexes are able to
bind both to single and double-stranded hepatoma cell DNA, but not
to RNA (28). If DNA is the true cellular site of receptor-steroid
complex binding, it seems most reasonable to suppose that the
action of the complex is to modulate gene transcription.

To gain further insights into the binding reaction between
receptor-dexamethasone complexes and their nuclear acceptor sites,
we have inquired whether such acceptor sites exist in the nuclei
of tissues which do not contain the glucocorticoid cytoplasmic
receptor (29). As I mentioned earlier, almost every tissue possesses such receptors. Fortunately, however, the immature rat
uterus appears to lack it, although of course, this tissue contains adequate concentrations of estradiol receptor molecules.
In any event, isolated uterine nuclei were prepared and tested
for their ability to accept both the homologous receptor-estradiol
complexes as well as heterologous receptor-dexamethasone complexes
prepared from hepatoma cell extracts. Rather surprisingly, we
have found that the uterine nuclei bind both dexamethasone- and
estradiol-receptor complexes with high affinity. The question that
immediately comes to mind is whether the acceptor sites for the
two different receptor-steroid complexes are identical?

Several types of experiments indicate that they are clearly
different. In the first place, estradiol-receptor complexes do
not prevent the nuclear binding of dexamethasone-receptor complexes, or vice versa. This lack of competition clearly indicates
that the two receptor steroid-complexes bind to topographically

different nuclear acceptor sites. Chemical studies have shown
that the acceptor sites for glucocorticoid receptors in uterine
nuclei are, as in hepatoma cells, destroyed on DNase treatment.
Surprisingly, however, this treatment does not prevent nuclei
from binding receptor-estradiol complexes. Other experiments as
well suggest that there are chemical differences between the two
sets of nuclear acceptor sites. Therefore, although both receptor-
dexamethasone and receptor-estradiol complexes bind to the nucleus, their nuclear acceptor sites must be spatially and chemically
different (29). Whether this difference implies differences in
the basic mechanisms of action of the two classes of hormones
remains to be seen.

To return to the hepatoma system, experiments using both
intact cells and extracts derived from them have shown that the
interaction of glucocorticoid-receptor complexes with their nuclear acceptor sites leads to an accumulation of messenger RNA
molecules active in coding for the synthesis of the inducible
enzyme, tyrosine aminotransferase (30,31). For the moment, our
evidence on this point is rather indirect, although much stronger
direct evidence has been obtained by other groups working with
estrogenic and progestational hormones in the chick oviduct. As
mentioned earlier, it seems reasonable to suppose that glucocorticoid receptor complexes function by altering gene transcription
and to conclude that the genes so affected are the structural
genes coding for the inducible enzyme. Unfortunately, evidence
for this conclusion is entirely lacking at the moment and there
are even reasons for doubting that it may be the case. In the
first place, whereas the nuclear acceptor sites are specific and
of high affinity, there are a great many of them, of the order of
4-5,000 per haploid amount of DNA (25). Thus in an ordinary di-
ploid cell, there are close to 10,000 nuclear acceptor sites.
This number is almost certainly much greater than the number of
proteins whose synthesis is directly affected by the hormones.

In addition, we have shown that there are unusual cytoplasmic
processes which promote messenger RNA inactivation (32). Quite
recently, this mechanism has been implicated in the regulation of
an estrogen-induced uterine protein, IP (33). In these cases,
although detailed understanding is lacking, it is known that
messenger inactivation requires the constant synthesis of RNA.
An hypothesis which we have entertained for some time has been
that the hormones might directly antagonize the action of the
degradative mechanism (34). Kinetic analysis of enzyme induction
carried out recently in our laboratory has, however, indicated
that hormones are more likely to play a role in stimulating the
accumulation of active messenger than in preventing its degradation (35).

Obviously, we are a long way from possessing the detailed knowledge about hormone action that we desire although significant progress has been made using the biochemical approaches I have discussed. The logical end point of these studies is the reconstruction, in an entirely cell-free system, of all the events involved in hormonal enzyme induction. Even if we achieve this goal, however, it will be necessary to correlate our findings with the events taking place in hormone-stimulated intact cells. To aid in this correlation, and incidentally to strengthen the more direct approach of biochemical analyses, we have recently begun to add the powerful techniques of genetic analysis to those more traditionally used in biochemistry and cell biology.

In these studies we take advantage of the fact that certain lines of cultured immunocytes contain specific cytoplasmic receptors which when complexed with the appropriate steroids bind specifically to nuclear acceptor sites. The physiological effect of this interaction is cellular death (27). Presumably this phenomenon is at least one of the bases of the immuno-suppressive action of the glucocorticoids. In any event, by studying the hormone-mediated death of cultured cells, we have been able to select a number of steroid-resistant variants. Although our studies are still rather preliminary, they indicate that resistant variants arise as a result of a random process, which can be accelerated by various classes of chemical and physical mutagens (36). We have used simple cell fractionation to classify our resistant populations and find, as mentioned above, that a significant number of them are missing the steroid receptor. More interesting from a mechanistic standpoint, however, is the finding that there are also receptor-containing resistant variants. One type possesses normal cytoplasmic receptors which do not associate with nuclear acceptor sites. A third class of resistant cells which we call "deathless", contain normal receptors which to all appearances, combine in the usual way with nuclear acceptor sites, but in which the events leading to cellular death do not take place (37).

It has been possible using irradiated Sendai virus to hybridize various types of steroid-resistant cells (e.g. 38), and although these experiments are still in rather early stages we have the impression that we shall be able to analyze cell-hormone action by a process analogous to genetic complementation, in which two cells, each defective in a different component of a complex biological process, are fused and the function of the hybrid studied.

Studies of this type using mutational and complementation
analyses can yield important information about a complex biological
process without the necessity for understanding its basic biochemistry. It seems clear that these techniques will prove to be
powerful additions to the already existing methodology for unravelling the complex and fascinating problem of hormone action.

REFERENCES

1. MAKMAN, R.S. & SUTHERLAND, E.W. (1965). J.Biol.Chem. 240, 1309.
2. CASHEL, M. & GALLANT, J. (1969). Nature, 221, 838.
3. TOMKINS, G.M. & GELEHRTER, T.D. In "The Biochemical Actions of
        Hormones" Vol. II, Ed. G. Litwack, Academic Press, New York,
        pp. 1-20 (1972).
4. FLAWIA, M.M. & TORRES, H. (1972). J.Biol.Chem. 247, 6873.
5. KONIJN, T.M., Van de MEENE, J.G.C., BONNER, J.T. & BARKLEY, D.S.
        (1967). Proc.Nat.Acad.Sci. USA, 58, 1152.
6. BARKSDALE, A.W. (1969). Science, 166, 831.
7. BALLARD, P.L., BAXTER, J.D., HIGGINS, S.J., ROUSSEAU, G.G. &
        TOMKINS, G.M. submitted for publication.
8. MOSCONA, A.A. & PIDDINGTON, R. (1967). Science, 158, 496.
9. For references see BAXTER, J.D. & FORSHAM, P.H. (1972).
        Amer.J.Med. 53, 573.
10. JACQUOT, R. In "Hormones in Development", Ed. M. Hambrugh and
        E.J.W. Barrington, New York, p.587 (1971).
11. YALOVSKY, V., ZELIKSON, R. & KULKA, R.G. (1969). FEBS Letters,
        2, 323.
12. MOOG, F. In "Hormones in Development", Ed. M. Hambrugh and
        E.J.W. Barrington, New York, p.143 (1971).
13. MOTOYAMA, E.K., ORZALESI, M.M., KIKKAWA, Y., KAIBARA, M.,
        WU, B., ZIGAS, C.J. & COOK, C.D. (1971). Pediatrics, 48, 547.
14. RAMALEY, J.A. (1973). Endocrinology, 92, 881.
15. For a recent review see BAXTER, J.D., ROUSSEAU, G.G., HIGGINS,
        S.J. & TOMKINS, G.M. In "The Biochemistry of Gene Expression
        in Higher Organisms", Ed. P. Benjamin, Australia and New
        Zealand Book Co., N.S.W. Australia, pp.206-224 (1973).
16. BALLARD, P. & TOMKINS, G.M. (1970). J.Cell Biol. 47, 222.
17. MANGANIELLO, V. & VAUGHAN, M. (1972). J.Clin.Invest. 51, 2763.
18. LIPPMAN, S., YANG, S. & THOMPSON, E.B. In preparation.
19. KULKA, R.G., TOMKINS, G.M. & CROOK, R.B. (1972). J.Cell Biol.
        54, 175.
20. LEVINSON, B.B., BAXTER, J.D., ROUSSEAU, G.G. & TOMKINS, G.M.
        (1972). Science, 175, 189.
21. BAXTER, J.D. & TOMKINS, G.M. (1971). Proc.Nat.Acad.Sci. USA,
        68, 932.

22. ROUSSEAU, G.G., BAXTER, J.D. & TOMKINS, G.M. (1972).
    J.Mol.Biol. 67, 99.
23. SAMUELS, H.H. & TOMKINS, G.M. (1970). J.Mol.Biol. 52, 57.
24. BAXTER, J.D., ROUSSEAU, G.G., BENSON, M.C., GARCEA, R.L., &
    ITO, J. (1972). Proc.Nat.Sci. USA, 69, 1892.
25. ROUSSEAU, G.G., BAXTER, J.D., HIGGINS, S.J. & TOMKINS, G.M.
    J.Mol.Biol. in press.
26. GEHRING, U., TOMKINS, G.M. & OHNO, S. (1971). Nature New
    Biol. 232, 106.
27. ROSENAU, W., BAXTER, J.D., ROUSSEAU, G.G. & TOMKINS, G.M.
    (1972). Nature New Biol. 237, 20.
28. ROUSSEAU, G.G., BAXTER, J.D., HIGGINS , S.J., WONG, K.Y. &
    TOMKINS, G.M. In preparation.
29. HIGGINS, S.J., ROUSSEAU, G.G., BAXTER, J.D. & TOMKINS, G.M.
    J.Biol.Chem. in press.
30. SCOTT, W.A., SHIELDS, R. & TOMKINS, G.M. (1972).
    Proc.Nat.Acad.Sci. USA, 69, 2937.
31. KLEIN, C., LEVINSON, B.B. & TOMKINS, G.M. submitted for
    publication.
32. TOMKINS, G.M., LEVINSON, B.B., BAXTER, J.D. & DETHLEFSEN, L.
    (1972). Nature New Biol. 239, 9.
33. DeANGELO, A.B., FUJIMOTO, G.I. (1973). Proc.Nat.Acad.Sci.
    USA, 70, 18.
34. TOMKINS, G.M., GELEHRTER, T.D., GRANNER, D.K., MARTIN, D.W.JR.,
    SAMUELS, H.H. & THOMPSON, E.B. (1969). Science, 166, 1474.
35. STEINBERG, R., LEVINSON, B.B. & TOMKINS, G.M. in preparation.
36. SIBLEY, C.H. & TOMKINS, G.M. (1973). Proc.Intl.Congress of
    Genetics, in press.
37. SIBLEY, C.H., GEHRING, U., BOURNE, H. & TOMKINS, G.M.
    Cold Spring Harbor Symp. in press.

EFFECTS OF OESTRADIOL ON DIFFERENT CELL TYPES

R.J.B. King and Jill Thompson

Hormone Biochemistry Department, Imperial Cancer Research
Fund, Lincoln's Inn Fields, London WC2A 3PX

INTRODUCTION

The steroidal oestrogens are produced primarily in the ovary
and are conveyed in the blood to their sites of action in different parts of the body. The blood transport is mediated by
attachment to plasma proteins (1,2). Hence it is legitimate to
think of these and other steroids as chemically defined serum
factors. Study of the mode whereby these steroids exert their
biological effect is of interest both from the aspect of ways in
which relatively simple molecules affect cell activity and as a
tool to see how the less well-understood serum factors work (3).

The title of this meeting contains the word "strategies"
which can be defined as "the art of devising plans to attain a
specific goal". Such a definition contains an element of fore-
sight; our paper will follow this definition and will discuss an
aspect of oestrogen action for which very little established data
is available but which we regard as one of the more important
questions to be answered in the coming years. The question to be
asked is "How do oestrogens affect different oestrogen-responsive
cells in dissimilar ways?"

The spectrum of effects produced by oestrogens varies from
the induction of DNA synthesis to the production of a limited
number of proteins (Table 1). The basic scheme whereby oestrogens
can affect cell function is depicted in Fig. 1; the oestrogen (E)
combines with a cytoplasmic receptor (R) and is transformed to a
complex ER* which enters the nucleus, combines with chromatin and

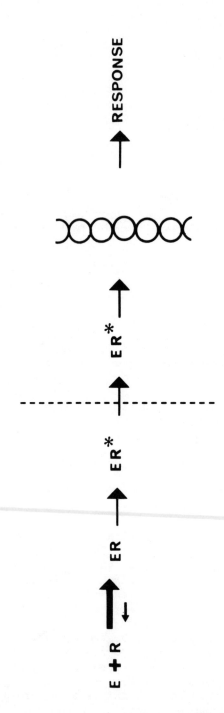

Fig. 1. Intracellular oestrogen (E) transport. R = cytoplasmic receptor; R* = transformed or nuclear receptor; --- = nuclear membrane; ⅗ = chromatin.

elicits the response characteristic of that cell type. The oestrogen binding data have been reviewed (3,4,5,6) and, although certain aspects of the scheme shown in Fig. 1 need further clarification, it will be used as the framework for the views presented
below. The biochemical events forming the basis of the term
"response" in Fig. 1 involve elevated RNA and protein synthesis,
and a topic which also has been quite recently reviewed (5,7,8).

TABLE   1

EFFECT OF OESTROGEN ON DIFFERENT ORGANS

Species	Tissue	Effect	Reference
Rat	Uterus	Cell division	9
	Kidney	Induction of two enzymes	10,11
	Hypothalamus	Synthesis/Release of polypeptides	12
Chicken	Oviduct	Ovalbumin production	13
	Liver	Phosphoprotein synthesis	14
Hamster	Kidney	Carcinogenesis	15

It is evident that there are three major ways in which a
different end-response to oestrogen might be achieved. 1) The
oestrogen affecting different cells might vary. 2) The binding/
transport process might not be identical in different responsive
cells, or 3) The biochemical responses may diverge at points dis-
tal to the oestrogen-chromatin interaction. This latter aspect
will not be discussed in this paper.

Biological Activity of Different Oestrogens

The vast majority of biological tests have been carried out
using uterine or vaginal responses as the end points and data for
the other systems included in Table 1 are scarce.

However, it is clear that save for a possible exception mentioned below, oestradiol-17β is the most potent of the naturally

occurring oestrogens in all of the systems studied (15,16). The exception just referred to is oestriol, which in terms of uterine water imbibition is as active as oestradiol, but which is appreciably less potent than oestradiol in increasing uterine dry weight (17,18). This anomaly can be explained by the shorter duration of nuclear retention of oestriol relative to that of oestradiol (18).

Thus there is no reason to think that different end-organ responses to oestrogen are due to different hormones although the paucity of data leaves ample scope for this statement to be disproved.

OESTROGEN-BINDING/TRANSPORT MECHANISMS

The scheme outlined in Fig. 1 has, in part, been shown to be operative in every oestrogen-sensitive cell type investigated with the possible exceptions of chick liver (19,20) and hamster kidney (21). The lack of binding in hamster kidney could readily be explained by the insensitivity of the detection methods, but on the data available at present, the chick liver is a candidate for a different type of binding process; no cytoplasmic receptor was found in this organ although a nuclear component soluble in Tris-buffer was readily detected (20).

Despite the near-universality of the binding/transport process, it is by no means ruled out that it is the only way in which oestrogen effects are mediated. Szego (22) has advocated effects via the lysosomes and Rabin and coworkers (23) have demonstrated oestradiol-binding sites on hepatic endoplasmic reticulum. Furthermore, explanations have to be found as to why 4-mercuri-oestradiol is a potent oestrogen which binds to cytoplasmic receptor but does not penetrate into the nucleus (24) and why pharmacologic doses of oestrogen can have the opposite effect to physiological doses (25).

With these reservations in mind, one can consider three ways in which different end-responses might be explained by variability in the binding/transport process; different responsive cells might have different R, R^* or chromatin acceptor.

Cytoplasmic Receptor

The cytoplasmic receptor R, has mainly been characterized by sucrose-gradient analysis, ligand specificity and its dissociation constant K_D. The data indicate that, with one exception, there are

no gross differences in receptor isolated from different cells
(reviewed in 2,26) but the methods used thus far are very crude
and there could easily be considerable differences in structure.
It is noteworthy that an antibody prepared against calf uterine
receptor did not cross react with receptor from pituitary gland
(27).

The exception is chick oviduct, which contains a receptor
somewhat larger (10S) than that reported for other cells and which
is not dissociated by 0.5 M KCl (19). If this finding can be confirmed, it would strongly indicate that different cytoplasmic
receptors exist in different cells. A further hint that different
types of cytoplasmic receptors exist comes from the experiment
depicted in Fig. 2. Uterine nuclei bound more uterine receptor
than did nuclei from oestrogen-responsive dimethylbenzanthracene-
induced rat mammary tumours but this effect was not evident when
tumour receptor was used. Because of the crudeness of the preparations used in these experiments, the possibility of artefacts
are high, hence the use of the word "hint".

Nuclear Receptor

Insufficient data is available concerning the transformation
of R to R* to warrant comment but, save in the chicken, all the
nuclear receptors isolated in hypertonic media have similar sedimentation (4-5S) characteristics (reviewed in ref. 2). Chick oviduct contains a 7S nuclear receptor (19) whilst the liver from
this animal contains a component soluble in Tris-buffer that, in
contradistinction to other oestradiol-responsive organs, will bind
oestradiol without the mediation of cytoplasmic events (20).

Comparison of the effects of oestrogen on different cells
(Table 1) would suggest that putative differences in R or R* would
be most readily found by comparing uterus with chick oviduct or
liver. The anomalous results reported for the chick tissues may
represent evidence for variable types of receptor. The greater
ease of extraction of nuclear receptor from DMBA-induced mammary
tumours than from nuclei of other oestrogen-responsive cells could
also be explained on the basis of different receptors (26).

Acceptor

One of the main problems in discussing this potential site of
discrimination is in deciding whether specific acceptors exist or
whether the only specificity is at the level of the oestrogen-
receptor complex. We believe, together with others (28,29,30,31)
that acceptor specificity does exist although this is not the

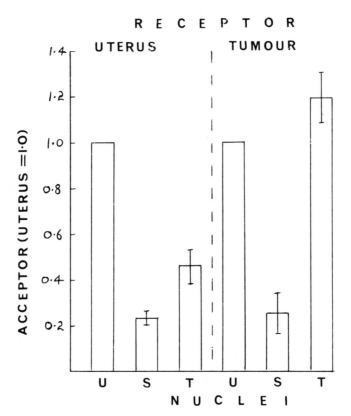

R E C E P T O R

UTERUS   TUMOUR

Fig. 2. Acceptor activity of nuclei from uterus (U), spleen (S)
or DMBA-induced rat mammary adenocarcinoma (T) for oestradiol
receptor from either uterus or T.
Nuclei were prepared from a 2 percent w/v homogenate of the tissue
in 0.25 M sucrose, 3 mM $CaCl_2$. The crude nuclear pellet, obtained
by centrifugation of the homogenate at 700 xg for 10 min, was resuspended in 2.1 M sucrose, 3 mM $CaCl_2$, layered over 2.1 M sucrose, and centrifuged at 20,000 rpm for 30 min in a SW27 rotor in
a Spinco L2-65B ultracentrifuge. All operations were carried out
at 4°.
Uterine receptor was prepared from 10 percent w/v homogenates in
10 mM Tris, 1 mM EDTA, 1.5 mM β-mercaptoethanol (TEM). After
centrifugation for 1 h at 39,000 rpm in a 50 Ti rotor, the supernatant was made 1 nM with respect to $[6,7-^3H]$ oestradiol and incubated overnight at 4°C. The 0-25 percent w/v ammonium sulphate-
insoluble fraction was dissolved in TEM.
Incubation of nuclei with receptor was carried out for 1 h at 4°C
- usually 100 μgm DNA with 2×10^4 dpm receptor. The nuclei were
precipitated by centrifugation at 700 xg for 10 min, washed twice
with 10 mM Tris, 3 mM $CaCl_2$, digested with 1 N NaOH and counted.

generally accepted view (32). Our original suggestion that specificity existed at the nuclear level came from the observation
that uterine nuclei from mature rats accepted more oestradiol-
receptor complex than did liver (28) or spleen (29) nuclei. This
difference disappeared seven days after ovariectomy (28), which
suggested that the specificity was controlled by ovarian hormones.
These studies have been extended to include data on nuclei from
other oestrogen-sensitive tissues (33). Figure 3 indicates the
acceptor capacity of nuclei from cell types of differing oestrogen
sensitivities obtained from mature animals, for the rat uterine
oestradiol-receptor complex. A range of acceptor levels exist
which bear only a superficial relationship to the oestrogen-sensi-
tivity of the cell of origin. Comparison of the data for uterus,
DMBA-induced mammary tumour, spleen and kidney type A tumour cells
would support the idea that nuclei from oestrogen-sensitive cells
can accept more receptor than nuclei from unresponsive cells, but
this conclusion is hard to justify when the hamster kidney type B
tumours are considered. Type A tumours, kindly donated by Dr. H.G.
Bloom and Mr. B.C.V. Mitchley from the Chester Beatty Institute,
were derived from oestrogen-induced, oestrogen-dependent primary
tumours by serial transplantation (15,34). They are relatively
autonomous and grow in both female and male hamsters, although
some degree of responsiveness is retained as growth is retarded by
orchidectomy and by antioestrogens (35). The type B tumours were
kindly donated by Dr. H. Kirkman of Stanford University; they were
derived from the same type of tumour as A, and grew equally well in
male and female hamsters (Kirkman, personal communication). It is
clear that the acceptor level is related to the sex of the animal
in which the tumour was growing, rather than to the oestrogen-
responsiveness of the tumour itself.

If chromatin is used instead of nuclei as the acceptor, differences between uterus and spleen are still found (Fig. 4 and
ref. 29); it is noteworthy that the chromatin acceptor sites in
spleen chromatin have similar binding contants to those in uterus
(Fig. 5 and Table 2).

It is obvious from the data presented above that much must be
done before the differences in acceptor levels can be graced with
the term specificity. Our belief that specificity does exist at
the nuclear level remains to be proven and at the present time it
is probably wiser to use the term "differences" rather than
"specificity". From the data presented in Fig. 3 and reference 28
it is tempting to think that the acceptor level is controlled by
ovarian hormones but how this suggestion can be related to the
biological effectiveness of oestrogens is obscure, as uteri both
from immature and ovariectomised, mature rats respond to exogeneous
oestrogen. The existing data do not preclude the possibility that

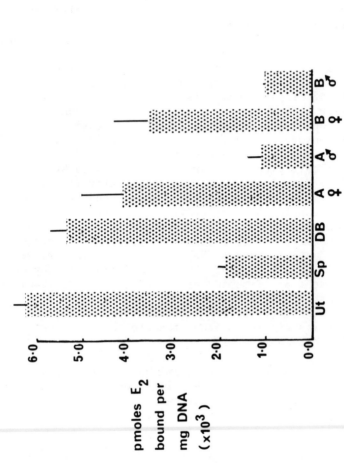

Fig. 3. Acceptor activity of nuclei from: rat uterus (Ut); spleen (Sp); DMBA-induced rat mammary adenocarcinoma (DB); unresponsive, oestrogen-induced hamster kidney tumour type A (A); and B (B) grown in male ($\male$) or female ($\female$) hamsters. Oestradiol-receptor was prepared from rat uteri. Assay conditions were described in Fig. 2.

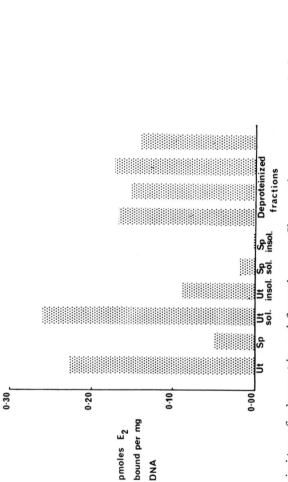

Fig. 4. Acceptor activity of chromatin subfractions. Chromatin was prepared from uterus (Ut) and spleen (Sp) by homogenization in 75 mM NaCl, 2 mM EDTA pH 7.4, filtration through cheesecloth and centrifugation at 700 xg for 15 min. The pellet was washed twice with 10 mM NaCl; once with 1 mM EDTA pH 7.0; once with 50 mM Tris-HCl pH 8.0; and twice with 0.4 M KCl. Finally the chromatin was sedimented through 1.7 M sucrose at 27,000 rpm in a Beckman-Spinco SW27 rotor. The chromatin pellet was digested for 1 h at 37°C with deoxy-ribonuclease II (125 μg enzyme per 250 μg DNA). After centrifugation at 30,000 xg for 20 min, 0.11 vol. of 1.5 M NaCl, 0.15 M sodium citrate pH 7.4 was added to the supernatant. The insoluble material (insol.) was sedimented at 30,000 xg for 20 min, resuspended in 10 mM Tris-HCl pH 8.0 and resedimented at 30,000 xg for 20 min. The material soluble in 0.15 M NaCl, 0.015 M sodium citrate pH 7.4 was centrifuged at 80,000 xg for 18 h on a cushion of 1.7 M sucrose. The sucrose layer plus pellet were dialysed against 10 mM Tris-HCl pH 8.0 to give the soluble fraction (sol.). All fractions were deproteinised by sedi-mentation through 6 M caesium chloride for 48 h at 105 xg. Reading from left to right, the four deproteinised fractions refer to material obtained from Ut. Sol., Ut insol., Sp. sol. and Sp. insol. respectively. Uterine oestradiol-receptor complex was prepared from rat uteri as described in Fig. 2. Acceptor activity was assayed as described in ref. 29.

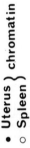

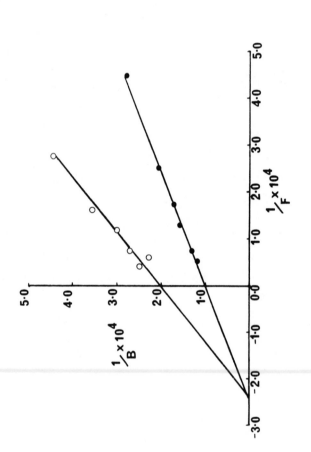

Fig. 5. Binding of uterine oestradiol-receptor complex to uterine (●) and spleen (o) chromatin. Preparation of the chromatins was as described in Fig. 4 up to the end of the first
centrifugation through 1.7 M sucrose. Oestradiol-receptor complex was prepared as described
in Fig. 2. Approx. 1 absorbance$_{260}$ unit of chromatin was incubated and assayed with
increasing levels of oestradiol-receptor complex ($2x10^3$ - $1x10^5$ dpm) as described in Fig. 4 .
Results are plotted as a reciprocal plot of bound (1/B) and free (1/F) receptor complex.

different quantitative responses to a given dose of oestrogen
might be elicited in ovariectomised and intact mature rats.

WHAT IS THE ACCEPTOR?

Part of the confusion surrounding differences between the
acceptor properties of different nuclei or chromatins is due to
the poor characterization of the acceptor. We believe that DNA
is the primary acceptor and that the non-DNA components of the
chromatin function to locate the receptor on the correct region of
the DNA. It should be stressed that this is a belief rather than
an established fact because most of the experiments have been
carried out in cell-free systems and the only way one can be sure
that such experiments are relevant to events occurring in whole
cells is by comparing the data obtained with the two types of experiment. From published data one can predict that the acceptor-
receptor interaction should have certain properties; it should be
dissociated in 0.4 M KCl, have a high affinity and low capacity
and the acceptor should bind ER but not E alone. DNA satisfies
each of these criteria and additionally deoxyribonuclease destroys
the acceptor (29,36); but there is no explanation for the differences in acceptor seen with different nuclei and chromatins
(Fig. 4 and refs. 28,29). The chromatin proteins impose a secondary level of selection; both non-histones and histones are important. If the histones are removed from uterine and spleen
chromatins, the differences still exist which indicates that the
histones are not the cause of the differences between these two
types of chromatin, but their removal exposes additional sites
(29). The same conclusion is reached from another type of experiment; when uterine and spleen chromatins are separated into his-
tone-poor (A) and histone-rich (B) fractions by deoxyribonuclease
treatment (37) B, has the lower acceptor level. Subsequent depro-
teinisation of the chromatin fractions with caesium chloride
exposes additional sites in fraction B without significantly affecting fraction A (Fig. 4). The DNA's from uterus and spleen
exhibit the same acceptor activity.

It is clear that the histones are blocking some acceptor
sites both in uterus and spleen, while the non-histone proteins
present in uterine and spleen chromatins are similar to that of
denatured DNA (Table 2). It is inferred that the acceptor sites
in whole chromatins, dehistoned-chromatin and DNA are similar.

This indicates to us that DNA is involved in the acceptor
mechanism and, on the premise that DNA is the primary acceptor,
the data could be explained by either of two general models. The

TABLE   2

AFFINITY OF ER FOR CHROMATIN

	K_D		n	
	$(Mx10^{10})$		(mole oestradiol/mg DNAx10^{12})	
	Uterus	Spleen	Uterus	Spleen
Chromatin	3.90	4.13	1.35	0.77

first scheme suggests that tissue-specific, non-histone proteins
determine which DNA sites are available in different responsive
cells without a direct interaction between the chromatin protein
components and receptor. The second model proposes that the receptor reacts with a tissue-specific, non-histone protein which
locates the receptor in the correct region of the genome; a
second reaction then occurs between receptor and DNA. A synthesis
of both schemes would be that the model 1-type reaction is followed
by a specific interaction with a non-DNA component of the chromatin.   In both schemes, some DNA sites are blocked by histones.
Although the term "non-histone protein" has been used in the above
discussion, it is a rather nebulous entity and could include other
components such as RNA.   Liao et al. (38) have presented evidence
that 80S nuclear ribonucleoproteins (RNP) will bind ER and the
RNP may facilitate attachment of ER to native DNA. All of our
data quoted above was obtained with chromatins that had been extracted with 0.4 M KCl which presumably would remove at least part
of Liao's factor.

Characterization of the Receptor-Binding Sites on DNA

     Despite the lack of specificity of ER for different types of
DNA, some specificity for certain conformations must exist because,
at saturation, only one receptor is bound per 10^7 nucleotides which
contrasts markedly with the attachment of small molecules like
actinomycin D (39), "reporter molecules" (40,41) or ethidium bromide (42) which have binding ratios of 1 ligand to fewer than 50
nucleotides and histones which bind at about 1 histone per 100

nucleotides (43). This difference between receptor and histone is not explicable on the basis of their respective sizes.

Single stranded DNA binds ER more efficiently than native DNA (29) which raises the possibility that the ER complex might be a DNA-melting protein. If so, it would be more likely to bind to A-T rich regions but our tentative conclusion is that this is not so. Denatured poly dG·dC binds ER as effectively as does denatured calf thymus-DNA (33). Furthermore, polyribonucleotides also bind ER in the following decreasing order of effectiveness rG>^+_hC>rU>rI. It would seem that guanine is important and, in particular the exocyclic amino group at position 6, as judged by the low binding to poly rI and to hydroxymethylated DNA (33). Attachment of R to guanine-containing polynucleotides prompted the idea that actinomycin D might block acceptor sites; this was not so as this antibiotic at concentrations between 10^{-5} - 10^{-4} M had no effect on ER uptake by uterine nuclei, chromatin or DNA. These results were not affected by the order of mixing the reactants and thus complement the earlier observations on the ineffectiveness of actinomycin on oestradiol uptake (44).

The type of binding involved in the receptor-DNA interaction is not known but it cannot be due solely to ionic interactions between R and DNA phosphate groups as R does not bind to phospho-cellulose (45).

In conclusion, apart from more detailed studies of receptors from different oestrogen-sensitive cells, one would very much like to know more about the nuclear events associated with receptor binding. What is the acceptor and are the differences in acceptor levels seen with different chromatins related in any way to biological function? It is to be hoped that some of the strategies mentioned here will help to answer some of these questions.

REFERENCES

1. WESTPHAL, U. (1971). In "Steroid-Protein Interactions", Monographs in Endocrinology, Vol. 4. Berlin, Springer-Verlag.
2. KING, R.J.B. & MAINWARING, I.W. (1973). In "Steroid-Cell Interactions". London, Butterworths.
3. Cell Division (1971). Ciba Foundation Colloquium. Ed. E.W. Wolstenholme and J. Knight. London, Churchill.
4. JENSEN, E.V. & DeSOMBRE, J. (1972). Ann.Rev.Biochem. 41, 203.
5. MUELLER, G.C., VANDERHAAR, B., KIM, V.H. & MATHIEU, M.L. (1972). Recent Prog.Horm.Res. 28, 1.

6. WILLIAMS, D. & GORSKI, J. (1972). Proc.Natn.Acad.Sci.(USA) 69, 3464.

7. HAMILTON, J.H., TENG, C-S, MEANS, A.R. & LUCK, D.N. (1971). In The Sex Steroids, p.197. Ed. K.W. McKerns, New York, Appleton-Century-Crofts.

8. GORSKI, J., DeANGELO, A.B. & BARNEA, A. (1971). In The Sex Steroids, p.181. Ed. K.W. McKerns, New York, Appleton-Century-Crofts.

9. MARTIN, L., FINN, C.A. & TRINDER, G. (1973). J.Endocr. 56, 133.

10. RYAN, K.J., MEIGS, R.A., PETRO, Z. & MORRISON, G. (1963). Science, 142, 243.

11. HERZFELD, A. & KNOX, W.E. (1968). J.Biol.Chem. 243, 3327.

12. FLERKO, B. (1966). In Neuroendocrinology, Vol. 1, p.613 Eds.L. Martin and W.F. Ganong. New York, Academic Press.

13. O'MALLEY, B.W., McGUIRE, W.L., KOHLER, P.O. & KONENMAN, S.G. (1969). Recent Prog.Hormone Res. 25, 105.

14. HEALD, P.J. & McLAUGHLAN, P.M. (1965). Biochem.J. 94, 32.

15. KIRKMAN, H. (1959). Natn.Cancer Inst. Monograph No.1, p1. U.S. Dept. of Health, Education and Welfare, Bethesda.

16. EMMENS, C.W. (1969). In Methods in Hormone Research. 2nd Edition, Vol. IIA, p.61, Ed. R.I. Dorfman. New York, Academic Press.

17. MERRILL, R.C. (1958). Physiol.Rev. 38, 463.

18. ANDERSON, J.M., CLARK, J.H. & PECK, E.J. (1972). Biochem. Biophys.Res.Commun. 48, 1460.

19. COX, R.F., CATLIN, G.H. & CAREY, N.H. (1971). Eur.J.Biochem. 22, 46.

20. MESTER, J. & BAULIEU, E.E. (1972). Biochim.Biophys.Acta. 261, 236.

21. STEGGLES, A.W. & KING, R.J.B. (1972). Eur.J.Cancer, 8, 323.

22. SZEGO, C.M. & SEELER, B.J. (1973). J.Endocrin. 56, 347.

23. BLYTHE, C.A., COOPER, M.B., ROOBOL, A. & RABIN, B.R. (1972). Eur.J.Biochem. 29, 293.

24. MULDOON, T.G. (1971). Biochemistry, 10, 3780.

25. HAYWARD, J. (1970). In Recent Results in Cancer Research, Vol.24, p.76, Ed. P. Rentchnick, Berlin, Springer-Verlag.

26. KING, R.J.B., BEARD, V., GORDON, J., POOLEY, A.S., SMITH, J.A., STEGGLES, A.W. & VERTES, M. (1970). In Advances in the Biosciences, Vol.7, p.21. Ed. G. Raspé, Oxford, Pergaman Press.

27. JENSEN, E.V., DeSOMBRE, E.R. & JUNGBLUT, P.W. (1967). In Endogenous Factors Influencing Host-Tumor Balance, p.15. Eds.R.W. Wissler, J.L. Dao and S. Wood, Chicago, University of Chicago Press.

28. KING, R.J.B., GORDON, J., MARX, JOANNA & STEGGLES, A.W. (1971). In Basic Actions of Sex Steroids on Target Organs, p.21, Eds. P.O. Hubinot, F. LeRoy and P. Galand, Basle, Karger.

29. KING, R.J.B. & GORDON, J. (1972). Nature, New Biology,
     240, 185.
30. O'MALLEY, B.W., SPELSBERG, T.C., SCHRADER, W.T., CHYTIL, F. &
     STEGGLES, A.W. (1972). Nature, 235, 141.
31. LIANG, T. & LIAO, S. (1972). Biochem.Biophys.Acta. 277, 590.
32. CHAMNESS, G.C., JENNINGS, A.W. & McGUIRE, W.L. (1973).
     Nature, 241, 458.
33. KING, R.J.B. (1972). In Effects of Drugs on Cellular Control
     Mechanisms, p.11, Eds. B.R. Rabin and R.B. Freedman, London,
     MacMillan Press.
34. BLOOM, H.J.G., BAKER, W.H., DUKES, C.E. & MITCHLEY, B.C.V.
     (1964). Brit.J.Cancer, 17, 646.
35. BLOOM. H.J.G., ROE, F.J.C. & MITCHLEY, B.C.V. (1967). Cancer,
     20, 2118.
36. SHYAMALA-HARRIS, G. (1971). Nature,New Biology, 231, 246.
37. MARUSHIGE, K. & BONNER, J. (1971). Proc.Natn.Acad.Sci.USA,
     68, 294.
38. LIAO, S., LIANG, T. & TYMOCZKO, J.L. (1973). Nature, New
     Biology, 241, 211.
39. KLEIMAN, L. & HUANG, R.C.C. (1971). J.Mol.Biol. 55, 503.
40. FARBER, J., BASERGA, R. & GABBAY, E.J. (1971). Biochem.
     Biophys.Res.Commun. 43, 675.
41. SIMPSON, R.I. (1970). Biochemistry, 9, 4814.
42. ANGERER, L.M. & MOUDRIANAKIS, K. (1972). J.Mol.Biol. 63, 505.
43. RICHARDS, B.M. & PARDON, J.F. (1970). Exp.Cell Res. 62, 184.
44. JENSEN, E.V., JACOBSON, H.I., FLESHER, J.W., SAHA, N.N.,
     GUPTA, G.N., SMITH, S., COLUCCI, V., SHIPLACOFF, D.,
     NEUMANN, H.G., DeSOMBRE, E.R. & JUNGBLUT, P.W. (1966) In
     Steroid Biodynamics, p.133, Eds. T. Nakao, G. Pincus,
     J.F. Tait, New York, Academic Press.
45. ARNAUD, M., BEZIAT, Y., BORGNA, J.L., GIULLEUX, J.C. &
     MOUSSERON-CANET, M. (1971). Biochim.Biophys.Acta, 254, 241.

SEQUENTIAL GENE EXPRESSION IN RESPONSE TO ESTRADIOL-17β

DURING POST-NATAL DEVELOPMENT OF RAT UTERUS

A. M. Kaye, Dalia Sömjen, R.J.B. King, G. Sömjen, I. Icekson and H. R. Lindner

Department of Biodynamics, Weizmann Institute of Science, Rehovot, Israel

INTRODUCTION

Hormonal model systems play an important role in the study of the control of protein synthesis (1) and of development (2). Thus the stimulation of nucleic acid and protein synthesis (3-5) in the immature rat uterus by treatment with estradiol-17β has received considerable attention. Our recent use of a developmental approach (6-9) to the mechanism of action of estradiol-17β provides a point of entry which complements and extends the current efforts through the study of receptor proteins and the control of RNA polymerase (10-12).

In this brief review, we should like to present our recent evidence for the sequential acquisition of responsiveness to estradiol by the rat uterus during the first month after birth. It is difficult to explain this developmental process on the basis of the known properties of the cytoplasmic and nuclear receptors for estradiol (10,11), and the chromosomal acceptor for the estradiol-receptor complex (14-17) found in the rat uterus. It seems necessary to postulate either heterogeneity of receptor (5) or acceptor sites or additional specificity-conferring factors in order to account for the selective responsiveness we have found at different stages of development.

The studies presented here followed roughly the same sequence as that found in biologic information transfer; DNA synthesis then RNA and protein synthesis. The stimulation of DNA synthesis by estradiol (18) has been previously studied in approximately 20-day-old rats. We have extended these studies by investigating the

effect of estradiol-17β in rats from 5 days before birth till the
age of 30 days (in our rat colony, the first estrous cycle begins
at about 32 to 34 days).

In our experiments, immature rats up to the age of 30 days
were given intraperitoneal injections of estradiol 17-β in dilute
ethanol (1 percent), or dilute ethanol alone, in amounts depending
on their ages. At specified times after injection, uteri were
explanted and incubated for 1 h in media containing radioactive
thymidine or amino acids, or examined for estradiol-binding
capacity.

Stimulation of DNA Synthesis by Estradiol-17β
During Postnatal Development (6)

During the period from the 16th day of fetal age until 30 days
after birth, the rate of incorporation of ^{3}H-thymidine into uterine
DNA declines by an order of magnitude in linear fashion (Fig. 1).
Estradiol has no influence on the rate of DNA synthesis through
the 15th day of life; only at 20 days or later is an estrogen
stimulated increase seen (Fig. 1). The non-responsiveness to
estradiol is not a matter of inadequate dose, since increasing the
dose at 15 days from 0.5 to 5 µg of estradiol has no effect; nor
does a series of two injections, at 13 and 15 days of age, each of
0.5 µg estradiol, lead to any increase in the rate of DNA synthesis.

Although uterine DNA synthesis is approximately doubled in
20-day-old rats 24 h after estrogen injection, it is still below
the rate found in fetal or newborn rats (>1000 cpm/µg DNA/h)
(Fig. 1), suggesting that estradiol's apparent stimulation of DNA
synthesis may actually reflect a partial release from inhibition,
possibly by a uterine chalone.

Throughout the rats' first ovulation cycle, administration of
exogenous estradiol does not raise the rate of DNA synthesis to
the level attained in estradiol-treated 30-day-old rats.   In
addition to the more rapid synthetic rate, the immature rat offers
another advantage for studying the mechanism of estradiol action,
in that all the tissues of the uterus respond to estradiol
(Table 1), whereas the stromal elements of the endometrium do not
respond to estradiol alone (19). This in fact may be a major
reason for the higher biosynthetic activity of immature as compared with castrate rats.

If one uses the less sensitive parameter, the content of DNA
in the uterus (8) rather than the rate of DNA synthesis, as a
measure of responsiveness to estradiol (Fig. 2), the classical

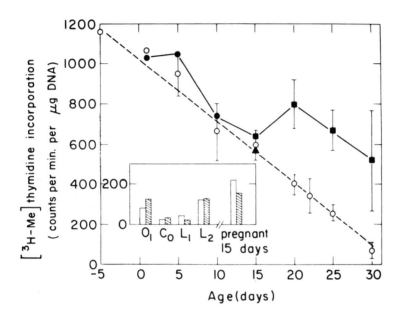

Fig. 1.   Responsiveness of rat uteri to estradiol-17β during post-
natal development measured by incorporation of [Me-^{3}H] thymidine
into DNA.   Twenty-four h after injection of estradiol the uteri were
removed and incubated for 1 h in 1 ml of medium 199 containing 3μC
of [Me-^{3}H] thymidine.   Sufficient uteri were used to have approximately 20 mg of wet tissue per incubation.   The point at 5 days
before birth (16-day embryos) represents the mean of duplicate determinations each made on a pool of the Wolffian and Mullerian duct
complexes from 10 embryos, weighing approximately 5 mg.   0---0
control rats; ●——● rats given 0.05 μg estradiol; ■ ——■ rats
given 0.5 μg estradiol; ▲ rat given 5 μg estradiol. Vertical lines
indicate 95% confidence intervals.   Inserted histogram O_1, proestrus;
C_0 estrus; L_1 metestrus and L_2 diestrus.   Open bars, control rats;
lined bars, rats given 5 μg estradiol.   The cycling rats were 40
days old, the pregnant rat was a multiparous adult. (From Ref. 6).

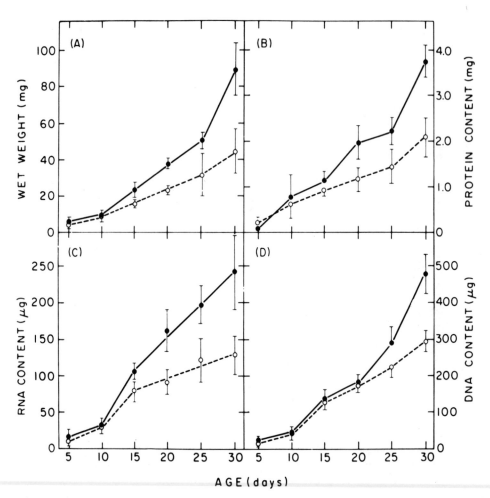

Fig. 2.   Responsiveness to estradiol-17β during post-natal development measured by increase in uterine weight and macromolecular
content.   Rats were given a single injection of either 1% ethanol
(control) or estradiol-17β on the day indicated and killed 24 h
later.   Rats 15-days or older received 0.5 μg estradiol, 10-day-
old rats 0.4 μg and 5-day-old rats 0.2 μg estradiol.   O----O, mean
value per uterus in control rats;   ●——●, mean value per uterus
in rats given estradiol.   Vertical lines indicate 95% confidence
intervals (Ref. 8).

TABLE 1

STIMULATION OF CELL DIVISION BY ESTRADIOL (a)

Dose (ng)	Epithelium	Mitotic Index (⁰/oo)		
		Gland	Stroma	Myometrium
0	3	1	10	8
5	66	3	69	60
5000	164	8	60	58

(a) 20-day-old rats were injected with estradiol-17β or with the dilute ethanol vehicle at time zero. After 24 h the rats were injected intraperitoneally with colchinine (1 μg/g) and killed at 28 h (Ref. 6).

contention that the content of DNA in the uterus does not increase within 24 h after estrogen injection into rats (18) is seen to be true for rats of 20 days of age but not for older rats. A significant increase in the uterine content of DNA after estradiol was found in 30-day-old rats.

Stimulation of Fluid Uptake,

Net Synthesis of RNA and Protein by Estradiol-17β (8)

Although DNA synthesis could not be stimulated in 15-day-old rats, the other classical parameter of estrogen action, gain in wet weight (20) is shown by 15-day-old rats, but not by 5 or 10 day old rats (Fig. 2A). The RNA content (Fig. 2C) shows the same response as the wet weight; the protein content also shows the same pattern, although the increase at 15 days is not significant as shown by the overlap of the 95% confidence intervals (Fig. 2B).

A more sensitive indicator of the action of estradiol on
protein synthesis is the rate of incorporation of labeled amino
acids into protein (7,9). The maximal rates of incorporation
(Fig. 3) into total protein occurred at 6 h, into acid soluble
nuclear protein at 12 h and into acid-insoluble nuclear proteins
at 3-4 h, preceding the synthesis of DNA, which shows a significant
increase by 18 h and reaches a peak at 24 h (Fig. 3). This asyn-
chrony of chromosomal protein and DNA synthesis has been observed
in other systems (21-23).

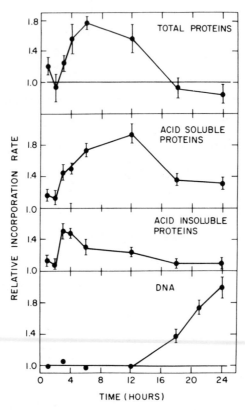

Fig. 3.   Time course of stimulation of incorporation of [3H]-labeled
amino acids into total nuclear proteins and of incorporation of
[3H] thymidine into DNA in uteri of 20-day-old rats after injection
of 0.5 µg of estradiol-17β.   The results are expressed as the ratio
between specific activity (cpm/µg DNA or mg protein) in the uteri
of treated animals and of rats given control injections of 0.1%
ethanol.   Vertical brackets indicate S.E.M. derived from 4-6
determinations (protein fractions), each on pooled uteri from
three rats, or 3-15 determinations (DNA), each on one uterus
(Ref. 9).

Since a significant increase in incorporation into total and nuclear proteins has taken place by 4 h after estradiol injection and the period from 3-4 h is the time of maximal incorporation into nuclear acid insoluble (non-histone) proteins, this time was chosen for the comparison of estradiol stimulation of incorporation rates into protein (Fig. 4).

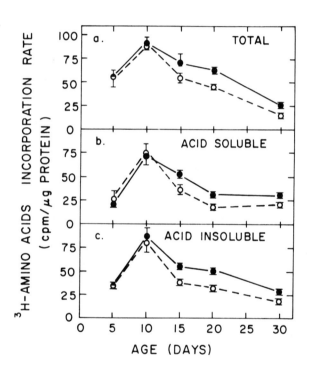

Fig. 4.   Rate of uterine protein synthesis: changes in responsiveness to estradiol during post-natal development. The incorporation of a mixture of ^{3}H-labeled amino acids into total protein, and acid-soluble and acid-soluble nuclear proteins, was measured 4 h after an intraperitoneal injection of estradiol-17β (0.5 μg to rats 15 days or older, 0.4 μg to 10-day-old rats and 0.2 μg to 5-day-old rats). ●——●, estradiol treated animals; O---O, rats given injections of 0.1% ethanol. Vertical brackets indicate the S.E.M. of the results from 6 or more incubations.

The rates of protein synthesis in all the three categories measured, as well as the protein content of the uterus, followed the same pattern. There was no stimulation by estrogen at the age of 5 to 10 days; but a significant stimulation was found in uteri from 15-day-old rats, an age at which DNA synthesis was not stimulated. Again, there is a high rate of incorporation into uterine protein at an early age, which declines during postnatal development in untreated rats and is capable of only partial restoration by estradiol-17β stimulation (Fig. 4). However, while DNA synthesis in control rats decreases linearly with age (Fig. 1), protein synthesis in the uterus during the period of 5 to 30 days after birth shows a peak at the age of 10 days. Whether this peak of incorporation into protein at 10 days of age is specific for the uterus and is significant for the development of uterine responsiveness to estradiol remains to be investigated.

Stimulation of Synthesis of a Specific Cytoplasmic

"Induced Protein" by Estradiol-17β

The results presented above refer at best to categories of proteins; we are more interested in specific proteins which are induced by estradiol. In 1966, Notides and Gorski (24) detected by starch gel electrophoresis a protein component in an extract of rat uteri in 0.05% EDTA, whose rate of synthesis was increased by estradiol. This protein was called "induced protein" (IP); its synthesis was found to increase within 30-40 min after estradiol administration (25,26) and it was inhibited by cycloheximide (24) and actinomycin (26,27). It is a cytoplasmic component with a molecular weight of 39×10^3/daltons (28) and an isoelectric point of 4.5 (Ref. 28). While its function in uterus and vagina (29) is unknown, Baulieu (11) has suggested that it may be the "key intermediate protein" which he postulates as a mediator of estrogen action.

In order to determine at what stage during postnatal development the IP first appears, we analyzed the supernatant fraction of uterine cells, after double labeling with ^{3}H and ^{14}C, leu, or ^{3}H and ^{35}S met, by "Cellogel" cellulose acetate electrophoresis as well as by the conventional polyacrylamide gel electrophoresis technique. The cellogel method suggested by Prof. L. Lewin proved faster and more sensitive than polyacrylamide gel electrophoresis (Fig. 5). This technique permitted a rapid and unequivocal demonstration that estradiol was capable of inducing the IP in the surviving uterus (11,26,30) (Fig. 6a); this was the first effect of estradiol to be clearly and reproducibly produced in a system not involving the intact rat. In order to improve our method for detection of IP, we fractionated the uterine high speed supernatant fraction with $(NH_4)_2SO_4$. The IP could be more sensitively identified in the fraction precipitated at 50-80% $(NH_4)_2SO_4$ saturation than in the

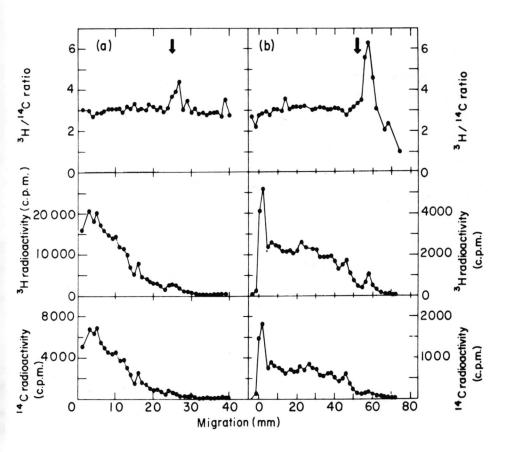

Fig. 5. Comparison of the electrophoretic migration of uterine soluble proteins in polyacrylamide gels and in Cellogel strips. Supernatant solutions (150,000 x g) from homogenates of uteri of 20-day-old rats collected 2 h after an injection of 5 μg of estradiol-17β and incubated for 1 h in either [3H] leucine (estradiol-treated) or [14C] leucine (controls) were combined and analyzed either on polyacrylamide gel (a) or on Cellogel (b). Arrows indicate the position of a bovine serum albumin marker. The direction of migration was from left to right, towards the anode (from Ref. 9).

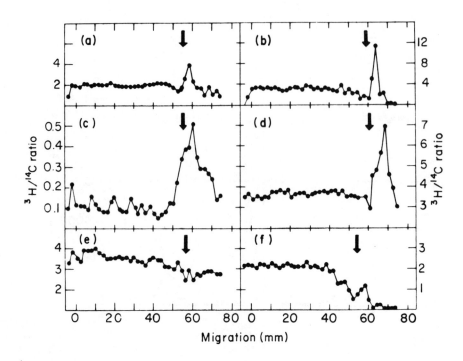

Fig. 6. Synthesis of specific estradiol-induced uterine cytoplasmic protein during post-natal development. The electrophoretic
distribution of uterine protein fractions on Cellogel (cellulose
acetate) strips runs in 0.04 M sodium barbitone, pH 8.6, at 20v/cm
for 70-75 min. (a) Soluble proteins from surviving uteri of 20-
day-old rats synthesized after 1 h incubation in 3 x 10^{-8}M estradi-
ol-17β in phosphate buffered saline. (b) $(NH_4)_2SO_4$ fraction
(precipitated at 50-80% saturation, 0^0) of soluble proteins from
uteri of 20-day-old rats synthesized 1 h after intraperitoneal
injection of 5 μg of estradiol. (c-e) Soluble proteins synthesized in uteri removed 1 h after injection of (c) 5 μg of estradiol
into 15-day-old rats, (d) 4 μg of estradiol into 10-day-old rats
and, (e) 2 μg of estradiol into 5-day-old rats; (f) $(NH_4)_2SO_4$
fraction (precipitated at 50-80% saturation, 0^0) of soluble proteins synthesized in uteri of 5-day-old rats removed 1 h after
intraperitoneal injection of 2 μg of estradiol. Arrows indicate
the position of a bovine serum albumin marker (from Ref. 9).

whole homogenate (Fig. 6b). With these techniques, we were able
to demonstrate the presence of IP after estradiol stimulation in
15-day-old (Fig. 6c) and 10-day-old rats (Fig. 6d), but not in
5-day-old rats (Fig. 6e) even in the 50-80% $(NH_4)_2SO_4$ fraction
(Fig. 6f). Thus, the cytoplasmic IP can be induced at an age when
no stimulation of general synthesis of protein can be detected
(Fig. 4). We therefore examined whether the induction by estradiol
of any specific nuclear protein could be detected by similar techniques.

A nuclear protein extracted by 0.15 M H_2SO_4 has been shown by
Barker (31) to be synthesized by rat uterus in response to estradiol. We analyzed extracts prepared by the method of Barker from
whole cells, nuclei and chromatin of rats at different ages using
a double-labeling technique (Fig. 7) and found that a specific
chromosomal protein appears in response to estradiol at 15 but
not 10 days after birth. It therefore falls in the category of
the bulk of nuclear proteins which show this developmental pattern
of responsiveness to estradiol.

Detection of Estradiol Nuclear Receptor

in Uteri of 1-Day-Old Rats

Although it is clear that the mere presence or absence of
estradiol receptor (s) (6-8) cannot provide a sufficient explanation for the sequential gene expression described in this review,
it is possible that total lack of nuclear receptor could explain
the complete absence of responses at the age of 5 days. Clark and
Gorski have reported on the ontogeny of the cytoplasmic estrogen
receptor (32); they found that it was present in the rat uterus as
early as at the age of 2 days, rose to a peak concentration (relative to DNA) at 10 days and that its concentration declined by 20
days. We posed the question whether there was a lack of entry of
estradiol into the nucleus (33, 34) in uteri of very young rats.
From the results of exchange binding (35) and sucrose density
gradient analyses we found that from the age of 1 day, nuclear
receptors for estradiol were present (Fig. 8) with the characteristic mobility in sucrose gradients (Fig. 9) of particles of approximately 5S. We showed that ontogeny of nuclear receptor (Fig. 8)
is parallel to that demonstrated by Clark and Gorski (32) for
cytoplasmic receptors, also showing a maximum at 10 days, followed
by a decline.

The decline in receptor concentration could result from the
differential multiplication of different cell types in the uterus.
Counts of the numbers of cells in transverse sections of uteri of
different ages (Fig. 10) show that there is a relative increase in

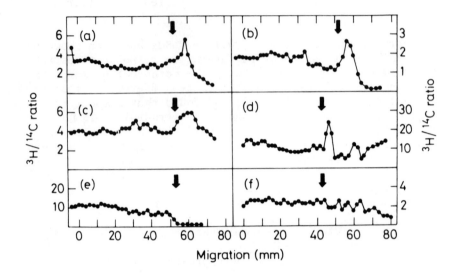

Fig. 7. Synthesis of a uterine nuclear protein in estradiol-treated rats during post-natal development. Rats were injected intraperitoneally with either estradiol-17β (5 μg for 15 and 20-day old rats, 4 μg for 10-day-old rats) or 1% ethanol and their uteri removed 4 h later. Uteri were incubated for 1 h in [³H] leucine (estradiol treated) or [¹⁴C] leucine (controls) and acid soluble proteins prepared from whole uteri, nuclei or chromatin according to Barker (31). Extracts were made from (a) uteri of 20-day-old rats; (b) chromatin of 20-day-old rats, (c) uteri of 15-day-old rats, (d) nuclei of 15-day-old rats, (e) uteri of 10-day-old rats, and (f) nuclei of 10-day-old rats. Electrophoresis was carried out on Cellogel strips in 0.9% acetic acid in the direction of the cathode. The arrows indicate the position of histone IIb-III markers (42).

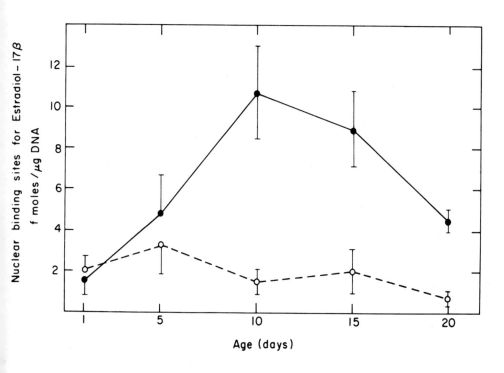

Fig. 8. Uterine nuclear binding capacity for estradiol-17β during post-natal development. Immature rats were given an intra-peritoneal injection of estradiol-17β (approximately 80 ng/g body wt) (●───●) or 0.15 M NaCl (O---O) 1 h before they were killed. The nuclear-myofibrillar pellets were incubated for 1 h at 37⁰ in the presence of 1.3 x 10⁻⁸M [³H] estradiol with or without the addition of 10⁻⁶M diethylstilbestrol. The number of binding sites for estradiol-17β (35) was calculated after subtraction of the corresponding value for the control incubated with excess diethyl-stilbestrol. The brackets indicate the S.E.M. of 5 to 8 deter-minations (from Ref. 9).

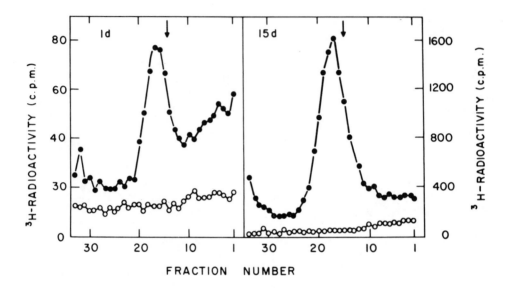

Fig. 9. Sucrose gradient analysis of nuclear estradiol-17β
receptor from uteri of 1-day and 15-day-old rats. The animals
were killed 1 h after an intraperitoneal injection of estradiol-
17β (approximately 80 ng/g body wt.). The nuclear-myofibrillar
pellets were incubated for 1 h at 37° in the presence of 1.0 x
10⁻⁸M [³H] estradiol (●——●) or 1.0 x 10⁻⁸M [³H] estradiol plus
1.0 x 10⁻⁶M diethylstilbestrol (0———0). Loosely bound and free
estradiol was removed by adsorption to dextran-coated charcoal.
The pellets were extracted with buffered 0.4 M KCl and the
extracts were centrifuged on 5-20% sucrose gradients containing
0.4 M KCl, in a Beckman-Spinco SW56 rotor at 46,000 rpm for
approximately 16 h at 0°. Arrows indicate the position of a
bovine serum albumin marker. The direction of sedimentation was
from right to left (from Ref. 9).

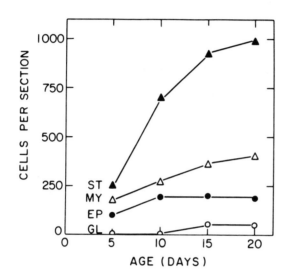

Fig. 10. Differential growth of cell populations during post-natal development of rat uterus. The middle third of each horn of immature rat uteri was placed on Millipore filter strips and fixed in Bouin's solution. Transverse paraffin sections (5 μm) were stained with hematoxylin and eosin and the number of each cell type per section was determined, using a magnification of 378 x and an occular reticule. Three uterine sections per rat and three rats per age-group were examined.

ST, stroma; MY, myometrium; EP, luminal epithelium; GL, stromal gland.

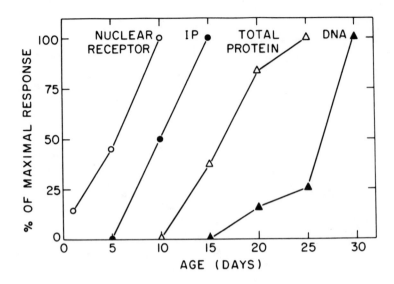

Fig. 11. Sequential acquisition of responsiveness to estradiol-17β during post-natal development of the rat uterus. Concentration of nuclear receptor per unit weight of DNA, 1 h after estradiol injection, was determined by a micro-modification (9) of the exchange binding method of Anderson, Clark and Peck (35); the rate of synthesis of the cytoplasmic "induced protein" (IP), 1 h after estradiol injection, by a modification of the isotope ratio method of Katzenellenbogen and Gorski (30) using electrophoresis on Cellogel; the rate of total protein synthesis, 4 h after estradiol injection, by incorporation of a ^{3}H-labeled amino acid mixture (9) into acid insoluble products; and the rate of DNA synthesis, 24 h after estradiol injection, by incorporation of [^{3}H-Me] thymidine (6) into DNA. For each parameter, the highest response observed during the first 30 days of life, at the time of maximum response after estradiol injection, was taken as 100%. Each point represents the mean value for 3-6 determinations.

the number of stromal cells during this period. However, there is no indication that these cells are poor in estradiol receptor.

In view of the fact that the estradiol receptor system is present even in one-day-old rats, it is possible that some response to estradiol could be found in the uteri of such young animals. We found that the induction of ornithine decarboxylase by estradiol (36,37) takes place as early as two days after birth

(38) to a level of specific activity which is not significantly lower than that attained by the age of 20 days.

Since the presence of a complete binding system for estradiol in uterine nuclei is not a sufficient condition for complete responsiveness to estradiol, during the period from 1 to 15 days of age, we have begun the search for additional control factors, for example for nuclear proteins which show increases in synthetic rates within an hour or two after estradiol injection. At least 3 or 4 candidates for such regulatory proteins can be detected (39) using double labeling techniques in conjunction with poly-acrylamide-SDS gel electrophoresis of the major chromatin fraction solubilized in guanidinium hydrochloride, according to the technique of Levy and Sober (40).

SUMMARY AND CONCLUSIONS

During the postnatal development of the rat, it was possible to distinguish a series of stages with regard to the response of the uterus to a single intraperitoneal injection of estradiol-17β (Fig. 11). Nuclear binding of [^{3}H] estradiol was present even at birth and induction of ornithine decarboxylase by estradiol was demonstrable at two days after birth. The response to estradiol by synthesis of the specific cytoplasmic IP developed between days 5 and 10 after birth, while estradiol stimulation of general protein synthesis and synthesis of nuclear proteins, including a chromosomal protein similar to that described by Barker (24), was first demonstrated between days 10 and 15. The capacity to respond to estradiol with increased DNA synthesis developed only between days 15 and 20.

A similar temporal sequence in the cellular response to the hormone, though on a shorter time scale, is seen in the uterus of the 20-day-old rat following a single injection of estradiol. Association of estradiol with cytoplasmic receptor and transport of this hormone-receptor complex into the nucleus takes place within minutes (41). The synthesis of IP is stimulated by estradiol 30-40 minutes after injection of the hormone (25-26). Stimulation of the rate of incorporation of radioisotope-labeled amino acids into the "Barker protein" and induction of ornithine decarboxylase is first found between 2 and 4 hours after injection, while incorporation into total and nuclear protein is maximal between 4-12 h. DNA synthesis is first detectable at 18 h and reaches its maximum at 24 h. Thus there may be a partial physiological recapitulation in the fully competent (20-day-old) rat of the sequence of gene expression observed during post-natal acquisition of responsiveness to estradiol.

The present analysis of sequential gene expression during post-natal development of the rat uterus shows that additional specificity, beyond that conferred by the presence of unique cytoplasmic and nuclear receptors and a single type of acceptor site on the chromatin is necessary to explain the sequential acquisition of responsiveness to estradiol. The analysis of sequential gene expression in the developing rat uterus provides a promising approach to the problem of the regulation of protein and DNA synthesis by steroid hormones.

ACKNOWLEDGEMENTS

This review includes work by D.S., G.S. and I.I. submitted in partial fulfilment of the requirements for the Ph.D. degree of the Feinberg Graduate School of the Weizmann Institute of Science. The work was supported by grants from the Ford Foundation and the Population Council, New York. R.J.B.K. was the holder of an EMBO Fellowship while on leave from the Department of Hormone Biochemistry, Imperial Cancer Research Fund, Lincoln's Inn Fields, London, U.K. A.M.K. is the Herbert Sidebotham Senior Research Fellow and H.R.L. is the Adlai E. Stevenson Professor of Endocrinology and Reproductive Biology at the Weizmann Institute of Science.

REFERENCES

1. DICZFALUSY, R. E., Ed. 6th Karolinska Symposium on Research Methods in Reproductive Endocrinology, Protein synthesis in reproductive tissue. Karolinska Institute, Stockholm, 1973.
2. HAMBURGH, M. & BARRINGTON, E. J. W., Eds. Hormones in development. Appleton Century-Crofts, New York, 1968.
3. HAMILTON, T. H. *Science 161*, 649, 1968.
4. GORSKI, J., DE ANGELO, A. B. & BARNEA, A. In: McKerns, K.W., Ed. The sex steroids: molecular mechanisms. Appleton-Century-Crofts, New York. pp. 181-195, 1971.
5. MUELLER, G. C., VONDERHAAR, R. K., KIM, U. H. & LEMAHIEU, M. *Recent Progr. Hormone Research 28*, 1, 1972.
6. KAYE, A. M., SHERATZKY, D. & LINDNER, H. R. *Biochim. Biophys. Acta 261*, 475, 1972.
7. SÖMJEN (SHERATZKY), D., KAYE, A.M., KING, R. J. B. & LINDNER, H. R. *J. Cell Biol. 55*, 246a, 1972.
8. SÖMJEN, D., KAYE, A. M. & LINDNER, H. R. *Develop. Biol.* (in press).
9. SÖMJEN, D., SÖMJEN, G., KING, R. J. B., KAYE, A. M. & LINDNER, H. R. *Biochim. J.* (in press).
10. JENSEN, E. V. & DeSOMBRE, E. R. *Ann. Rev. Biochem. 41*, 203, 1972.

11. BAULIEU, E. E., ALBERGA, A., RAYNAUD-JAMMET, C. & WIRA, C. R. *Nature New Biology 236,* 236, 1972.
12. GLASSER, S. R., CHYTIL, F. & SPELSBERG, T. C. *Biochem. J. 130,* 947, 1972.
13. KING, R. J. B. & MAINWARING, I. W. Steroid-cell interactions, Chapt. 7 and 9. Butterworths Scientific Publications Ltd. London, 1973.
14. KING, R. J. B. & GORDON, J. *Nature New Biology 240,* 185, 1972.
15. O'MALLEY, B. W., SPELSBERG, T. C., SCHRADER, W. T., CHYTIL, F. & STEGGLES, A. W. *Nature 235,* 141, 1972.
16. CHAMNESS, G. C., JENNINGS, A. W. & McGUIRE, W. L. *Nature 241,* 458, 1972.
17. KING, R. J. B., *Adv. Exp. Med. Biol.* 18th Oholo Biological Conference, "Strategies for the control of gene expression". This volume, 1973.
18. MUELLER, G. C., HERRANEN, A. M. & JERVELL, K. F. *Rec. Progr. Hormone Res. 14,* 95, 1958.
19. TACHI, E., TACHI, S. & LINDNER, H. R. *J. Reprod. Fert. 31,* 59, 1972.
20. ASTWOOD, E. B. *Endocrinology 23,* 25, 1938.
21. STELLWAGEN, R. H. & COLE, R. D. *Ann. Rev. Biochem. 38,* 951, 1969.
22. SMITH, J. A., MARTIN, L., KING, R. J. B. & VERTES, M. *Biochem. J. 119,* 773, 1970.
23. STEIN, G. S. & BORUN, T. W. *J. Cell Biol. 52,* 292, 1972.
24. NOTIDES, A. & GORSKI, J. *Proc. Nat. Acad. Sci. U.S. 56,* 230, 1966.
25. BARNEA, A. & GORSKI, J. *Biochemistry 9,* 1899, 1970.
26. MAYOL, R. F. & THAYER, S. A. *Biochemistry 9,* 2484, 1970.
27. De ANGELO, A. B. & GORSKI, J. *Proc. Nat. Acad. Sci. U.S. 66,* 693, 1970.
28. SÖMJEN, D., KING, R. J. B., KAYE, A. M. & LINDNER, H. R. *Israel J. Med. Sci. 9,* 546, 1973.
29. KATZMAN, P. A., LARSON, D. L. & PODRATZ, K. C. In: McKerns, K. W. Ed. The sex steroids: molecular mechanisms. Appleton-Century-Crofts, New York, pp. 107-147, 1971.
30. KATZENELLENBOGEN, B. S. & GORSKI, J. *J. Biol. Chem. 247,* 1299, 1972.
31. BARKER, K. L. *Biochemistry 10,* 284, 1971.
32. CLARK, J. H. & GORSKI, J. *Science 169,* 76, 1970.
33. SHYAMALA, G. *Biochem. Biophys. Res. Commun. 46,* 1623, 1972.
34. CLARK, J. H., CAMPBELL, P.S. & PECK, E. J. Jr. *Neuroendocrinology 77,* 218, 1972.
35. ANDERSON, J., CLARK, J. H. & PECK, E. J. Jr. *Biochem. J. 126,* 561, 1972.
36. COHN, S., O'MALLEY, B. W. & STASTNY, M. *Science 170,* 336, 1970.
37. KAYE, A. M., ICEKSON, I. & LINDNER, H. R. *Biochim. Biophys. Acta 252,* 150, 1971.

38. KAYE, A. M., ICEKSON, I., LAMPRECHT, S. A., GRUSS, R., TSAFRIRI, A. & LINDNER, H. R. *Biochemistry*, (in press).
39. KAYE, A. M., KING, R. J. B., SÖMJEN, D. & LINDNER, H. R.   Abs. 9th Inter. Congr. Biochem., 1973.
40. LEVY, S., SIMPSON, R. T. & SOBER, H. A. *Biochemistry 11*, 1547, 1972.
41. WILLIAMS, D. & GORSKI, J. *Proc. Nat. Acad. Sci. U.S. 69*, 3464, 1972.
42. KAYE, A. M. & SHERATZKY, D. *Biochim. Biophys. Acta 190*, 527, 1969.

PANEL DISCUSSION

Participants:

Y. Aloni, H. Aviv, E.K.F. Bautz, M. Bizunski, F.Conconi,
V. Daniel, D. Elson, M. Herzberg, H.Inouye, A.M. Kaye,
R.G.B. King, M. Kotler, R. Kulka, P. Lengyel, B.J.
McCarthy, M. Revel, K. Scherrer, W. Szybalski, Y. Teitz,
G. Tomkins, A. Traub, G. Yagil, A. Zaritsky

Tomkins: We shall commence the discussion by asking the members of
the panel to say what they will be doing, or would like to be doing
in the somewhat non-foreseeable future. Are we going to look for
more initiation factors? What will happen to protein synthesis?
What is phage good for? and so on.

Bautz: For several years I have been thinking of changing my
approach to something more closely related to humans than to
bacteria. When I was planning my sabbatical leave at the Weizmann
Institute, the sigma factor came along, so I postponed going to
Israel and turning to the study of higher organisms.

        Now we have done all the easy experiments on sigma, but
we still do not know enough and there is yet a limited amount of
things to do. The people who work on mammalian polymerases are
very often in trouble, even more so than we are. So we feel that
before getting ourselves into trouble by switching to mammalian
polymerases, perhaps we might find answers through the bacterial
systems which will illuminate the problem of transcription in
general.

        We do not know yet whether in mammalian polymerases there
are factors missing - e.g. there is no evidence yet for sigma
factors, etc. Bacterial polymerases are large, so people started
working on smaller polymerases, like the T3 enzyme, but not much
can be done on regulation with these small polymerases and the
major problem in transcription is the regulatory part of it. It
is very easy to understand how chains are made, but it is not so
easy with initiation. We have still a lot of work to do in bac-

403

teria. We are now looking for temperature sensitive mutants and
hope that it will be possible to isolate outside suppressors to
these mutants. These may be either missense suppressor tRNA mutants or, hopefully, mutations in regulatory proteins that will
interact with the polymerases so as to make them non-temperature
sensitive. This is the way of picking up some factors (and not
artifactors) that are truly connected with the transcription of the
E. coli chromosome. Such work may eventually help put people on
the right track in their work on higher organisms.

Szybalski:First, I must say that at present I am happily married
to phage lambda and plan to stay faithful to her. In 1958-1964 I
had my fling with higher organisms, that is, the genetics of human
cell cultures. This was very instructive and even productive but
the remaining years of my scientific life I plan to devote to a
simpler system, which I hope can be analyzed in complete fine detail. We plan to determine the sequence, structure and function of
all the recognition sites on the phage DNA, which serve as the signals for (1) initiation of gene expression, (2) its termination
or antitermination, (3) binding of repressors or transcriptional
factors, (4) initiation of DNA replication and (5) many other
functions. The structure of the corresponding polymerases and of
the controlling factors also have to be elucidated.

In discussions with my scientific friends I frequently
hear two "pessimistic" comments. One is that the complete details
of all phage controls will probably become unravelled within the
next few years, since they should be rather simple, and second
that research in the phage field will be finished and cease to be
interesting very soon. Let me comment on these views.

When lecturing, I often try to give an impression that
developmental controls in phage lambda are basically simple, but I
know that this is not really true since there is a whole network of
interlocking controls that are barely amenable to complete analysis.
At this stage of our studies I feel that we have only scratched the
surface, but fortunately we have also learned how to design future
experiments in the next phase of our research. I reassure you
that it is tough going to understand all aspects of the controls
of as small a creature as lambda, and it is a long way to achiev-
ing the same degree of understanding of larger viruses and then of
bacterial cells, which have a hundred times more DNA than lambda.
I hesitate to contemplate the difficulties in the way of total
understanding the controls in eukaryotic cells, the genomes of
which contain 10^5 more DNA than does lambda. Thus, for some time
to come we will have to use viruses to gain complete insight into
the detailed mechanisms of control, before even hoping to attempt
similar studies with higher organisms.

Let me make one more comment about complexity versus the simplicity of phage lambda. I emphasized that the controls of lambda are quite complex and still hard to fully understand. But actually they are perhaps much simpler than the controls of such man-made products as color television or the 747 jet liner which brought me here. But a specialist in electronics fully understands how television works, although a molecular biologist who for the first time encounters a color TV receiver might say that it is too complex an "organism" to comprehend its complete mechanism.

Tomkins: It would be difficult to get mutants of a color TV set.

Szybalski: Actually not. I am frequently faced with lethal or par- tially lethal mutations in my 10-year old TV set and trying to re- pair these "mutations" I learned quite a bit about the mechanisms controlling this electronic "organism".

Let me now comment on the question "what next". Up to now we are working on the descriptive phase of molecular biology. We are unravelling and describing the viral control mechanisms as found in nature. But the real challenge will start when we enter the synthetic phase of research in our field. We will then devise new control elements and add these new modules to the existing ge- nomes or build up wholly new genomes. This would be a field with an unlimited expansion potential and hardly any limitations to building "new better control circuits" and "new better lambdas", or finally other organisms, like a "new better mouse" instead of a better mouse trap. I am not concerned that we will run out of exciting and novel ideas, first in the descriptive and then in the synthetic phase of lambdology.

Lengyel: I shall continue to study the control of the expression of genetic information. My major effort will be devoted in the near future to the understanding of the molecular basis of the interferon defense mechanism. Exposure to interferon apparently "teaches" cells to distinguish between a virus-directed biosynthe- sis and a host-directed biosynthesis, and enables cells to block the replication of viruses. This "knowledge" is lacking in cells not exposed to interferon. Elucidation of the basis of the se- lective antiviral action of the interferon system will shed further light on aspects of virus-cell interactions and may provide the basis for developing a chemotherapy of viral diseases.

Aloni: The question of symmetric versus asymmetric transcription seems to be extremely important. As a consequence of the results that have already been obtained, much of the work in the field of genetic expression of mitochondrial DNA in higher cells and of the DNA tumor viruses SV40 and polyoma in lytically infected cells, had to be reassessed.

Using model systems that mainly involve the various interactions between SV40 polyoma and the cells, we shall examine the questions whether these viruses are transcribed symmetrically in transformed cells and whether the cellular DNA sequences that are covalently linked to the viral DNA are also transcribed symmetrically. In addition, we shall study whether the mode of symmetrical transcription occurs from "normal" genes. If post-transcriptional regulation of gene expression proves to be a widespread phenomenon, the aspects of how selective RNA degradation is achieved will be studied. Finally, we shall study the biological implications of symmetrical transcription in relation to the occurrence of double-stranded RNA in infected and transformed cells.

Daniel: We have shown that we can effectively transcribe the polynucleotide chains of a tRNA molecule. It seems however that we get precursor molecules of a larger size than of mature tRNA. All the work done till now concentrated on tyrosine tRNA. We should like, therefore, to extend the work to other tRNA genes and see if similar precursors are obtained. The in vitro transcripts of tRNA will be used also to study the specific modification reactions, like methylation, thiolation, etc. Finally, since we are able to isolate small DNA fragments carrying a tRNA gene, we will try to do sequential analysis of the transcription product.

Elson: It was obvious from the beginning that ribosomes are very complicated, and as information accumulated it became apparent that they are even more complicated than we had thought at first. Not only do they contain three species of RNA and over fifty different proteins but it now seems likely that certain specific inorganic cations are also true structural components which occupy specific sites in the active particle. In addition, it is becoming evident that the ribosomal structure is not fixed, but is flexible and changing; and it may well be that the ribosome goes through a cycle of structural transitions when functioning. However, we have now reached a stage at which it is becoming possible to make sense out of at least some of this complexity. Many techniques are being brought to bear on this problem -- biochemical, chemical, genetic-- and others, not yet fully exploited, are available. We shall therefore continue for the foreseeable future to study the ribosome, probably with increased emphasis on the use of chemical techniques for elucidating structure.

Revel: I want to make a case for continuing the investigation of the biochemical mechanisms of gene expression. We shall continue to work with cell-free systems to verify if we can reproduce in vitro the controls of gene expression and devise ways to repair them if necessary. Here an overall scheme is not enought, details about each of the molecules involved are required.

We would like to work back from the protein synthesis apparatus to the DNA genome and to obtain for eukaryotic cells the same type of DNA-dependent protein synthetizing system that we have in prokaryotic cells. Eventually, we hope to put together the pieces obtained from such molecular dissection and create a synthetic (reconstituted) cell or genetic unit.

One of the most intriguing aspects of regulation of protein synthesis is to understand how signals received at the cell membrane can affect transcription and translation of genes and end up in the synthesis of a new protein. We should not neglect, nevertheless, studies of gene expression in whole cells and the use of genetic mutants, of somatic cells, many of which have now becomes available and are sometimes connected with human genetic diseases.

Traub: Although extensive experimental evidence has accumulated on the inhibition of cellular RNA and protein synthesis during infection with picorna viruses, the molecular mechanisms responsible for these events are not known. The progress made in the understanding of the mechanism of RNA and protein synthesis, which was reviewed in this symposium, emphasizes the essential role of a number of soluble protein factors which are in constant equilibrium with main synthesizing centers (such as core RNA polymerase or ribosomes). The maintenance of this rather delicate equilibrium is essential for the operation of the RNA and protein synthesizing systems. In the near future, we would like to examine the hypothesis that infection with a picornavirus leads to a disruption of the equilibrium state, and hence to inhibition of these host functions. According to this view, an early function of the viral RNA, which penetrates the cell, is to serve as messenger for the synthesis of protein(s) with high affinity for the soluble factors. An interaction between a virus-coded protein(s) and a cellular soluble factor will decrease the optimal concentration of the soluble factor and will result in a decline in the activity of the biosynthetic system in which it plays an essential role. The inhibition by a viral protein product is visualized as occurring not as a direct action of the protein on the inhibited system, but rather by elimination of an essential protein constituent from the affected system through the formation of a stable complex between two proteins. As a first step in this direction we plan to isolate the replicase of EMC virus and characterize its sub-unit constitution with respect to origin (cellular or viral) and function.

Yael Teitz:We know quite a lot about direct transcription (from DNA to RNA) in which the DNA-dependent RNA polymerase (transcriptase) plays a central role. The direct transcription process involves four well defined steps: (a) binding of the enzyme to the template; (b) the initiation of polymerization; (c) elongation of

the RNA chain on the template, and finally (d) termination accompanied by release of the nascent RNA molecule and liberation of
the enzyme for reinitiation of another cycle. Each subunit of polymerase has a specific function in this process. The core enzyme
(lacking sigma factor) can bind to DNA and synthesize RNA but less
efficiently and with little specificity. The specificity of this
direct transcriptase can be changed by (a) modification of the core
enzyme in one or more of its subunits so that it will interact
only with a new, specific sigma factor; (b) by the appearance of
a completely new polymerase.

I would like to devote my attention in the future to the
elucidation of the enzymatic steps involved in reverse transcription, to attempt to define the functions of each of the enzyme's
subunits and to characterize protein factors which might influence
the specificity and the efficiency of the enzyme. In addition, I
have always been intrigued by the possibility that viruses have
some enzymes different from their host cells. The RNA-dependent
RNA polymerase in naked RNA virus and the reverse transcriptase in
RNA tumor viruses are present only in viruses. In view, however,
of the recent reports that reverse transcriptase activity was also
detected in uninfected animal cells, it would be interesting to
find whether or not this is a specific viral product or not.

King: Looking ahead, I would focus my research on three topics.
1. Purification of receptors from different oestrogen-sensitive
cells. This is essential for any subsequent work on the relationship of receptors to the mechanism of action of steroids.
2. The use of certain well-defined hormone-responsive tumor cells
in culture to study the mechanism of action of steroids. Such
tumors progress from a hormone-responsive to the unresponsive
state. The mechanism whereby this progression occurs is not known
but could be due to changes in receptor, acceptor or a post-
acceptor event. 3. At present there are a very limited number of
experimental systems that can be used for studying steroid action
in vitro. This aspect of hormone action requires more intensive
study.

Kaye: Since the word hormone comes from hormeo, ("I arouse"),
perhaps one way of looking at the problem of hormone action is to
try to determine whether apparent stimulation of synthesis by hormones is in truth a result of simple induction or derepression as
in bacterial systems, or whether, one can think of hormonal stimulation as perhaps having more of the character of restoring the
capacity of a cell to synthesize protein(s) at the higher rate
characteristic of its embryologic existence or of a former physiological state and which is inhibited in the absence of sufficient
hormone. Estradiol action on the uterus is a case in point. To
test theories of regulation of gene expression in the uterus,one

of the practical things which has to be developed for the future
is some cell or organ culture system. Work is being done in our
department on this problem. The second area which has to be developed is to clear up the uncertainty due to lack of definition
of the non-histone portion of the chromatin. Since there are
proteins which have a physiologically important interaction with
DNA or nucleoprotein and which are not histones, the best available definition of the non-histone proteins today perhaps would be
in terms of enzymatic activity or hormone receptor activity. In
this field of chromosomal protein activity, we have plans to
examine some of the enzymes. If one has these tools, I believe we
will see a development in our understanding of the non-histone proteins as great as has occurred in the last generation in terms of
the histones. I foresee very rapid progress in this area, and I
suspect that whatever name will finally be found for the non-
histone proteins which associate meaningfully with chromatin it
will be part of the title of very many symposia in the future.

McCarthy: In the last few years the study of biochemistry of
the cell nucleus has become much more intensive. The whole field,
especially chromatin chemistry, was vaguely disreputable largely
because of the absence of methodology to do good experiments and
ask important, significant and quantitatively answerable questions.
Now, however, histone chemistry is on a solid footing,histone:
DNA interactions are being understood and, as Scherrer has pointed
out, giant nuclear RNA seems now to be a tractable problem.

        With the availability of purified messengers, eukaryotic
RNA polymerases and sensitive hybridization and translation assays,
it appears to be possible to define transcription control mechanisms in eukaryotes. One may also hope to purify small segments of
chromosomes.

        Two further extrapolations from present day understanding
of chromosome chemistry may be made. Although the specificity of
chromosome synapsis can be described on the genetic and cytological
level, the biochemical mechanisms are as yet undefined. Similarly,
the basis for temporal control of DNA synthesis in the multiple
replicons of a eukaryotic chromosome remains to be defined. Considerable progress may be anticipated in both these not unrelated
areas.

Conconi: The future development of our research program will
basically deal with the problem of β-Thalassemia and, more generally, with the factors specifically controlling mRNA translation
in higher organisms.

        The induction of β-globin synthesis in Ferrara homozygous
βzero-thalassemic subjects, occurring after blood transfusion, is a

clear indication that the normal inducer, present in transfused red
blood cells may cross the cell wall of thalassæmic erythrocytes
and turn on β-globin mRNA translation. On the basis of this
finding, we plan to purify from the blood of normal adult individuals the specific inducer of β-globin synthesis and eventually
try to use it "in vivo" in Ferrara thalassemic patients. The
characterization of the purified molecule and the identification
of its site of action in the protein synthesizing process could
be useful in the clarification of the mechanisms through which
specificity of messenger translation is achieved.

        We believe that the pathogenesis of Ferrar β-Thalassemia
may apply to other human hereditary diseases, caused by mutations
of genes coding for translation-specific proteins. Consequently,
one of the future developments in human pathology may be the identification of such diseases, and the isolation from normal individuals, for therapeutic purposes, of the missing translation-
specific inducers.

Aviv: The problem that we face is not what to do but rather
what not to do. Now that we have a way to measure messengers for
specific gene products chromatin transcriptional studies are entering a new stage. In the near future many genes will be transcribed
from chromatin, and probably control elements regulating transcription will be isolated and defined.

        I had the impression from Tomkins that hormones are the
secret of life. I think that this is misleading. As a father of
a 3-month old baby I am impressed by embryology, by the ways a
single cell differentiates into many various and specific directions. I cannot see how the hormones mentioned by Tomkins can induce a cell to develop into different directions. These hormones
probably activate preset programs.

        We still lack good systems to study specific inducers
of development. We know that specific inducers for embryonic
differentiation do exist but we do not have good experimental systems to study them in biochemical terms. Since we have now the
technology to study specific gene expression from transcription
to translation, I hope that we will be able to tackle the molecular
aspects of differentiation.

Scherrer: What is important to do and what one would like to do
may be not the same. I have a predilection for problems which
Brian (McCarthy) defined as "non-reputable"; problems such as the
giant RNA story of five years ago. Thus I should probably move
out of this by now reputable field; however it is not easy to
abandon ones 10-year old child. I shall therefore continue to
investigate why a cell synthesizes a giant RNA molecule as an inter-

mediary to a little piece of globin messenger, representing only
a few percent of its precursor.

It will be necessary to identify biochemically all the
steps in intra-cellular information transfer and to delineate the
regulation of this process. Moreover, I feel that we are missing
completely another system of control not directly linked to
mRNA; however, at this point, we do not know where in the cell to
search for this hypothetical additional system of regulation.

In my judgement, it will be important to study in detail
the interactions between proteins and nucleic acids. Sequencing
the 30,000 bases of a given pre-mRNA will not be possible. Hence
one should analyse the sites within the RNA that are important,
those sites where proteins associate in a protective or regulatory
fashion. This should enable us to identify the programming code -
directing the fate of mRNA in the cell - which is superimposed and/
or added to the coding sequences in nucleic acids.

Another interesting problem of the future is intra-cellular movement, an area of research that is completely out of focus
at present. People talk about the cell's "architecture" as if it
were as stable as the Parthenon that has been standing for the last
2,000 years. However, in the cell everything moves; every second
the structure changes. These movements most likely represent communication mechanisms within the cell or between cells. Much could
be learned about the regulation of phenotypic expression by studying the movements of particles and membranes in the cell. I do not
know how this can be investigated, but I think that this will become an interesting field of research in the future.

Tomkins: Having heard the respective programs of the panel members, it is clear that in biology not all is over, as Gunther Stent
implied, and people seem to be still interested in what they are
doing.

Now let us turn to questions from the audience.

Kulka: I find there is a certain polarization. People work either on the simplest viruses and bacteria or on the most complex
organisms such as mammals. I wonder why none of the participants
of this conference has thought of working with systems of intermediate complexity like simple eukaryotes, the genetic analysis of
which is well developed.

Szybalski:One could imagine two classes of "intermediate" organisms.
One class would comprise the simple eukaryotes found in nature, of
the kind you describe, and the best examples would be Neurospora
or yeasts, which are subjects of active study. But the second

class could be artificially created by inserting into a phage or
viral genome a block of eukaryotic genes and then studying their
own or virus-supplied controls in this isolated form, supported
by the synthetic machinery of the prokaryotic or eukaryotic host,
in vivo , or in cell extracts. This second approach would be most
promising for studying the detailed control mechanisms for spe-
dfic eukaryotic genes. It again stresses the importance of phages,
like lambda, in the study of controls not only in prokaryotic but
also in eukaryotic systems.

Kaye: If one speaks of simpler systems, perhaps one may include
avian as compared to mammalian ones. I am thinking for example
of O'Malley's work on the hormonal control of development in the
chick oviduct. He and his colleagues found that the application of
oestrogen for several days to the immature chick resulted in the
differentiation of morphologically characteristic cells in the
oviduct and in the specific synthesis of ovalbumin. Moreover,
when cells from oviduct were treated for several days with oestrogen and then secondarily subjected to treatment with progesterone,
there was a specific synthesis of avidin. Working on the mechanism of these inductions, for which the avian system has some technical advantages over the mammalian system, will provide a fertile
field for future work.

Kulka: I did not mean why don't people move up from simpler
systems, but rather why don't they move down from more complex
ones. For example, why is not more work done on hormones in
Neurospora which has good genetics and shows some interesting hormone effects. In Neurospora, unlike mammalian cells, one knows
whether one has a mutant or a phenotypic variant.

Scherrer: This discussion about simple and more simple systems
sounds to me like "Ein Streit um Kaisers Bart". It was relatively
simple to identify mRNA in bacteria; however, it was much easier
to discover polyribosomes in animal cells than in bacteria. In
working with Neurospora there are some practical difficulties
which do not exist in animal cells, even though genetic studies
are simpler in Neurospora. It is crucial, however, that we examine
a full range of systems and choose among these the one suiting a
particular problem.

McCarthy: I should like to endorse Scherrer's views. Because
human beings are bigger than bacteria and the amount of DNA per
human cell is 700 times that of E. coli it does not necessarily
follow that regulation is more complicated. I am not convinced
that control of the synthesis of an enzyme in human cells is going
to be more complicated than regulation in lambda. Therefore one
should not be frightened by multicellularity or large genomes.

Herzberg: The problem is that even if one takes apart the whole cell machinery and isolates its elements it will not be a cell. Let us take something relatively simple, such as protein synthesis in rabbit reticulocytes. If one separates polysomes and supernatant the system is not yet a cell. One has around the cell a membrane, and this membrane has functions, even if one speaks only of active transport. The membrane gets signals from outside which have to be taken care of from inside. We have therefore to understand better the membrane functions and how the signals are interpreted by the machinery for protein synthesis, and what is the difference between protein synthesis in a test tube and protein synthesis in a finite environment surrounded by the membrane.

Zaritsky: One important problem which was not discussed here is ribosomal biogenesis. That is, the coordination between ribosomal proteins and rRNA synthesis and the proper assembly of the two components to make a mature ribosome. We ought to tackle this problem by much more direct in vivo experimentation than is being done to date.

          The importance of this question stems from the involvement of the ribosomes in translation on the one hand and the involvement of both translation and transcription in ribosomal production on the other.

Scherrer: I cannot stress enough the important area of the study of ribosome biosynthesis in animal cells. If rRNA synthesis is quite well understood, relatively little is known about the biogenesis of the ribosome as a ribonucleoprotein and the accompanying regulation processes. Relatively few people work on this problem. However, ribosome synthesis represents one of the relatively simple systems to study regulation. The regulation of ribosome biogenesis is not only transcriptional; cases are known of cells in which ribosome synthesis stops, but the transcription of the precursors continues. This represents a clear example of post-transcriptional regulation. Moreover, rRNA synthesis represents a relatively simple function and, thus is much easier to study than mRNA.

Revel: As to ribosome biogenesis, the theme of this conference is to ask how it can help gene expression. It could help it either by increasing or decreasing protein synthesis. I believe there are many controls in the pathway of ribosome formation, or on the level of RNA synthesis and we have already heard a detailed account from Dr. Lengyel of what is known about the role of ppGGpp on ribosome RNA synthesis in prokaryotes.

Tomkins: I should like to mention the persistent observation by Harris' group that nucleoli are required for the expression of genetic information.

Kotler: Since nobody touched on the problem of DNA synthesis in
the cytoplasm of eukaryotic cells perhaps one of the panelists
would refer to this matter?

McCarthy: The primary issue is that the proponents of the informational DNA theory must show that DNA found in the cytoplasm is a
non-random part of the genome. Experiments have been reported by
several groups which show that this DNA is indistinguishable by
the C_ot analysis and by density gradient analysis from total DNA.
So, until one can show that cytoplasmic DNA represents a specific
part of the cellular DNA I do not think that the hypothesis is
particularly viable.

Yagil (to Tomkins): As to the 30 s RNA of Harris, is there any
evidence that you have new nucleolar particles?

Scherrer: As long as the cell is in a steady state, ribosome synthesis is not necessary for messenger transport. We can label mRNA
in Hela polyribosomes for hours in the presence of agents which
completely block rRNA synthesis. However, it seems to me that
whenever the physiological state of the cell is changed, ribosomal
RNA synthesis becomes necessary. For example, in the temperature
shift experiment of Penman, all polyribosomes are destroyed in
5-7 minutes; about 70% of the original polyribosome reform within
another 10 min. thereafter. This restoration of protein synthesis
does not occur when ribosomal RNA synthesis is blocked. The
Harris experiment in which destruction of the nucleolus blocked
the appearance of a surface-antigen, can be explained in the sense of re-programming of the translational machinery rather than in
terms of simple mRNA transport. This suggestion is based on the
observation that whenever a cell changes its physiological state
(implying the translation of a new and other message) nucleolar
function must be intact.

Concerning cytoplasmic DNA synthesis: to my knowledge
there are no conclusive reports indicating clear differences between cytoplasmic DNA and nuclear DNA. However, "where there is
smoke, there is fire". For example, there are clear-cut examples
of cells which are not in S-phase but which synthesize DNA. S.
Modak in our laboratory has found that erythroblasts incorporate
TdR at a stage when no further cell division occurs. However, we
also have not been able thus far to define a straight-forward
difference between nuclear and cytoplasmic DNA. This is a field
that demands closer investigation.

Bizunski (to Tomkins): Why does the viral genome lead to transformation in some cases, but not in others?

Tomkins: I can only speculate. In the case of DNA viruses, it is not clear whether they contain the "oncogenes" or merely activate host or other latent RNA viral genes, which are oncogenes.

It may also be important where the virus is integrated. It was believed at first that a large number of DNA viral genomes are integrated, but later hybridization experiments showed that only a few may in fact be so.

It seems to depend on the clone of cells examined. It is not known whether the viral genomes are integrated in the same site in each cell and it is conceivable that the site of integration can make a difference.

As to the action of hormones: it is possible that host or viral oncogenes have no other function than to alter either the production of, or response to, the cyclic nucleotide.

In transformation, there is perhaps an alteration in the way a cell handles cyclic nucleotides. The main problem seems to be whether such an alteration in cyclic nucleotide metabolism might be the basis of the malignant phenotype. Transformed cells have less cyclic AMP than normal. In the experiments of Pastan with temperature-sensitive RNA (Rous) virus, at one temperature the cAMP is low and cells are transformed and at another temperature, the cell is not transformed and cAMP is high. Recent experiments of Torres from Argentina indicate that lowering cAMP concentration in non-transformed BHK cells with the aid of insulin (which is an inhibitor of adenyl cyclase) stimulates cells to express various aspects of the malignant phenotype, such as lack of density inhibition and growth of colonies in agar.

The fact that a given gene in a given place does or does not work, can be explained by a number of models, e.g. like that of lambda.

Inouye (to Szybalski, Bautz, Revel): One view of the current situation of the code in prokaryotes seems to me unsatisfactory. We know the vocabulary, but not the grammar. Without grammar it is difficult to find out what the words mean. We know that grammatically important signals, like termination or initiation signals exist, but not how they organize information.

Szybalski: Does your question refer to the punctuation system?

Inouye: Not only to the individual punctuation signals but also
to their mutual relationship and their relationships to the structural genes. For example, punctuation signals should not be present
in structural genes. These things are mutually exclusive, because
if a punctuation signal is in the structure of the gene, it must,
by definition, punctuate.

Bautz: We do understand the crude aspects of the code - but we
do not know the fine details, the fine print, that gives instruc-
tions how genes are regulated. In RNA phages there are certain
regions between the termination and initiation signals which are
important in making the ribosomes fall off and go on. Similarly
there are in the DNA regions which have signals for regulatory
proteins. I believe that in the near future we shall know a lot
more about the primary structure of operators and promoters.

Tomkins: Do you also mean why can AUG appear in the middle of a
cistron and not affect translation? It seems as though no termination signals can occur in the middle of a cistron without stopping polypeptide synthesis. Another "grammatical" question might
be "what determines the arrangement of genes on chromosomes?"
In phages, one can see developmental reasons: for example, the
linear gene sequence must be related to temporal expression in a
sophisticated way. It also seems reasonable that salmonella and
coli have a very similar gene order.

Scherrer: What you refer to as "grammar", one may also call a program. Accompanying the message there must be a program that de-
fines in time and space the fate of the coding information. Concerning your statement of mutual exclusivity of coding and programming information, this may not necessarily be so. Superimposed
on the genetic code there may exist another type of information
which is expressed by the secondary structure of the mRNA per se.
It is theoretically possible that a particular primary sequence
leads to a particular secondary structure in the RNA; such specific
sequences could be recognized by specific proteins. Thus "grammar",
"print" or "program" may be superimposed directly on the primary
sequence of the coding RNA. However, I certainly agree that programming sequences must also exist outside the message. Poly(A)
is a good candidate for such a sequence.

Revel: Dr. Inouye asked about the possibility that there is a
correspondence between the RNA termination and protein termination signals. The same question is posed regarding their respective initiations. Probably, evolution started with RNA and DNA
appeared later. Did the punctuation first appear on RNA and only
then in the DNA? It is, however, most probable that the signals
on RNA and DNA are very different. There are apparently many

examples of waste,pieces which are lost, or added; the initiation
signal of transcription may be remote from the initiation signal
of translation.

       Concerning the role of secondary structure of ribosome
in RNA recognition, one error is to focus on RNA phages. They are
peculiar systems that have to survive in an environment containing
RNAse and they may have a tertiary structure that protects RNA,
which E. coli mRNAs do not have. We need more information about
ribosome binding to mRNA transcribed from DNA in order to get some
idea of where the signal might be.

Lengyel: The problem of the recognition of peptide chain initiation signals by ribosomes and initiation factors reminds me of the
problem of the recognition of transfer RNAs by aminoacyl-tRNA
synthetases. There are many different aminoacyl-tRNA synthetases
and each recognizes only one or a very few tRNA species. Consequently, mutations that change the recognition between one of these
enzymes and its substrates might be tolerated by the organism.
Thus it is conceivable that different aminoacyl-tRNA synthetases
recognize different regions in their substrate transfer RNAs. The
only restriction is that the recognition within a given cell or
subcellar organelle should not be too ambiguous. The same considerations may apply to peptide chain initiation signals in mRNA.
If all recognition signals are not recognized by the same set of
proteins, then we do not have to expect the emergence of a general
rule. Again, the only restriction is that the recognition should
not be too ambiguous.

Kaye: A mammalian system may not necessarily be more complex
in regulation than a bacteriophage system. Perhaps we should postulate not necessarily more complex, but different, and as yet
unknown, regulating mechanisms which occur in the eukaryote, which
are a result of evolution of the chromosome from the naked DNA
of the prokaryote.

Szybalski:The prokaryote DNA is not really naked. It is at least
partially covered by repressors, polymerases, various factors,poly-
amines and other goodies.

Kaye: A sort of Bikini clad DNA.

Szybalski:In eukaryotes the DNA appears to be more prudish, but
prokaryotic DNA can also be wrapped into tight nucleoid bodies or
even become fully packaged.

McCarthy: The question has been raised, why do eukaryotes bother
to have histones? Why don't they have naked DNA? There is not

yet a tenable hypothesis to answer this question. They are simply
there. They don't represent specific gene regulators, nevertheless
the eukaryotic organisms find it useful to have them for reasons
that elude everyone at the present time. Perhaps we could have
profitably discussed chromosome models during the meeting, but at
this late hour, it is impossible to deal adequately with problems
such as single stranded ss-regions of DNA in chromosomes, whether
chromosomal proteins bind to such single stranded regions and so
on. In any case there are already too many chromosome models, considering the paucity of facts.

Scherrer: I understand your feelings about the complexity of the
regulatory systems; certainly it would be understating the case to
pretend that regulation in eukaryotic cells may not be more complex than in prokaryotes. Obviously, more information has to be
controlled in the former; however, the complexity of the regulative
system may not necessarily increase proportionally, for the system
could be simplified by organization. It is not "more complex" in
a "mystical" sense but the regulatory system of eukaryotic cells
may simply be the expression of a higher degree of integration of
information processing. Concerning chromosomal models? I feel
that we must accumulate more experimental facts before making
concrete models.

Aviv: I think that it is premature to advance models for chromatin structure and function. If you want to understand the relation between structure and function, you have to be able to assay
function before you go on to understand structure. Structure without function is not too meaningful to me. My feeling at this stage
is that when methodological tools have been developed to study
function for specific genes, this information will lead to more
intelligent models. Another aspect which was not mentioned here is
gene inactivation. The cell has not only the problem what to do,
but also the problem what not to do.

Bautz: Higher organisms are in some cases much less complicated
than bacteria. There is no E. coli mutant that produces only one
product like some eukaryotic cells. In theory, therefore, it
should be much easier to study cells of higher organisms that make
only one product like hemoglobin. The cells have ways of shutting
off all genes except one. Biochemically it is unfortunate that
this one gene does not multiply. The cell can go along with only
one or few copies and get enough information. If it had more
copies it would be more amenable to biochemical analysis. This is
why bacterial or phage systems which are very complicated, are
still simple to study biochemically.

Zaritsky: Two brief remarks. The first refers to punctuation. The mutual exclusiveness, which was mentioned here before, is implied by the basic grammatical rule we all know. That is, the non-over-lapping of the genetic code.

The problem of ribosomal biogenesis is directly relevant to gene expression. One act of transcription of the rRNA set makes enough RNA for one ribosome only, whereas one act of trans-cription of the ribosomal-protein genes results in 30 to 50 copies of each of these proteins. The redundancy of rRNA genes in bac-teria (because they exist in 4-6 copies per genome) may explain only part of this disparity. Therefore, the frequency of trans-cription of a rRNA gene must be about 10 fold higher than that of a ribosomal protein gene. If they are under the same control ele-ment a much higher affinity of the promoter of the rRNA is implied. Unfortunately, we can say very little concerning this problem.

Tomkins: In order to conclude the discussion I should first like to thank the organizers and express our gratitude for the opportu-nity to be here.

One can see from the comments of the members of the panel that there are a number of different ways of doing science; every-body does it in his own image. Some like to see the things in tre-mendous detail, others who look for general philosophical rules are happy with block diagrams, and call E. coli and eukaryotic cells similar since they use the same genetic code. It is obvious that all of these approaches are necessary and it depends on the evolution of a subject what particular type of contribution will be the most valuable. Individuals do not seem to change from one style of research to another.

I should like to argue, as a philosophical generalization, that rules exist which override the complexities of biological or-ganization. Before it is sensible to look for such rules, other problems must be solved: like what determines the differentiation decision? I don't believe that hormone molecules contain enough information to tell the cells what to do. They are only signals which call out programmes, and we do not understand how those pro-grammes are organized, how they are called, whether they are sub-routines of other programmes,etc.

Very often the "classic" way in which a problem is phra-sed is incorrect. For example, why do bacteria have naked DNA while eukaryotes have very complicated chromosomal structure? Everybody working in the field "knows" that the chromosomal organi-zation is very different, yet, recent work has shown that bacterial chromosomes have three dimensional structure held together by pieces of RNA and perhaps even protein. Perhaps the bacterial

chromosome is not a simple one dimensional circle, but also has
some kind of complicated organization. For example, Dr. Szybalski
discussed data concerning untranslated regions and processing in λ.
Making hybrids between animal viruses and λ DNA can also give some
useful clues.

We all know the established pathways, and we talk about
what we shall do in the future based on these ideas. But, some
apparently unlikely and even impossible things will turn out to be
true. The history of science is remarkable in that respect. In
the twenties it was believed that there could be no molecules with
a molecular weight higher than a few hundreds. Proteins were
thought to be loose aggregates and not defined macro-molecules.
The first man to synthesize a macromolecule, Staudinger, was drum-
med out of scientific meetings as being irresponsible.

I would like to close with a plea of clemency for danger-
ous lunatics. Let us keep open minds.

LIST OF PARTICIPANTS

ACS, GEORGE
    Institute for Muscle Disease, New York, U.S.A.
AHREN, KURT
    University of Goteborg, Sweden
ALONI, YOSEF
    Weizmann Institute of Science, Rehovot, Israel
AMIR, RIVKA
    Faculty of Agriculture, Rehovot, Israel
ARGOV, SHMUEL
    Tel-Aviv University, Ramat-Aviv, Israel
ARONOVICH, JACOB
    Hebrew University-Hadassah Medical School, Jerusalem, Israel
ASHKENAZI, ORINA
    Tel-Aviv University, Ramat-Aviv, Israel
AVIV, HAIM
    National Institutes of Health, Bethesda, Maryland, U.S.A.
BACHRACH, URIEL
    Hebrew University-Hadassah Medical School, Jerusalem, Israel
BARZILAI, ERGA
    Kimron Veterinary Institute, Beit-Dagan, Israel
BARZILAI, ROY
    Hebrew University-Hadassah Medical School, Jerusalem, Israel
BAUMINGER, SARA
    Weizmann Institute of Science, Rehovot, Israel
BAUTZ, EKKEHARD K.F.
    University of Heidelberg, Germany
BAUTZ, FRIEDLINDE
    University of Heidelberg, Heidelberg, Germany
BECKER, YECHIEL
    Hebrew University-Hadassah Medical School, Jerusalem, Israel
BECKMANN, JACQUES
    Weizmann Institute of Science, Rehovot, Israel
BELFORT, MARLIN
    Hebrew University, Jerusalem, Israel
BEN-DAVID, AMNON
    Israel Institute for Biological Research, Ness-Ziona, Israel

BEN-PORATH, EDNA
    Aba Khoushi School of Medicine, Haifa, Israel
BEN-ZEEV, IVRI
    Hebrew University, Jerusalem, Israel
BERDICEVSKY, ISRAELA
    Aba Khoushi School of Medicine, Haifa, Israel
BERISSI, HANNA
    Weizmann Institute of Science, Rehovot, Israel
BINO, TAMAR
    Israel Institute for Biological Research, Ness-Ziona, Israel
BIZUNSKI, NOEMI
    Tel-Aviv University, Ramat-Aviv, Israel
BLEIBERG, ILAN
    Tel-Aviv University, Ramat-Aviv, Israel
BRAND, GABRIELA
    Israel Institute for Biological Research, Ness-Ziona, Israel
BUSTIN, MICHAEL
    Weizmann Institute of Science, Rehovot, Israel
CANAANI, DAN
    Weizmann Institute of Science, Rehovot, Israel
CHEN, LOUISE
    Weizmann Institute of Science, Rehovot, Israel
COHEN, AMIKAM
    Hebrew University, Jerusalem, Israel
COHEN, SARA
    Israel Institute for Biological Research, Ness-Ziona, Israel
CONCONI, FRANCESCO
    University of Ferrara, Ferrara, Italy
CONCONI, Mrs.
    Ferrara, Italy
DANIEL, VIOLET
    Weizmann Institute of Science, Rehovot, Israel
DAVIES, BERNARD
    Harvard Medical School, U.S.A.
DECKEL, DROR
    Tel-Aviv University, Ramat-Aviv, Israel
DE GROOT, NATHAN
    Hebrew University, Jerusalem, Israel
DISKIN, BLUMA
    Israel Institute for Biological Research, Ness-Ziona, Israel
DUVDEVANI, NURIT
    Israel Institute for Biological Research, Ness-Ziona, Israel
DYM, HAVIV
    Weizmann Institute of Science, Rehovot, Israel
EISENSTADT, AUDREY
    Yale University, U.S.A.
EISENSTADT, JEROME
    Yale University, U.S.A.

ELIZUR, ERELA
    Hebrew University-Hadassah Medical School, Jerusalem, Israel
ELSON, DAVID
    Weizmann Institute of Science, Rehovot, Israel
ELSON, PNINA
    Weizmann Institute of Science, Rehovot, Israel
EVENCHIK, ZIGMUND
    Israel Institute for Biological Research, Ness-Ziona, Israel
EYLAN, EMANUEL
    Tel-Aviv University, Ramat-Aviv, Israel
FRENKEL, AYALA
    Weizmann Institute of Science, Rehovot, Israel
FRENKEL, GERALD
    Weizmann Institute of Science, Rehovot, Israel
FRENKEL, NIZA
    Weizmann Institute of Science, Rehovot, Israel
FRENNSDORFF, ASHER
    Tel-Aviv University, Ramat-Aviv, Israel
FRISCH, AMOS
    Hebrew University, Jerusalem, Israel
FUCHS, PINHAS
    Israel Institute for Biological Research, Ness-Ziona, Israel
GAZIT, ARNONA
    Tel-Aviv University, Ramat-Aviv, Israel
GERSHON, DAVID
    Israel Institute of Technology, Haifa
GERSHON, H.
    Israel Institute of Technology, Haifa
GINZBURG, CHEN
    Volcani Agricultural Center, Beit-Dagan, Israel
GINZBURG, IRITH
    Weizmann Institute of Science, Rehovot, Israel
GIVOL, DAVID
    Weizmann Institute of Science, Rehovot, Israel
GOLDBERG, GREGORY
    Weizmann Institute of Science, Rehovot, Israel
GOLDSMIT, LEAH
    Kimron Veterinary Institute, Beit-Dagan, Israel
GOLDWASSER, ROBERT
    Israel Institute for Biological Research, Ness-Ziona, Israel
GORDIN, MENACHEM
    Hebrew University-Hadassah Medical School, Jerusalem, Israel
GREEN, RESA
    Bar-Ilan University, Ramat-Gan, Israel
GREENMAN, BENJAMIN
    Weizmann Institute of Science, Rehovot, Israel
GRESSER, JONATHAN
    Weizmann Institute of Science, Rehovot, Israel

GROSSMAN, LAWRENCE
    Bar-Ilan University, Ramat-Gan, Israel
GROSSOWICZ, NATHAN
    Hebrew University-Hadassah Medical School, Jerusalem, Israel
GRUSS, ROSEMARIE
    Weizmann Institute of Science, Rehovot, Israel
GUTNICK, DAVID
    Tel-Aviv University, Ramat-Aviv, Israel
GUTTER, BEZALEL
    Hebrew University-Hadassah Medical School, Jerusalem, Israel
HAGILADI, AMIR
    Tel-Aviv University, Ramat-Aviv, Israel
HALMANN, MIRJAM
    Israel Institute for Biological Research, Ness-Ziona, Israel
HALPERIN, BILHA
    Israel Institute for Biological Research, Ness-Ziona, Israel
HALPERN, YEHESKEL S.
    Hebrew University-Hadassah Medical School, Jerusalem, Israel
HAY, JACOB
    Israel Institute for Biological Research, Ness-Ziona, Israel
HEFTER, ALINA
    Sick Fund Central Laboratory, Haifa
HELLER, EMANUEL
    Hebrew University-Hadassah Medical School, Jerusalem, Israel
HERSHKO, ABRAHAM
    Aba Khoushi School of Medicine, Haifa, Israel
HERZBERG, MAX
    Bar-Ilan University, Ramat-Gan, Israel
HIZI, AMNON
    Weizmann Institute of Science, Rehovot, Israel
HOCHMAN, JACOB
    Weizmann Institute of Science, Rehovot, Israel
HOFMAN, JUDITH
    Rogoff Institute, Beilinson Hospital, Petah Tikva, Israel
HONIGMAN, ALEXANDER
    Hebrew University-Hadassah Medical School, Jerusalem, Israel
HORNSTEIN, LEA
    Sick Fund Central Laboratory, Haifa
HOROVITZ, AVIVA
    Hebrew University, Jerusalem, Israel
HUBERMAN, ELIEZER
    Weizmann Institute of Science, Rehovot, Israel
ICEKSON, ISAAC
    Weizmann Institute of Science, Rehovot, Israel
INOUYE, H.
    Weizmann Institute of Science, Rehovot, Israel
ISRAELI, EYTAN
    Israel Institute for Biological Research, Ness-Ziona, Israel

JACOB, KARL
    Weizmann Institute of Science, Rehovot, Israel
JACOBY, MIRIAM
    Hebrew University, Jerusalem, Israel
KALMAR, ELISABETH
    Kimron Veterinary Institute, Beit-Dagan, Israel
KATZ, DAVID
    Israel Institute for Biological Research, Ness-Ziona, Israel
KATZ, EHUD
    Hebrew University-Hadassah Medical School, Jerusalem, Israel
KAUFMANN, ELISHEVA
    Israel Institute for Biological Research, Ness-Ziona, Israel
KAUFMANN, GABRIEL
    Weizmann Institute of Science, Rehovot, Israel
KAUFMANN, YAEL
    Weizmann Institute of Science, Rehovot, Israel
KAYE, ALVIN
    Weizmann Institute of Science, Rehovot, Israel
KAYE, MYRA
    Israel Institute for Biological Research, Ness-Ziona, Israel
KEYNAN, ALEXANDER
    Hebrew University, Jerusalem, Israel
KESSLER, GANIA
    Weizmann Institute of Science, Rehovot, Israel
KEYDAR, JAFA
    Tel-Aviv University, Ramat-Aviv, Israel
KIMCHI, ADY
    Tel-Aviv University, Ramat-Aviv, Israel
KIMHI, YOSEF
    Weizmann Institute of Science, Rehovot, Israel
KINAMON, SIMHA
    Ministry of Defence, Israel
KINDLER, SHMUEL H.
    Tel-Aviv University, Ramat-Aviv, Israel
KING, R.G.B.
    Imperial Cancer Research Fund, London, England
KIRSCHMANN, CHAVA
    Rogoff Institute, Beilinson Hospital, Petah Tikva, Israel
KLEINBERG, DANIELA
    Israel Institute for Biological Research, Ness-Ziona, Israel
KOHN, ALEXANDER
    Israel Institute for Biological Research, Ness-Ziona, Israel
KOHN, CHANA
    Sick Fund Central Laboratory, Rehovot, Israel
KOLAKOFSKY, DANIEL
    Institute of Molecular Biology, Geneva, Switzerland
KOTLER, MOSHE
    Hebrew University-Hadassah Medical School, Jerusalem, Israel

KUHN, JONATHAN
    University of the Negev, Beer-Sheba, Israel
KULKA, RICHARD
    Hebrew University, Jerusalem, Israel
KUNIN, SARA
    Weizmann Institute of Science, Rehovot, Israel
LACHMI, BAT-EL
    Hebrew University-Hadassah Medical School, Jerusalem, Israel
LAHAV, MICHAL
    Weizmann Institute of Science, Rehovot, Israel
LAHAV, MIRA
    Sick Fund Central Laboratories, Tel-Aviv, Israel
LAPIDOT, YEHUDA
    Hebrew University, Jerusalem, Israel
LASKOV, REUVEN
    Hebrew University-Hadassah Medical School, Jerusalem, Israel
LAVIE, GAD
    Weizmann Institute of Science, Rehovot, Israel
LAVI, SARA
    Weizmann Institute of Science, Rehovot, Israel
LEHRER, SHOSHANA
    Israel Institute for Biological Research, Ness-Ziona, Israel
LENGYEL, PETER
    Yale University, New Haven, Conn., U.S.A.
LEVANON, AVIGDOR
    Israel Institute for Biological Research, Ness-Ziona, Israel
LEVISOHN, REUBEN
    Tel-Aviv University, Ramat-Aviv, Israel
LINDNER, HANS R.
    Weizmann Institute of Science, Rehovot, Israel
LITTAUER, URIEL
    Weizmann Institute of Science, Rehovot, Israel
LIVNAT, SHMUEL
    Weizmann Institute of Science, Rehovot, Israel
LOEWENSTEIN, JAMES
    Tel-Aviv University, Ramat-Aviv, Israel
LOYTER, BARAHAM
    Hebrew University, Jerusalem, Israel
MARGALITH, CHAVA
    Hebrew University-Hadassah Medical School, Jerusalem, Israel
MARKS, PAUL A.
    Columbia University, New York, N.Y., U.S.A.
MASHIAH, PNINA
    Tel-Aviv University, Ramat-Aviv, Israel
McCARTHY, BRIAN J.
    University of California, San Francisco, Calif., U.S.A.
MERZBACH, DAVID
    Aba Khoushi School of Medicine, Haifa, Israel

MESSER, YAEL G.
    Bar-Ilan University, Ramat-Gan, Israel
MIRSKY, NITZA
    Israel Institute of Technology, Haifa, Israel
MISKIN, RUTH
    Weizmann Institute of Science, Rehovot, Israel
MOAV, NEOMI
    Tel-Aviv University, Ramat-Aviv, Israel
MOLDAVE, KIVIE
    University of California, California, U.S.A.
NACHTIGAL, DAVID
    Weizmann Institute of Science, Rehovot, Israel
NEGREANU, JACOB
    Israel Institute for Biological Research, Ness-Ziona, Israel
OLSHEVSKY, UDI
    Hebrew University-Hadassah Medical School, Jerusalem, Israel
OREN, RACHEL
    Israel Institute for Biological Research, Ness-Ziona, Israel
OPPENHEIM, AMOS
    Hebrew University-Hadassah Medical School, Jerusalem, Israel
OPPENHEIM, ARIELLA
    Hebrew University-Hadassah Medical School, Jerusalem, Israel
PATCHORNIK, ABRAHAM
    Weizmann Institute of Science, Rehovot, Israel
PATERSON, BRUCE
    Weizmann Institute of Science, Rehovot, Israel
PAYES, BENJAMIN
    Israel Institute for Biological Research, Ness-Ziona, Israel
PERETZ, HAVA
    Weizmann Institute of Science, Rehovot, Israel
PLUZNIK, DOV
    Bar-Ilan University, Ramat-Gan, Israel
POLLACK, JAAKOV
    Weizmann Institute of Science, Rehovot, Israel
PRIVES, CAROL
    Weizmann Institute of Science, Rehovot, Israel
RAANANI, HAVA
    Tel-Aviv University, Ramat-Aviv, Israel
RABINOWITZ, ZELIG
    Weizmann Institute of Science, Rehovot, Israel
RAFAELI, DEVORAH
    Aba Khoushi School of Medicine, Haifa, Israel
RAMOT, BRACHA
    Chaim Sheba Medical Center, Tel-Hashomer, Israel
RAVEH, DINA
    Weizmann Institute of Science, Rehovot, Israel
RAVID, ZOHAR
    Hebrew University-Hadassah Medical School, Jerusalem, Israel

REVEL, MICHEL
        Weizmann Institute of Science, Rehovot, Israel
ROBERTS, BRYAN
        Weizmann Institute of Science, Rehovot, Israel
ROIZMAN, BERNARD
        University of Chicago, Chicago, Illinois, U.S.A.
RON, ELIORA
        Tel-Aviv University, Ramat-Aviv, Israel
RON, GILA
        Israel Institute for Biological Research, Ness-Ziona, Israel
ROSENBERG, EUGENE
        Tel-Aviv University, Ramat-Aviv, Israel
ROZENSZAIN, ARIE
        Bar-Ilan University, Ramat-Gan, Israel
SAAR, MICHAEL
        Israel Institute for Biological Research, Ness-Ziona, Israel
SACHS, LEO
        Weizmann Institute of Science, Rehovot, Israel
SARID, SARA
        Weizmann Institute of Science, Rehovot, Israel
SCHAYN, RUTH
        Hebrew University, Jerusalem, Israel
SCHEPS, RUTH
        Weizmann Institute of Science, Rehovot, Israel
SCHERRER, KLAUS
        Swiss Institute for Experimental Cancer Research,
        Lausanne, Switzerland
SCHMITT, HENRI
        Weizmann Institute of Science, Rehovot, Israel
SENIOR, ARIELA
        Israel Institute for Biological Research, Ness-Ziona, Israel
SHALITA, ZAMIR
        Israel Institute for Biological Research, Ness-Ziona, Israel
SHANI, AHUVA
        Israel Institute of Technology, Haifa, Israel
SHANI, MOSHE
        Weizmann Institute of Science, Rehovot, Israel
SHAPIRA, ADAM
        Israel Institute for Biological Research, Ness-Ziona, Israel
SHATKAY, ADAM
        Israel Institute for Biological Research, Ness-Ziona, Israel
SHENBERG, ESTHER
        Israel Institute for Biological Research, Ness-Ziona, Israel
SHLOMAY, JOSEPH
        Hebrew University, Jerusalem, Israel
SIMANTOV, ROBI
        Weizmann Institute of Science, Rehovot, Israel
SIMON, EDWARD
        Hebrew University, Jerusalem, Israel

SIMON, GAD
    Israel Institute for Biological Research, Ness-Ziona, Israel
SINAI, JUDITH
    Israel Institute for Biological Research, Ness-Ziona, Israel
SINGER, ROBERT
    Weizmann Institute of Science, Rehovot, Israel
SMETANA, OFIRA
    Tel-Aviv University, Ramat-Aviv, Israel
SOMJEN, DALIA
    Weizmann Institute of Science, Rehovot, Israel
SOMJEN, GIORA
    Weizmann Institute of Science, Rehovot, Israel
SOMPOLINSKY, DAVID
    Bar-Ilan University, Ramat-Gan, Israel
STARK, AVI
    Tel-Aviv University, Ramat-Aviv, Israel
STAVY, LARY
    Weizmann Institute of Science, Rehovot, Israel
STAVY, RUTH
    Weizmann Institute of Science, Rehovot, Israel
STEIN, ADINA
    Volcani Agricultural Center, Beit-Dagan, Israel
SZEINBERG, ARIE
    Chaim Sheba Medical Center, Tel-Hashomer, Israel
SZYBALSKI, WACLAW
    McArdle Laboratories for Cancer Research, University of
    Wisconsin, Madison, Wisconsin, U.S.A.
TEITZ, YAEL
    Israel Institute for Biological Research, Ness-Ziona, Israel
TOMKINS, GORDON
    University of California, San Francisco, California, U.S.A.
TORTEN, MICHAEL
    Israel Institute for Biological Research, Ness-Ziona, Israel
TRAUB, ABRAHAM
    Israel Institute for Biological Research, Ness-Ziona, Israel
UMIEL, NAKDIMON
    Faculty of Agriculture, Rehovot, Israel
URETSKY, STANLEY
    The Mount Sinai School of Medicine, New York, U.S.A.
VELAN, BAROUCH
    Israel Institute for Biological Research, Ness-Ziona, Israel
WINOCOUR, ERNEST
    Weizmann Institute of Science, Rehovot, Israel
YAFFE, DAVID
    Weizmann Institute of Science, Rehovot, Israel
YAGIL, GAD
    Weizmann Institute of Science, Rehovot, Israel
YANKOFSKY, SAUL
    Tel-Aviv University, Ramat-Aviv, Israel

YORAV, HANOCH
     Israel Institute for Biological Research, Ness-Ziona, Israel
ZAHAVI, AMALIA
     Israel Institute for Biological Research, Ness-Ziona, Israel
ZAMIR, ADA
     Weizmann Institute of Science, Rehovot, Israel
ZARITSKY, ARIEH
     University of the Negev, Beer-Sheba, Israel
ZASLAVSKY, ZEEV
     Weizmann Institute of Science, Rehovot, Israel
ZELCER, AARON
     Weizmann Institute of Science, Rehovot, Israel
ZELLER, HANNA
     Weizmann Institute of Science, Rehovot, Israel
ZILBER, ILANA
     Tel-Aviv University, Ramat-Aviv, Israel
ZYDON, ELISHEVA
     Ramat-Gan, Israel
ZYDON, YAAKOV
     Israel Institute for Biological Research, Ness-Ziona, Israel
ZYLBER, ESTHER A.
     Hebrew University-Hadassah Medical School, Jerusalem, Israel

SUBJECT INDEX